Eating Puerto Rico

A BOOK IN THE SERIES LATIN AMERICA IN
TRANSLATION / EN TRADUCCIÓN / EM TRADUÇÃO

Sponsored by the Consortium in Latin American Studies at the
University of North Carolina at Chapel Hill and Duke University

Eating Puerto Rico

A History of Food, Culture, and Identity

CRUZ MIGUEL ORTÍZ CUADRA

Translated by RUSS DAVIDSON

The University of North Carolina Press Chapel Hill

Translation of the books in the series Latin America in Translation / en Traducción / em Tradução, a collaboration between the Consortium in Latin American Studies at the University of North Carolina at Chapel Hill and Duke University and the university presses of the University of North Carolina and Duke, is supported by a grant from the Andrew W. Mellon Foundation.

Designed by and set in Quadraat types by Rebecca Evans
Manufactured in the United States of America

Originally published in Spanish with the title *Puerto Rico en la olla, ¿somos aún lo que comimos?*, © 2006 Cruz Miguel Ortíz Cuadra, Ediciones Doce Calles, S.L., Madrid.

The paper in this book meets the guidelines for permanence and durability of the Committee on Production Guidelines for Book Longevity of the Council on Library Resources. The University of North Carolina Press has been a member of the Green Press Initiative since 2003.

Library of Congress Cataloging-in-Publication Data
Ortíz Cuadra, Cruz M.
[Puerto Rico en la olla. English]
Eating Puerto Rico : a history of food, culture, and identity /
Cruz Miguel Ortíz Cuadra ; translated by Russ Davidson.
pages cm.—(Latin America in translation)
"Originally published in Spanish with the title Puerto Rico en la olla."
Includes bibliographical references and index.
ISBN 978-1-4696-0882-2 (cloth: alk. paper)
1. Food habits—Puerto Rico. 2. Diet—Puerto Rico.
I. Davidson, Russ, translator. II. Title.
GT2853.P83O7713 2013   394.1′2097295—dc23   2013011560

17 16 15 14 13   5 4 3 2 1

To my father, Humberto Ortíz Gordils,
and mother, Providencia Cuadra García

Contents

Figures and Tables

TABLES

Foreword

For centuries now, the analysis of culture—of all that we create, shape, and do, to borrow the wording of Roman Guardini—has tried to *distinguish* humankind from nature. The book before you—*Eating Puerto Rico: A History of Food, Culture, and Identity*—fits within an emerging genre that might be called ecological humanism: a form of social-historical analysis that breaks down the artificial barriers between human beings and the universe in which they exist, between mind (or soul . . . or spirit) and body, between chemistry and economy, biology and culture. After all, what more animal and, in its way, cultural act can there be than eating?

By pursuing multiple angles and through a rigorous and imaginative use of a wide variety of documentary sources—customs house logs and records; inventories of provisions stocked by hospitals, monasteries, and landed estates; travelers' accounts and literary writings; interviews with shopkeepers, housewives, and cooks serving school cafeterias; the menus for prison inmates and of diners, restaurants, and fast food establishments; cookbooks; recipes; agricultural statistics; oral history records; nutritional and food chemistry studies; studies focusing on international politics, business, and commercial practices; and much more—Cruz Miguel Ortíz Cuadra draws us into this enticing feast of research and analysis on the history, anthropology, and sociology of Puerto Rican cookery and of what he quite correctly calls "the memory bank of our palate." This feast, cooked up on a slow burner by Ortíz for years, is made richer still by the dialogue he carried on with a far-flung network of scholars. His notes provide the most complete bibliography yet that I have seen on the anthropology and history of cooking and food consumption in an international context. It is a feast celebrated at the outset of the new millennium on "the enchanted island," but one whose guests hail from widely varying places and times. Like our salsa music—which we began dancing in Borinquen and the Bronx but which aficionados of dance around the world now revel in—*Eating Puerto Rico* is a feast that Puerto Ricans will doubtless enjoy in concert with readers everywhere who are interested in the dynamic relationship between ecology, gastronomy, and society.

The book that you are poised to read, with its various appetizers, many main dishes, and a selection of side dishes and desserts,[1] is at once both erudite and refreshingly accessible. Ortíz takes pleasure in the object of his research. He displays a wide smile—though from time to time his brow will be knit—as he carefully goes about unearthing dusty documents in the national archives, tries out recipes in his kitchen, or, beer in hand, chats with people attending one of the many food fests held in Puerto Rico. Several spring to mind, among them: the *Festival de la Pana* (breadfruit) in the Mariana de Humacao district; the *Festival de la Cocolía* (a small crab) in Dorado; and the festivals of *Hojaldre* (puff pastry) in Añasco; of *Macabeo* (a small fritter made with grated taro root and other ingredients) in Trujillo Alto; of the *Piña Cabezona* (king pineapple), which takes place, I believe, in Valle de Lajas; of "*Platos típicos*" (typical Puerto Rican dishes) in Loíza; and of the *Patita de Cerdo Guisá* (stewed pig's feet) in Guaynabo. Both for the general reader and for the most demanding specialist, *Eating Puerto Rico* is a feast prepared by one devoted to his "topic" and his "task," by one who combines—in a most exceptional way—solid historiography with a special liking and talent for tasting and cooking dishes both simple and elaborate, dishes based on traditional, quite involved recipes, as well as those drawing their inspiration from the most sophisticated *nouvelle cuisine*.

But do not be lulled into thinking that Ortíz is inviting us to a frivolous feast, to just another cute production of a light postmodernism. No, you will quickly come to a different realization. True, the book is a hedonistic blowout—and why not!—but it is also intelligent and searching. It is a work of scholarly rigor aimed at examining one of the central themes of contemporary historical and social scientific inquiry: the thorny problem of the dynamic of collective identity. Are we still what we ate?

Grounding himself in the daily biological struggle to survive, to feed oneself, Ortíz examines—with methodological soundness and with what C. Wright Mills termed the sociological imagination, one of the most powerful collective social identities of recent centuries: national identity, and the different faces that it wears. This shaping of national identity, resting far more on material than on imagined determinants (the former are the point of departure for the latter), is a process both contentious and contradictory, as well as one deeply felt. Thus Ortíz's book is not meant only for those whose interest lies in gastronomy. On the contrary, it stands as one of the strongest and most creative contributions I have read in recent decades—and I have read many, from any number of countries—to what at the beginning of the twentieth century Otto Bauer called "the national question,"[2] and what at the beginning of this century Gervasio García (Ortíz's former teacher) analyzed as the fundamental and problematic "horizon of feelings."[3]

Nor does Ortíz's history follow a traditional chronological sequence. Shadowing the trajectories left by the core elements of Puerto Rican cooking and cuisine, it ranges freely across the five centuries that have molded this Antillean community into one that, by periodically transforming itself, has avoided hardening into a fixed national state. Like the best cultural studies, the book examines ruptures and continuities while emphasizing—in terms of who we are as a people today—the undervalued Afro-Caribbean "first floor," whose central importance was so insistently stressed by José Luis González in his El país de cuatro pisos.[4] What we ate and what we eat, this is something we Puerto Ricans owe to an idiosyncratic welter of influences reflecting the colonial past and ethnic inheritances, as well as the interplay of gender and social class. Yet behind all these separate strains lies a central core, defined, as I analyzed it for music,[5] by the capacity for creative adaptability—this arte de bregar (art of toiling and winning through) that, more than any other group, the descendants of the African population have imprinted on the culture of the Caribbean.

In addition, then, Eating Puerto Rico advances an antiracist, democratic argument with respect to the central role played by popular culture in the formation of Puerto Rican national identity. It is a feast filled from beginning to end with new information and findings that, in turn, open up many new avenues for additional study and research.

Let me not detain you any longer in sampling the pleasures of this stimulating and delightful book.

¡Buen provecho!

ÁNGEL G. QUINTERO RIVERA
Old San Juan

Acknowledgments

While researching and writing this book, I sampled many of the dishes mentioned in it, taking care to follow exactly each step called for in the old recipes. My use of traditional ingredients and methods, however, does not mean that this is a recipe book or even a historical study of food with old recipes as its foundation. More than anything, it represents an attempt—in terms of theme, method, and theory—to put into perspective how and why in Puerto Rico we came to eat what by and large we do eat; to understand why and how for the majority of Puerto Ricans what they eat remains so familiar to them in the midst of all the changes and adaptations occurring, often with great rapidity, in our contemporary food habits and practices.

In writing this book, I have had assistance from many people, in particular:

Professors Astrid Cubano Iguina, Juan Giusti, Antonio Mansilla, Carlos Pabón, and Fernando Picó, who read the initial version of the manuscript and offered useful comments and suggestions.

Professor Sidney Mintz, who kindly entered into a rich and fruitful critical dialogue during the translation of the book.

Ángel Quintero Rivera who, in the best tradition of the master teacher, made a series of worthy suggestions based on more than a dozen critical readings of the text; Edgardo Rodríguez Juliá, who urged that I observe the mestizo "interplay" of Caribbean dishes.

The faculty of the Humanities Department of the University of Puerto Rico in Humacao—the philosophers Carlos Rojas Osorio, Joaquín Jimenez, Edward Rosa, and Rubén Soto; the historians José M. García Leduc, Pablo García Colón, Luis López Rojas, Luis Sánchez Longo, and Jerry Piñero; the art critics and curators Nelson Rivera Rosario, Rubén Moreira, and José Rojas; the artists Daniel Lind and Vilma Maldonado; the foreign language specialists Lourdes Suárez and José Eugenio Hernández; the writer Zoe

Jimenez Corretjer; the theater person and dancer Gradisa Fernández; the musicians Rubén López and José Hernández; the filmmaker and documentalist Reynaldo Álvarez—all of whom listened to my litanies about the relevance of studies on food and eating habits both as a field of interdisciplinary scholarship and as a way of understanding the patterns of food consumption in contemporary Puerto Rican society.

I am grateful as well to Pilar and Glorimar—secretaries in the Department of Humanities—for maintaining order in my correspondence during my absences; and to Jennifer Cintrón, my research assistant, for her frankness in alerting me to some passages that needed livening up and her adeptness in helping me avoid several blind alleys of research.

My thanks, too, to my siblings—Humberto, Carlos, Gerardo, Vanessa, and María Carolina—for their steady encouragement and unsuspected interest in the history of food and Caribbean cooking and cuisine. I could not have written a line were it not for the mediating effect of their gastronomic sensibilities on my thinking.

Special recognition goes to my wife, Anita. Everything that I have brought to fruition in my work on this topic during the past several years I owe to the sacrifices she has made. The encouragement she gave me in difficult moments enabled me to carry on to the end. Daily, she persevered in listening to some dry anecdote about the cooking ways of old and was intrepid in trying hoary dishes that, from the moment they went on the stove, looked unpromising and indeed turned out to be indigestible. On such occasions, Anita always consoled me with her pronouncement, "it's all really tasty," a gesture that often allowed me to overcome my frustrations and quickly recover my air of the historic chef.

To all,

Thank you

University of Puerto Rico, Humacao campus

Eating Puerto Rico

Introduction

When the Puerto Rican newspaper El Nuevo Día interviewed several public figures in 1999 regarding their favorite meal, Orlando Parga—a leading proponent of what has been labeled anexionismo jíbaro[1]—replied, "corned beef with fried ripe plantains." For Senator Norma Burgos, it was "chicken fricassee with white rice and pega'o (rice with the crisp, slightly charred scrapings off the bottom of the pot)." Longtime activist and Puerto Rican Independence Party leader Rubén Berrios confessed to a liking for "viandas (starchy root vegetables) with salted codfish (bacalao)." Renán Soto (the then president of the Puerto Rican Teachers Federation) chose "dry salted beef with potatoes and rice and beans." The comedian Raymond Arrieta answered that he favored "rice and beans with pork chops." Senator Velda González was more expansive, declaring "Oh, my goodness, that's a really difficult question. I love chicken with rice, salted codfish, pasteles (resembling tamales, pasteles are made of plantain dough that are filled with meat and other ingredients and boiled in salted water). . . . There are so many things I like"; and—shying away from naming one dish over others—the singer Ricky Martin declared "Puerto Rican food."[2]

How should we take these statements? Should we interpret them as the surface expressions of something deeper, more rooted, lending credence to the idea that people, regions, societies, and nations are in fact defined by their respective palates, by what is consumed at mealtime? On one level, food is simply the indispensable element that sustains our physical, social, and material well-being and that enables the human species to reproduce and carry on. On another level, however, food—and the various ways in which we cook and consume it—also reveals and measures how people, groups, and societies interact among themselves, negotiate and experience strange or different cultural traits, and, in the broadest sense, relate to the world. As such, food shapes modes of representing social reality, helping to stamp onto it structures and hierarchies laden with powerful symbolic overtones.[3]

Thus the maxim "tell me what you eat and I'll tell you who you are" has always been a prime factor when it comes both to delineating social and material differences between people and groups and to contemplating or imagining the culinary dimensions of ethnicities, nations, and cultures scattered across the planet. As Massimo Montanari asserts, food and cooking are a great vehicle for self-representation, communication, and the protective covering of identities, while also constituting "the principal outlet for entering into contact with different cultures."[4] Broadly speaking, food, cooking, and diet have polyvalent meanings.

In all the responses elicited by El Nuevo Día, however, two aspects stand out with particular clarity. First, there is the association between food and identity, in this case national identity. Although today in Puerto Rico one can readily sample cuisine and styles of cooking from various countries and regions around the world, and though the experience may be "the principal outlet for entering into contact with different cultures," since, as Montanari further states, "food opens up cookery to all kinds of inventions, exchanges, and influences,"[5] I am confident that the newspaper's interviewees gave the aforementioned dishes as their preferences, rather than others, because they know that the powerful metaphor of "Puerto Ricanness" attaches to them, especially in contemporary Puerto Rico. In contrast to how things were in the past, food and cooking have become categories of national identity, of loyalty to country, and of social pluralisms. In responding as they did, these individuals registered their desire to be identified as Puerto Ricans.[6]

Second, there are "the palate's memories," the formation of a kind of intimate bond with food and diet molded by material circumstances, a mother's cooking, the frequent repeating of various dishes and meals, and the "principles of taste."[7] This bond speaks to and evokes memories and emotions (good and bad), fixations on flavors and tastes, and—at times— sensations of estrangement. Put another way, societies and the inhabitants of particular regions also eat "what they have been," that is, their own history. As Montanari reminds us, "man is what he eats . . . but the opposite is no less true, man eats what he is: his own values, choices, and culture."[8]

Focusing less on examining the important and complex symbolic dimension of food, cooking, and eating—which constitutes the first constellation of meanings revealed by the interviewees' responses—this book instead explores the possible conditions constituting the second dimension, that of the "palate's memories." What happened in the past that led these people to say that such and such food and dishes were their preferred ones? Why, if today certain traditional food shares a culinary stage that embraces variety, are there still some people who prefer the traditional over the new, or the different? Or—phrased differently—why do some Puerto Ricans still eat what we (all) ate in the past? Moreover, in the midst of the contemporary food scene, in which a shift in culinary rules and performance is evident and we are everywhere flooded with information and notions about our current food and diet, is it really so strange that Puerto Ricans should be inclined to hold fast, nostalgically, to images of their past diet?

In the pages that follow, I intend to pursue these questions by looking at texts that discuss types of food we still find familiar, or—short of that—of food that still evokes the sensation and taste of traditional home cooking, at least for the generations of Puerto Ricans born before and during the 1950s. These are rice; beans; corn, in particular cornmeal and its derivatives; salted codfish; tubers (including the plantain), root vegetables and fruits, collectively known in Puerto Rico as viandas; and, of course, pork and beef. I further intend to consider such additional questions as:

What is it that underlies Puerto Ricans' identification with certain kinds of food? What is the path over time of those foodstuffs that are still recognized as definitive of Puerto Rican cooking? Why, in Puerto Rico, should we have developed such a close relationship with these particular types of food?

Rice, for example, is not native to the agriculture of the region, yet it has come to be central to our diet. Indeed, for some it is the most central ingredient in what is considered a complete meal. What are the drivers behind a culinary rice culture here that differs from its counterparts elsewhere in the world? Why do we cook rice "piled up" rather than "spread out" in a pan, as the Spanish do, for example? When did we begin to prefer grains that are short and polished? What expectations do we have when it comes to eating rice?

Cod is not fished in warm waters, such as those of the Caribbean, where—in contrast—*chillo* (red snapper, *Lutjanus vivanus*), *mero* (grouper, *Epinephelus guttatus*), *jurel* (mackerel, *Caraus hippos*), and *colirrubia* (pompano, *Diapterus olisthostonus*) are all found in abundance. Under what circumstances was salted codfish introduced, and when did it become a basic food item in Puerto Rico? What were the qualities that turned it into a "peripheral" food? Why was it viewed as a poor man's food, and what is its status today within the broader patterns of Puerto Rican food consumption?

The *yautía* (tannier) is called "yautía," and the *batata* (sweet potato) "batata" when—as part of a meal—they are the only food of their kind on the table. Yet when they appear together with other rhizomes or *frutas hervidas* (boiled bananas, plantains, and breadfruit) they are called "viandas." Why? What properties make them "good to eat?" What role did viandas play as part of a simple diet of accessible food?

For a long period of time pigs and cows roamed across wild land, and the possibility of killing and eating them was not confined to the privileged few, a limitation first imposed during the mid-1700s and one that lasted until the middle of the twentieth century. How did the rural environment change so that access to this culinary resource began to be differentiated along class lines? What role did the state play in this dynamic? On the other hand, why does eating roast pig today generate a party atmosphere and a feeling of community solidarity, in contrast to the ambience—now as in former times—surrounding the consumption of beef that is roasted? Why is it that we now eat so much meat?

Kidney beans, also known as *colorás*, always yielded the smallest crop in home plots and gardens, were the most costly, and had the least amount of nutritional value. Did they, then, possess some other qualities that people recognized as being superior to those found in white or black beans? Why did the majority of Puerto Ricans come to prefer "dry colorás?"

How have these foods typically been cooked and prepared? What beliefs and opinions have accompanied them into the kitchen? What changes can be discerned in these today, and how have they evolved over time? The answers to such questions can help shed light on why these types of food were eaten in the past, why they were prepared in certain ways, and whether—despite all the observed changes—people still have the same ideas about them and continue to prepare and consume them as before.

Each type of food is treated in a separate chapter, with the term "food" used first in the sense of "object of production," "edible object," object of "sustenance," what human beings take in on a daily basis in order to subsist, obtaining it from farming, hunting, scouring the land, raising animals, and via the agroindustrial market. The term is also used in the classic sense, as being what gives us the strength to live and maintain life.

The spectrum of food, however, does not stop there. I also include edible varieties of the main foodstuffs, such as the many varieties of beans and viandas, as well as food that is derivative—the cassava from the yuca plant, for example, or the cornmeal made from corn.

In sum, the book makes specific reference to the following: rice, beans, corn, cassava, tannier, sweet potatoes, plantains and bananas, yams, pork, beef, and salted codfish. At some juncture, each of these became a standard food item, one that appeared unfailingly on menus, or at the very least was a familiar sight on the dining tables of Puerto Rican homes—hence their designation as the basic or core foods of the Puerto Rican population.

Although these can all be obtained today from a variety of outlets and sources (global agroindustry, *hipermercados* [big-box supermarkets], corner groceries, restaurants offering local or native fare, "caterers," "casual diners," "fast food" establishments, and street cart vendors), they achieved their status in a preindustrial food-consuming context dominated by farming, hunting, gathering, and domestic animal raising, on the one hand, and the dietary limitations imposed by rigid exportation and importation markets, on the other. The exportation of food products obeyed a monoculture and their importation followed a very restricted, colonial model.

In this context, which characterized Puerto Rico until the middle of the twentieth century, the basic food items—to borrow Marvin Harris's phrase—became "good to eat,"[9] and as their potential benefits (in particular those belonging to the "original foods," which were passed on from the island's indigenous inhabitants to the Spanish and African populations) increasingly became known, so the indigenous and African populations in turn discovered the dietary value of the cattle and pigs that had been introduced from Europe. In addition, several new crops, having adapted easily to the agro-ecological environment, became "complements" of the original foods.[10] Later still salted codfish was brought in and became a "supplement," thereby fulfilling certain specific functions.[11]

Over time, and after many experiments, the basic foods formed a "matrix" that was organized on the lines of "core-fringe-legume." The "core" consisted of cereals and tubers that were a source of complex carbohydrates; the "fringe," of meat, fats, and also spices and condiments which—even more than being a source of protein—enhanced the taste of food; and the "legumes," of beans and all types of green leafy vegetables that helped lengthen the nutritional arc by adding proteins.[12]

To properly study the basic or key foodstuffs, I have found it necessary to acquaint myself with their characteristics in the fullest sense, from knowing their botanical and bromatological qualities and their capacity to survive as agricultural products, to the manner in which we interact with them—handle, plant, gather, buy them in the market and cook them—to the distinct ways in which we serve and eat them.

It is also necessary to consider different features of food and cooking in relation to agro-ecology, the food importation market, social and economic differences among human groups, large-scale farming, changes in the agricultural landscape, and state policy making. Another set of factors, visible and variable in some cases, concealed and fleeting in others, and whose potential Puerto Ricans have always wanted—and on many occasions have managed—to exploit, must likewise be taken into account. Formed around a practical knowledge and understanding of foods growing in the wild, these factors included deciding what is viable to plant and eat, working it successfully into a diet and taking full advantage of certain nutritional qualities, combining ingredients and flavors, and assigning different meanings to particular foodstuffs and dishes. As Puerto Ricans sustained these initiatives over time, they contributed to the formation of what can be defined as "Puerto Rican culinary culture." The British historian and sociologist Stephen Mennell states it thus:

> I use "culinary culture" only as a shorthand expression for a whole complex of matters relating to food . . . culinary culture, by extension, includes everything that we mean by "cuisine" of society or social group, but a lot more besides. It refers not just to what foods are eaten and how they are cooked—whether simply or by increasingly elaborate methods—but also to the attitudes that are brought to cooking and eating. Those attitudes include the place of cooking and eating in people's patterns of sociability (eating out, in company, or in private); people's enthusiasm or lack of it towards food; their feelings, conversely, of repugnance towards certain foods or methods of preparation; the place of food, cooking and eating in a group or a society's sense of collective identity, and so on.[13]

This definition of culinary culture is the sum of many interrelated parts that come into play in the matter of food and diet. It thus follows from Mennells's definition that cuisine is but one feature of the "culinary culture" of a region, nation, ethnic group, or special community.

What, then, is this "cuisine" to which he refers? What is meant by that expression "everything that we mean," which for Mennell constitutes the "cuisine" of a society or social group? Is it the act of turning foodstuffs into a meal in a place called the kitchen, that is, the purely physical aspect of cooking and no more; or is it a mélange of products and ingredients, recipes, menus, and social behaviors regarding the meal? Mennell does not elaborate, but perhaps he is referring to the outcome of multiple, extended, and varied human experiences realized in the encounter between nature, on the one hand, and the social, economic, and political circumstances of people, on the other. These experiences give "cuisine" its distinctive personality; they endow it with character and meaning.

In light of the foregoing, I have opted for two different definitions of "cuisine," definitions at once more specific and broader than Mennell's. One is Claude Fischler's the other Sidney Mintz's. Fischler puts it this way:

> "Cuisine" is usually defined as an amalgam of ingredients and techniques used in the preparation of meals. But "cuisine" can be understood in a different and at the same time more wide-ranging and yet more specific sense: [as] representations, beliefs, and practices that are associated with it and are shared by individuals who form part of a culture or group within that culture. Each culture possesses a specific [type of] "cuisine" which implies classifications, particular taxonomies, and a complex set of rules that apply not only to the preparation and combination of foodstuffs but also to their cultivation, harvesting, and consumption. It possesses, too, meanings which are closely tied to the way in which culinary rules are applied.[14]

Fischler's definition emphasizes several points worth bearing in mind when envisioning the evolution of what is understood today as "cuisine." First, there is the element of familiarity that operates in respect to foodstuffs, techniques, and rules within a community or group having common interests. Second, the environment that surrounds the actions involved in cooking and the application or non-application of rules is suffused with beliefs and representations. For example, in the case of Puerto Rican cooking, to use *azúcar moscabado*, or very dark, unrefined sugar, was synonymous with African or black cooking, or cooking done by the poor; to toss out the *sofrito* (a sautéed marinade of herbs, ham, and vegetables) was to be guilty of producing flat, insipid, or even un–Puerto Rican food; to cook meat during Lent was sinful; raw meat was synonymous with illness; cold food was not food at all; damp *mofongo* (mashed plantains combined with seafood, meat, or vegetables) was the equivalent of Dominican *mangú* (a mash of boiled plantains), and so on. Third, partly following the formulation of

Claude Lévi-Strauss, Fischler's definition casts light on the idea that ways of preparing food—cooking it, boiling it, leaving it raw—can signify levels of complexity or simplicity in the culture, in communities, or in groups under study.[15] And fourth, different beliefs, representations, and culinary practices are found within specific cultures. More directly, several cuisines can coexist—although not necessarily harmoniously—within such cultures.

Fischler's observation about the meanings that flow from the application or non-application of rules in the act of cooking is very helpful in discovering some of the elements that were shaping "Puerto Rican" culinary culture, in the sense that Mennell ascribes to it and, within it, to "cuisine" per se.

All the same, the meanings about which Fischler speaks suffer from a kind of rigidity. These meanings, it seems, come to light because they exist a priori and are immutable. In this sense, Fischler's "cuisine" fails to take into account the evolutionary stages and special circumstances and conditions through and under which the rules were solidifying and taking on their meanings. This book elucidates these particularities, identifying elements that, over time, slowly and gradually helped to set in place, or disrupt, or replenish the culinary "actions" (the rules about which Fischler speaks) and their meanings. These rules, subject to constant renewal, were to trace out the features of what eventually crystallized into a more or less shared or commonly accepted definition of the term "Puerto Rican cuisine."

What is understood, then, to be "Puerto Rican cookery and cuisine?" Here Mintz's definition comes into play: "People using ingredients, methods, and recipes on a regular basis to produce both their everyday and festive foods, eating the same diet more or less consistently, and sharing what they cook with each other . . . active producing of food and . . . opinion about food, around which and through which people communicate daily to each other who they are."[16]

Mintz has grounded the meaning of "cuisine" less in rules and structures than in a world of experiences, of pragmatic human abilities and capacities to use what is available, in order to try things out, mark off differences, and make judgments.[17] This practice is active, continuous, and open, but in time it becomes familiar, becomes common to a community. As Mintz writes: "I mean to argue . . . that what makes up cooking is not a set of recipes aggregated in a book, or a series of particular foods associated with a particular setting, but something more. I believe a cuisine requires a population that eats that cuisine with sufficient frequency to consider themselves expert on it. They all believe, and *care* that they believe, that they know what it consists of, how it is made, and how it should taste. In short, a genuine cuisine has common social roots; it is the food of a community—albeit often a very large community."[18]

Puerto Rican cooking, like that of the Caribbean as a whole, was developed and continued to be refashioned by immigrants who introduced their culinary traditions into new or largely unfamiliar agro-ecological environments and also faced the challenge of surviving in a colonial and slave society.

Just as in Puerto Rico, a defining feature of cuisine on the other islands of the Caribbean is the diverse origin of its central foods. Mintz, however, does not isolate this factor, since such diversity of origins has generally characterized cooking and cuisine from one side of the planet to the other. In the specific case of the Caribbean, and clearly in that of Puerto Rico, what matters is how foodstuffs, the way in which foodstuffs—both original and new—have been employed over time. In a colonial and slave environment, not to speak of one that was altogether new, foodstuffs that were freely available had to be used. According to Mintz, the resulting cuisine was a "bricolage," a medley, made out of what was available, designed to recreate—in a new way and using new ingredients—different and discrete culinary traditions. In this "bricolage-cuisine" the role played by slaves was decisive, since the great majority of them were directly connected to the production, distribution, and processing of food. They were at the heart of things culinary, even to the point of molding the food preferences of their masters.[19]

Mintz claims more than once, quite correctly it seems to me, that it makes more sense to speak of "regional cuisines" than of "national cuisines"—the latter, after all, are an aggregate of the particular foods and methods of preparation of the former—and he likewise believes that food need not serve in any strict way to validate group membership on the social or the community level.[20] Nevertheless, his definition is ultimately governed by the recognition that a cuisine is made up of "distinctive cultural products" that work to establish group or community identity, as well as to define places, societies, nation-states, cultural practices, and ethnic origins.

Viewed from this angle, his definition helps solidify the idea not only of "ethnic cuisine" but of a "local cuisine" that—when measured against a recipe book, or against ethnic and national restaurants within and outside Puerto Rico—strikes us as definitely Puerto Rican. It is the recognition that assails us when, for example, a serving of mofongo is contrasted to a serving of mangú or of fufu (mash of yams and plantains with other ingredients), even though the three are all prepared with plantains—one of the classic foods in regional cooking.

As I wrote the book, I decided to arrange the chapters according to how frequently particular foods are eaten by the majority of people in Puerto Rico. Rice therefore comes first, since it is the undisputed king of the daily diet, and meat comes last, for despite being almost as important as rice, the possibility that it will be eaten day in and day out is quite new to the island. The book concludes with two chapters covering the special features of cooking and diet in contemporary Puerto Rico.

The historiography of food and dietary patterns during the last quarter of the twentieth century and the initial years of the twenty-first is marked by three points of rupture and renewal. The first (to describe them in broad outline), dating to the beginning of the 1960s, was inspired by the concerns of the historians of the French *Annales* school to reinvigorate historical methodology and writing. This initiative was characterized by studies that focused on regional geographic contexts and by an interest in highlighting the material, biological, and nutritional aspects of food and diet.

The second point of renewal coincided with the 1986 founding of the journal *Food and Foodways: Explorations in the History and Culture of Human Nourishment*. This phase was characterized by an interdisciplinary approach and by a strong desire to explore the history of food and associated topics in terms of mental attitudes and feelings, incorporating the contributions of disciplines—anthropology and sociology in particular—that had developed a deeper theoretical foundation to the study of food and diet. In general, while important studies emphasizing physiological and material factors continued to appear in this period, the orientation championed by the *Annales* school lost some of its prominence.

In the Caribbean, the development of this second phase reached new heights with the publication of such works as Mintz's *Tasting Food, Tasting Freedom: Excursions into Eating, Culture, and the Past* (1996) and Barry Higman's "Cookbooks and Caribbean Cultural Identity"—an influential piece of research that, among other things, drained cookbooks of their apparent textual innocence.[21]

These studies signaled the opening of a third phase, in which the search for new source material branched even further afield to encompass literature and literary theory; ethnography; cultural anthropology; gender, urban, and environmental studies; chemistry; nutritional medicine; and many other disciplines in addition to history.[22] Creative as it was, this multidisciplinary initiative, which fell under the rubric of food studies and to which historiography was but an appendage,[23] nonetheless exhibited, in many cases, what Warren Belasco diagnosed as a preoccupation with research unrelated to food, a preoccupation in which food, cooking, and eating ceased to be the object of study and instead became simply a means to investigating other issues and concerns.[24]

In this book, by contrast, I have aligned myself more with the intent and purposes of the second phase of study, the phase that emphasized the interdisciplinary study of the history of food and nutrition.

The majority of those who have tried to engage this subject in Puerto Rican historiography have experienced frustration because of the difficulty of prizing out useful archival material on it. While the archives hold documentation that affords insight into the economic and productivity sides of food and cooking, they seem at first glance to have little if any data concerning the social and cultural aspects of these pursuits. Yet when perceived multidimensionally, or "crosswise," to use Montanari's term, the picture changes significantly.[25]

When read, for example, not only as production statistics but also as indicators of dietary preferences and food consumption, many local and regional records take on deeper meaning and mark new avenues for research. For Puerto Rico, such records include the list of food purchases, found in the archdiocesan archive of San Juan, made by the Carmelite nuns during the mid-1860s, and a similar list belonging to the Municipal Hospital in Caguas; the microfilmed *Balanzas Mercantiles* (account books, or logs), which provide a running list of all of the products imported by ship into Puerto Rico during the nineteenth century, housed in the University of Puerto Rico's Centro de Investigaciones Históricas (CIH). These are complemented by requests to evaluate food consumption and to assess municipal taxes, also held on microfilm in the CIH; the reports of the Department of Home Economics regarding its curriculum of cooking courses, stored in the University of Puerto Rico's central archive; and police files, located in Puerto Rico's Archivo General, which document cases of food theft in the early 1930s.

Above all, however, I have attempted to subject well-known texts in

Puerto Rican historiography—documentary collections and historical accounts in particular—to new readings and interpretations.

Moreover, in consulting works covering Puerto Rican social and economic history from the sixteenth century to the nineteenth, I have noted that some aspect or feature of food and nutrition is often treated somewhere in them; in quoted material, for example, or in the authors' footnotes or interpretive comments, or in illustrations or documentary appendices. These forms of corroboration, as scarcely noticed as they are valuable, serve as textual material in their own right, allowing one to cast a second light on the issues lying at the heart of this book.

I have found Berta Cabanillas's work, *El puertorriqueño y su alimentación a través de su historia*, exceptionally valuable. A pioneer in recognizing that any full-scale historical treatment of food and diet must go beyond the limits of nutrition and home economics, Cabanillas expended much time and energy combing Spanish archives for primary source material relevant to the subject. Without her work and its rich documentary appendix, I would have found many fewer openings to explore.

Manuals of hygiene, cookbooks, menus (relatively scarce on the whole), treatises on agriculture and botany, travel accounts, writings on local customs and folkways, the literature of home economics and nutrition, the highly valuable studies of food consumption sponsored by federal authorities during the Depression and the Second World War, advertising by the food industry, Department of Agriculture compilations on the importation and consumption of food, and contemporary gastronomic writing have all proved indispensable to comprehending the historical phenomenon of selecting, cooking, and consuming food in Puerto Rico, as they have to understanding—as Montanari puts it—ways of "thinking," or construing, food.[26]

Throughout the book, personal biography, the traditional methods of historical research, language, and the conventional ways of representing the continuum of "past-present" have posed—because they are necessarily interconnected—a tricky but alluring problem. How does one write about a subject at once so concrete, ordinary, and unavoidable and also so human, personal, and pleasurable, without creating disequilibrium between academic expression, a voice that preserves the simple and the unembellished, and the writing of the enthusiast? To elude the dilemma, I have actively woven personal experiences, oral testimonies, culinary events, and recipes and names of different foods and dishes into the narrative, keeping three central objectives in mind: to make all these elements contributors to history, to inject life into the writing and tone of the book, and to advance the book's hypotheses.

With the exception, perhaps, of the last two chapters, the arrangement and organization of the text also flow out of this intentional intermeshing of the popular and the scholarly, not in the form of themes falling into firm and uniform chronological divisions, but, instead, of distinct foods following a chronological sequence of their own and, in the process, manifesting particular gastronomic features and qualities. I have confined the more academic explanations to the notes and to the two concluding chapters. Tables and figures, too, are inserted more for illustrative than for closely argued scholarly purposes.

On the other hand, I have not set out to study the differing usages, written and spoken, that have governed the production, use, and consumption of foodstuffs in Puerto Rico. When I do appeal to them, it is with reference to specific ideas, for example, the representation of the plantain in the agronomic paradigms of the eighteenth and nineteenth centuries or the beliefs that took shape toward meat and its consumption at the end of the nineteenth century. Nor have I tried to document the economic history of each type of food under discussion; instead, I refer to tables and figures whenever they help (as they often do) to illustrate the rise or decline of particular edibles in wholesale and retail markets, or their nutritional value. To a considerable extent, eating, cooking, and selecting which foods to consume depended heavily on these factors.

In sum, my aim in this book is to trace the dynamic arc of food and culinary experience in Puerto Rico within the context of the ideas expounded thus far and, within this scheme, to pose various answers to the core questions: why did we eat what we ate and why do we still eat it, and where, when one examines contemporary Puerto Rican cookery, do we observe both changes and continuities in this pattern?

In Puerto Rico today, the experience of food and diet—and all the dimensions of which it is composed—mimic what Montanari notes as operative in societies enjoying an abundance of food and a flourishing food scene, namely, a powerful attraction to the subject of eating, cooking, and selecting different foods. What is the reason for this attraction? Is it because, in the words of Lee Dawdy, "[historically we] were driven to think about food in [the] daily fight against hunger,"[27] so that, to again quote Montanari, "our attitudes and behavior are still marked by the fear of famine?"[28] Whatever the answer(s), I hope in the end that this book will promote wider reflection on the subject of food and society from multiple perspectives: gender and cultural studies, sociology, clinical nutrition, food chemistry and engineering, the culinary arts, and—it goes without saying—history and its vantage points.

1 | Rice

> In Puerto Rico we are used to a diet centered on rice, and
> so accustomed are our digestive systems to it, that on a day
> when we miss rice, it seems as though we haven't eaten.
>
> —ELÍAS GUTIÉRREZ, Superintendent of the San Sebastián
> Demonstration Farm, Agricultural Experiment Station, 1938

Perhaps the most effective introduction to the topic of rice is a personal anecdote. One night in July 1989, while I was staying in Sisikon—a town in the Swiss canton of Uri—it turned out that my only option for having supper was the restaurant of a local hotel. A first look at the hotel confirmed that winter, not summer, was presumably its busiest season. An attentive waitress led me to the dining room, where—lost among the wooden posts and columns of a large hall—four couples were enjoying their meals.

Detecting that I was a foreigner, the waitress went out of her way to wish me a pleasant evening and to warn me that the restaurant offered only a single, fixed menu for dinner. In response, I asked her if it included rice, to which she replied, quite cheerfully and encouragingly, that—yes—it did.

To this point, everything had unfolded with the propriety and customary orderliness of a Swiss restaurant that catered to locals. However, when I proceeded to inform thirty-five students—who were waiting in the entryway for tables to be set up—that the first course would consist of rice, the atmosphere of quiet decorum instantly dissolved. My news set off a buzz of commotion, and as the students spilled into the dining hall, exclaiming "at last, at last"—for they had spent weeks eating regional dishes accompanied by vegetables, greens, pastas, and whole wheat bread—they expressed the hope that the rice might also be accompanied by stewed beans. Ever since, this vivid spectacle—the students' fervent reaction—has keyed many of my questions about the history of Puerto Rican food and culinary customs.

The sentiment quoted at the beginning of this chapter dates to 1938, but it is still frequently voiced by Puerto Ricans of all ages. Rice continues to be an essential part of the daily intake of food for the majority of the Puerto Rican population. A new breakdown adopted by the island's Nutrition Assistance Program (PAN) in fact recognizes rice as a basic food in its promotional graphics. These show a plate of food, split into two parts, which together illustrate how the 429,000 families that, as of 2001, were program recipients should expend the funds provided them for the purchase of food: of the monies awarded to individuals, 25 percent is to be used for meat and vegetables, and 75 percent for rice and beans.[1]

In the most venerable little eateries and restaurants of metropolitan San Juan, or of the city's Tejas de Humacao neighborhood, it is enough simply to read the menu to assure oneself that Elías Gutiérrez's dictum still applies. Gracing the menu are white rice, rice with salted cod, rice with sausages, rice with pig's feet, rice with fatback, rice with chicken, rice with land crabs, and rice with beans. Or similarly, one could flip through the recipe books for the cuisine known as *puertorriqueña de navidades* (traditional Puerto Rican Christmas treats and dishes) and find: rice with coconut, rice cornmeal pudding, rice *pasteles*, and rice with pork and pigeon peas. In addition, although they are remnants of an older fried cuisine, one will also encounter *granitos* and *almojábanas* (fried rice flour infused with cheese, and cheese-flavored rice flour fritters, respectively) in certain Puerto Rican municipalities. Such is the predilection for rice that servings of it will even be accompanied by "*pega'o*," for which there is usually a craving at the moment it is cooked.

All of this leads one to ask, why does it occupy such a central position in our diet? Why do we have these expectations of it? Why—given all the smart, clever ways we now have to shape our diet, do we continue preparing rice with fatty pieces of meat in it? Furthermore, why do we expect that a portion of rice must in itself be a major part of meals, while at same time thinking of rice as indispensable for turning a serving of food into a true "meal?" But what in a way is most curious and compelling is that, as is increasingly the case with other foods that define cooking and meals in contemporary Puerto Rico, rice is not produced anywhere in the country.

To answer these questions we need to consider certain background factors: the ready adaptation of rice to our agro-ecological zone, its capacity to grow and yield harvests, the practical wisdom in agricultural and culinary matters already accumulated by the various groups that came to constitute society on the island, the role of foods that were capable of bolstering intake during periods of food insecurity, the ability of rice to mix well with other foods—above all fats—and the place it occupied in the fixed diet of certain population blocs, such as plantation slaves or soldiers stationed on the island. Bound up with these and related factors, a series of expectations took hold in daily life with regard to how much rice to consume, when to consume it, and how to cook it. Before examining them, however, the original trajectory of rice in the country's agriculture needs to be explained.

The Scattering of Rice over Wetlands

If there is one ironclad certainty in the culinary history of Puerto Rico it is that rice was introduced by the Spanish. The records of the Royal Treasury uphold this fact.[2] What will never be known, however, is who, exactly, took charge of its rapid planting as a crop in the extensive coastal wetlands of the island. Prior to the arrival of Europeans in the Caribbean, rice did not exist in the agricultural system developed by the indigenous Arawak population and was thus absent from their diet. Even the wettest areas of the coastal valleys and plains, which later proved so propitious for the cultivation of rice, were used by the native inhabitants in food-gathering ways far removed from agriculture. They were exploited for fishing, collecting crabs, and hunting birds and lizards. Consequently, in terms of the agricultural knowledge of the native population, rice—like other foodstuffs brought over, planted, and successfully adapted to the local terrain—struck the Indians as highly strange. It is therefore likely that if indigenous communities participated in the development of systematic rice cultivation, they did so very minimally.

Yet as far as the expansion of agriculture on the island was concerned, everything seems to indicate that the participation of the Spaniards, who before setting out for the New World had grown and eaten the *Oryza sativa* variety of cereal, was also minimal. The loads of rice that they brought with them were quite limited in quantity, fluctuating between eight and fifty pounds.[3] This detail, and the fact that they were intermixed with grape seeds for wine, batches of honey, pots and kettles, cumin, coriander seeds, cloves, quince jelly, and many additional provisions contained in personal luggage, leads one to think that the settlers were more concerned with assuring their own food supply during the first months after their arrival than they were with beginning the cultivation of rice as an agricultural or commercial enterprise. Alonso Manso, the first bishop appointed to serve in the newly conquered land, had brought, as part of his own cargo of food, the largest quantity of rice, and that amounted to no more than fifty pounds.[4]

The lack of interest in fomenting a broad-scale agriculture that would guarantee food for the newly settled population stemmed from the preoccupation on the part of many Spaniards with acquiring gold and other precious metals. They devoted themselves—at least in the early years of colonization—to searching for gold in the island's rivers and streams, commandeering the native population as a labor force. Under these conditions, agriculture and the growing of foodstuffs remained in the hands of the indigenous population. In addition, the failure of some European crops to adapt to the agro-ecology of the island reinforced the importance of certain foods, such as corn and cassava, which the native inhabitants had learned to cultivate successfully. For fear of dying from starvation, the first wave of colonists made both cassava and corn a central part of their diet. Both also became a standard part of the crops cultivated on newly explored land.

Thus, in terms of the relationship that obtained between human beings and the agricultural environment, it appears that during this initial phase neither Spaniards nor Indians took up the systematic cultivation of rice, the former because they treated it more as an item of food than as a seed for planting, the latter because they did not know how to grow it. If in some fashion rice began to be planted during the period of the conquest, this must have occurred only when another people—the Africans—who like the Spanish had known about, cultivated, and consumed rice before the discovery of the Caribbean, began to arrive on the island as enslaved labor.

In contrast to the Spanish, however, and under the socioeconomic realities that now pressed down on them, the Africans immediately had to involve themselves in agriculture. In addition to this direct participation, many other factors make it likely that it is the Africans to whom we owe the dissemination of a cereal that no more than a century later was commonly found on almost all the colony's dining tables.[5]

According to specialists in the field, the cultivation of rice (the species known as *Oryza glaberrima*) extends back nearly 3,500 years in certain regions of West Africa. More specifically, in those areas out of which the present-day nations of Senegal, Sierra Leone, Liberia, and the Ivory Coast were formed, areas which supplied a large number of the Africans who arrived in the Caribbean in the sixteenth century, a rice civilization existed that antedated the Spanish conquest of the Americas.[6] The cultivation of rice both along the banks of the Niger River and within various coastal zones of West Africa sometime between the eighth and the sixteenth century was commented on by travelers who visited these regions and recorded their impressions.[7] The mark of rice's evident importance in these regions is that, for all the displacements that eventually occurred in the role of certain food products by virtue of the exchanges set in motion by the conquest (for example, cassava and corn in the direction of Africa and the yam and plantain in the direction of the Americas), the New World cassava—which over time displaced the yam as a principal crop in other parts of Africa— did not displace rice as a crop and primary food in the regions cited above. Moreover, the *glaberrima* species of rice was also planted, prior to the Spanish conquest, in the regions comprising present-day Ghana, Togo, Benin, and Nigeria, in all of which the transplanted cassava eventually replaced the yam as a crop and basic food.[8]

The enslavement and importation of Africans to work in agriculture coincided with what has come to be called, in Puerto Rican history, the first sugar era, that is, the period that roughly falls between 1535—by which time the extraction of gold had dried up—and 1580. It was during this period that Africans hailing from the rice cultures of West Africa began to arrive in large numbers.[9] Quite possibly, furthermore, it was during this initial sugar era that the cultivation of rice on the island (whether of the *glaberrima* or *sativa* species) was begun on a wide scale by African slaves. If such was indeed the case, it was due to the interplay of several factors.

First and foremost, the Africans' strong association with certain foods that conserved well and required minimal preparation—such as the yam and, of course, rice—enabled the slave traders to use them as rations for the captured Africans during their passage to the Americas. During the first decades of the African slave trade, the use of yams and rice must have been paramount, since the yuca and its derivative, the cassava, as well as corn— all of which later became basic food on the slave ships that left Africa—had yet to make a strong impact on African agriculture and on the cooking of different ethnically based rice dishes.

In these circumstances, in which rice was not only an essential food but also among the few food items provisioned to the imprisoned Africans on slave ships (in contrast to the diverse range of foodstuffs contained in the personal cargo of the Spanish colonists) the cereal and its grains that came off the ships and into the ports had a central, recurring function—to serve as a basic food for the slave population. It is also plausible, as Mintz has suggested, that some Africans brought it for its value as a seed in the face of uncertainty over the prospects of one day returning to their native land or because they looked ahead to the possibility that they would face a shortage of food, outlooks which contrasted with the thinking, or presumed thinking, of slaves and colonists who could see in the trade with Seville the possibility of provisioning themselves with the foods they were accustomed to eating.[10]

The Africans' long-standing familiarity with rice cultivation, the ubiquity of rice on the slave ships, and the close connection that slaves would have to agricultural labor during the initial stage of sugar production must have given rise to the first experiments with rice cultivation on both land that was used for subsistence farming on sugar plantations and in the encampments, or maroon communities, established by runaway slaves on the periphery of the nascent settler towns.

Another factor supportive of the instituting of rice cultivation by the African population during these years was the location of the first sugar plantations, or at least of the most prosperous operations, which were situated close to the wetlands and marshy areas of Puerto Rico's northern coast. This meant that the Africans lived in island-based agro-ecological zones that were very similar to the areas in West Africa where for centuries they had grown and harvested rice. To cultivate it, the Africans had developed water management techniques, such as closing off marshlands by building mud embankments and constructing small canals to retain or drain off water in keeping with climatic conditions or the flow of tides and sea.[11] What is more, in their native lands the Africans had cultivated rice in paddies that had high salinity and were located in areas subject to drought during one part of the year and to torrential rainfall and floods during another. Since the conditions they encountered in Puerto Rico were very similar, they already knew how to succeed in growing a crop that had been central to their diet for hundreds of years in this new (but familiar) agro-ecological zone. The Spanish, too, had integrated rice into their agriculture and diet centuries before, but for them it was just one more food and of secondary importance.

Brought over by the slaves themselves, the *glaberrrima* species of rice was quite possibly the first to be planted on the island. This species offered better resistance to the saline conditions of marshlands, and it was more resistant to both drought and flooding than the *sativa* species,[12] which had been planted and consumed by *Peninsulares* since the time of the Moors.

Other strains of *sativa* reached the island in subsequent periods, and gradually—due to phenotypical changes—adapted to the environment.[13] During the eighteenth century, at least one observer noted the importance of rice cultivation to heavily populated communities of African origin, which typically sat in low-lying coastal areas that had excellent conditions for growing rice.[14] By this time, the island's rice fields produced a yield of 2 million pounds, or—if considered in terms of individual consumption—an annual yield of about twenty-six pounds of rice per inhabitant.[15] The colony's total population was estimated to be 72,000.

The Bounty in the Cereal of the Marshlands

In 1772, Domingo Estévez, a resident of Aguada (a coastal valley community located on the western side of the island), proclaimed that the rice fields worked by slaves could produce a harvestable crop all year round. Of course he also acknowledged that such a boon almost never happened, since—according to him—the Africans did not take "the trouble to go into these wetlands, or lagoons, to clear the water of its undergrowth of weeds, which smothered the rice."[16]

As we see, Estévez makes two points in his assertion: first, that the environment—the wetlands, lagoons, and marshy areas that get clogged up with weeds—lends itself to growing rice, and second, that the African population is not motivated to exploit the rice-growing potential of the land to its fullest. Pointedly, Estévez's contention about the work ethic of slaves makes no allowance for the illness and disease that are the constant companion of those who labor in these fertile wetlands and suffer from the prevalence of mosquito bites and the ill effects of tramping barefoot through the mud and ooze of the marshes. In the rice fields, the threat of infection rises after the time of planting, which takes place once the water level has dropped. An extended period of rainfall then ensues; the humid flat lands reflood, at which point the newly planted rice begins to shoot up.

As soon as his crop has been planted and is growing, the rice farmer's concern shifts from the care of the land to the prospect of harvesting food for himself and his family. He does go into the steamy lowlands to make important adjustments, such as altering the position of the flood guards that regulate the water levels of the wetlands. But as soon as the grain shafts are in flower, the relationship between the plant and the field hands turns more on the question of food security than on the technicalities of farming per se. In the words of our eighteenth-century observer: "[If] they made the effort to go into these wetlands, or lagoons, to clear away the weeds which spring up with the water, and smother the rice, it would continue to produce harvestable grain throughout the year, and he who frets over the considerable mud and muck found in the soil of these lagoons would not elicit any admiration."[17] The rice field, given the real possibility of succumbing to disease or of falling ill, was a place one went into and left quickly, with the sole purpose of planting and reaping, and not of removing weeds or of extending oneself to cut and clear away other noxious growth, as some late eighteenth-century farmers wanted, primarily those of a more scientific bent who were more removed from the seasonal burdens of planting and harvesting. The colony's blacks only prolonged the time they spent in the wetlands on two occasions, each of which—according to Fray Iñigo Abad y Lasierra—occurred three times a year: when they needed to broadcast the seed and when they were ready to cut and collect the grain.

Only two methods for planting rice existed in the eighteenth century, two methods that had been known about and used since antiquity. In areas of natural flooding, the oldest and most common was that of broadcasting the seed and covering it over with wet, muddy earth. The other entailed cultivating seed plantings in separate beds or nurseries and later replanting these in plots that were flooded artificially.[18] It is worth emphasizing that broadcasting was the method that Africans had always used, just as it was used—as late as the mid-nineteenth century—on some of the rice plantations in the American South.[19] It quite possibly was also the method used on the island colony. Broadcasting first involved preparing a mixture of mud and water in a barrel until it attained the consistency of molasses. This mixture was then spread over rice seeds that had been scattered on the ground, following which the seeds were "enfolded in mud" by male and female field hands using their bare feet. The mud-covered seeds were later mounded up into separate piles, and these were left to soak until the following morning. The piles were then thrown onto plots, which at that point were no more than damp. The last step in the process was to open the small "gates," or barriers, through which water running down from the mountains was allowed to flow, thereby flooding the plots up to a level that was not to exceed twelve centimeters. The mud covering played a critical role, since the seeds—balled up in a damp muddiness—now stuck to the mud plots, in this way countering the possibility that they would simply float on the surface of the water and become nothing but nourishment for the birds.[20] If the rains did not produce any setbacks, an initial harvest would be realized four months later.

Abad y Lasierra's observations, made some two centuries after rice was first introduced into the wetlands and had—by his day—become part of the daily diet, highlight one of its most fruitful characteristics: its capacity to yield grain more than once a year. Rice plants act in this way because during their reproductive phase, the stem of the leaves or stalks produces a primary spikelet, from which sprout secondary and tertiary spikelets.[21] Although each of the spikelets remains attached to the plant, every one begins to produce stems of its own. Thus under normal circumstances, the more skilled harvesters can collect the primary spikelets while leaving the secondary and tertiary ones for later. However, even in circumstances in which they opt to collect all the spikelets—as during periods of galloping famine—they can still elect to make a high cut, a cut that is next to the spikelets, thus leaving two thirds of the plant in the ground.[22] In this way, the stalks would continue to sprout spikelets for several years, especially in rice fields that received decanted natural water flowing down from the mountains. Such water was rich in organic material and did not carry much sediment with it. By following this process, the local population could help assure itself of a steady supply of food. Or, to view the matter from the opposite angle, in places where the irrigation of the fields did not depend on lugging in supplies of water and where the level of flooding could be controlled without undue effort—as was the case in Puerto Rico—the growth of the rice stalks ceased being annual and became multiyear.[23]

In addition, rice also had the virtue of conserving well if, after being cut and left to dry, it was threshed so that the grain was rid of any remaining straw or other impurities, and the bran was not detached from the grain during the husking. Rice seeds of any species have a cuticle with two distinct strata or layers, one of which—the bran—acts as a protective layer for three of the seed's most vital elements, among them the pericarp, a thin delicate layer of cells that is impermeable to oxygen, carbon dioxide, and water. When preserved intact, it protects the grain kernel against fungus and the breakdown of enzymes.

When stored in dry containers kept in a fresh place, and if not deprived of the bran, rice preserved even longer. This quality, together with its potential to be harvested more than once a year, turned rice into one of the most available and dependable foods on the island. As with tubers, it became a staple in people's diets.

From the Marshes to the Kitchen

The desire to eat rice was one thing, but rendering it edible another. As we have seen, before it could be eaten, rice had to be husked. Husking was either accomplished by beating the rice with a mallet or by milling it. Initially, the former was the method most frequently used. The grains were first placed in a huge wooden basin, after which they were transferred onto a sieve or some other sifting device, where the grain was separated from the husk by hand. At that point what remained on the surface of the sieve were coarse grains, opaque in color and broken or cracked as a result of the mallet blows. At the same time, however, these grains were more nutritive, because they had not been subjected to excessive friction, such as occurred when they were husked between millstones. When the process was done by hand, the bran was preserved.

The second method was used in the kitchens of the most prosperous. Milling was done with two wheels placed on top of one another. The top wheel was serrated and the bottom wheel covered with a fine layer of cork. The objective was to reduce the chances of getting grains that were crushed and tiny. If the operation was carried out carefully and skillfully, the reddish pericarp was eliminated, leaving a slightly polished, shiny grain, a grain that agronomists call "pearled" or "bleached."[24] It is important not only to draw but to understand this distinction, because in the twentieth century, the preference of most Puerto Ricans was for rice of short, white, polished grains. This rice had the least nutritional value, but its shiny appearance as well as other qualities made it the favorite of those of lesser means.

At the end of the nineteenth century, husking and polishing via millstone wheels was not the method typically used, and not because millstones were unavailable or because people preferred rice that still had the pericarp, but rather because in contrast to other cereals, such as wheat, it was the rice grains themselves that people wanted to eat, not the flour produced from them. Furthermore, and this was on people's minds as well, one ultimately got a greater yield of food by cooking or boiling rice than by doing the same with a mixture of rice flour and some other pulpy substance.

Well and good, but if the slave cook on a plantation, or the cook in someone's home, or the cook in a little eatery, or, let us say, an emancipated former slave woman who sold rice fritters in the market decided to cook rice, how would they treat it to make it edible? They would go to the storeroom or pantry, located in a dry, ventilated part of the house, remove the top of a barrel—a *dita* perhaps (vessel made from a coconut), or a tin that had once contained crackers—and grab some rice. It was not as simple, however, as just blindly collecting a handful of rice. One had to choose, by looking closely to find the cleanest, most intact grains. These had then to be placed on the sieve to eliminate the residual matter that always remained after the first sifting. All of this work was done by hand: "First the rice is to be selected, removing from it any grains with pieces of husk," wrote the anonymous author of the first cookbook published in Puerto Rico, in 1859.[25]

Then, to ensure that one would be eating clean rice, it was rinsed twice: "Wash it once and then a second time, scrubbing it so that it sheds the dust and straw on it, until the water comes out clean."[26] A sharp eye and careful touch were essential.

The Cooking of Rice

Bearing in mind three key historical variables or markers about rice—that it was disseminated across the island starting in the middle of the sixteenth century, that the techniques for cultivating it were known and mastered by the colony's continually growing population, and that its particular properties allowed it to yield several harvests and to preserve well once it was cut—it is not surprising that in 1770 Abad y Lasierra would see fit to put rice on the same footing as foodstuffs that were central to the islanders' diet: "Their food comes down to a pot of rice or of sweet potatoes, yams, squash, or all of them together."[27]

The continuing, vibrant relationship between the colony's inhabitants and rice fueled the development of different ways of using the cereal once it was husked, sifted, and rinsed, different ways, that is, of cooking and exploiting it. The specific forms and patterns of use varied according to the inherited traditions of those who came into contact with it in what for all—Africans, Spaniards, and the mixed-race (mestizo) and mulatto descendants of the aboriginal population to a lesser extent—was a new social and agricultural context. Many factors came into play: the availability of agricultural resources, the varying conditions underlying and affecting its use, the economic and material circumstances of those cooking it, the quality of the rice itself, and the human-social element—for whom was it being prepared and on what occasions. These factors, while they differed and were sometimes exclusive of each other, nonetheless nurtured the formation of a unified, coherent "Puerto Rican culinary rice culture," the elements of which—when it is time to cook and then eat the food—are familiar to all: that the rice is brought to the table clean and shiny, that it have a loose, grainy texture, that it be a major and central component of a full meal, that it be flavorful, that it either be combined with other ingredients or come accompanied by legumes, and, last but not least, that it not be devoid of the crisp rice scrapings from the bottom of the pan.

This shared sensibility has various points of origin, many of them intertwined with old and venerable ways of cooking whole rice that, as we will see, were designed to take full advantage of environmental resources and to follow recipes for preparing rice dishes that varied according to the occasion and the guest list. Without dwelling overly on the changes that gradually affected ways of cooking rice in the decades leading up to 1950, it is instructive to examine them briefly and to review selected early cookbooks that make reference to rice. The first element to consider is the *remojo*, the soaking of rice in water.

SOAKING THE RICE

Picture a cookbook reader living at some point between the end of the eighteenth century and the period preceding modernization in Puerto Rico. The rice has been husked, sifted, selected, and rinsed. Having been cleaned, it is ready to undergo "soaking," the first in a series of treatments that will make it edible. This step would be skipped if the grains were not especially coarse or if the dish to be prepared did not require that the rice first be steeped in liquid. The next step was to cook the rice, plunging it into boiling water. Depending on the economic circumstances of a particular home and its kitchen, the vessel holding the boiling water might be a humble clay pot, an iron kettle, or a more elegant glazed casserole dish. From this point on, the options for seasoning, preparing, and presenting the rice were varied.

THE SEASONING OF WHITE RICE

The most common method of seasoning this rice was to add a little salt to the water and—later on—to sprinkle over it a bit of lard in which several cloves of garlic had been fried. The garlic cloves came apart, and the lard was spread over the rice just before it was fully cooked.

Another seasoning technique was to avoid the salt itself and instead fry pieces of salted fatback in the cauldron, lightly frying the rice in the fat before adding the water, all the while keeping the bits of fried fatback in the mixture. This detail is important, because in the kitchens of those of more modest means, the seasoning was almost never done by adding salt, but instead by sautéing the rice in the fatback drippings. It was preferable to save the salt and use it to preserve meat. By the middle of the nineteenth century, by one means or another, a recipe for cooking *arroz blanco criollo*, or a locally inspired version of white rice, was commonly known and used. The recipe entailed the following: "Put a little more than one pitcher of water in a casserole with an appropriate amount of salt, heat it, and once it is boiling, throw in the rice—not to exceed a measurement of one pound— well washed according to earlier instructions: let it cook until all of the water is gone; separately, fry four cloves of garlic in four tablespoons of fat, remove them when they are golden brown, pour the fat on the rice only when it has been cooked per above, always making sure it is fully cooked with a light texture; only then does white or criollo rice come out right."[28]

The recipe's insistence that the merits of the dish depend on the rice being fully cooked and smooth helps explain the expectation that still reigns in Puerto Rico just before white rice is eaten, the expectation that it come out fluffy and not *amogolla'o*, or gummy.

The sprinkling of the fried lard over the rice at the end of its preparation, or sautéing the rice in lard before adding the water, is what gives flavoring and sheen to white rice. The addition of fat drippings came to be the norm when serving rice. When this ingredient was lacking, the reaction of those eating white rice was that it had not been properly cooked. Lydia Roberts, a nutritionist, was surprised to discover this reaction during field work that she carried out on the island in the midst of the Second World War: "The dependence on lard was brought home to me by the case of a maid in a home I visited. Lard in those days was totally unavailable at the time, and the woman of the house explained that she was having great trouble in feeding the maid because of it. The maid could not eat rice because there was no lard to 'season' it, and without lard she couldn't eat beans, for rice and beans are indispensable complements of each other."[29]

Today, vegetable oils are used, but the preparation of rice with lard or fatback, which still occurs in the kitchens of those who are less in tune with more progressive ideas on nutrition, now has about it the nostalgic overlay of a simpler but tasty and inviting way of cooking.

White rice—still picked out and washed in the old way—reappears in twentieth-century cookbooks,[30] even though a cleaner, more polished imported rice was frequently found on the shelves of Puerto Rican markets between the end of the nineteenth century and the 1950s.

RICE CASSEROLES

The procedures described above were also necessary to make rice casseroles (*arroces compuestos*), or dishes into which local meats, poultry, shellfish, fish, or legumes were incorporated. Yet in this case, too, rice continued to be the main ingredient, and while a little less water was used, boiling was also a key feature in the preparation of these dishes.

Seasoning was more important for the casserole than for plain white rice, since the aim was to produce a really tasty form of rice. To this end, wild herbs (coriander), chili peppers (sweet and hot), and various condiments (paprika, cumin, garlic, and onions) were used. As a rule, these ingredients, or some combination of them, were ground up in a mortar and sautéed over the flame with lard or bits of salted fatback with the oil from annatto seeds, since—with casseroles—the objective was, as it remains, "to paint the grain," that is, to add color to the dish.

Depending on availability, pork or dried salted cod, pigeon peas or land crabs, pig's feet and garbanzos, pig's head, hen, and the like would be mixed with the rice and broth. The process of sautéing herbs, chili peppers, and condiments as a way of seasoning the fat was also used in making legume-based stews or casseroles with ingredients like beans, pigeon peas, or chickpeas, which generally accompanied helpings of rice. Over time, this seasoning—eventually known by the name *sofrito*, became iconic to Puerto Rican cooking, its most indispensable complement.[31]

In the preparation and perfecting of mixed rice dishes, the experiences and knowledge bases of different traditions intermixed and came together to produce a uniquely Puerto Rican form of cooked rice. Beyond the highly defined role played by the ingredients themselves, a number of elements rooted in the tastes and cooking practices of the discrete populations making up Puerto Rican society came into play.

These included organoleptic factors, such as the intense smell of the coriander leaf or of sweet chili pepper coming into contact with sizzling fat; the flavor that the plantain leaf gives to rice when it is used as a covering for *arroz apastela'o* (a rice casserole mixed with pork, lardoons, pigeon peas or chickpeas, flavored and colored with a strong sofrito and garnished with shredded green plantain and then covered with plantain leaves); the reddishness of sautéed annatto or paprika; and the sensation to the palate of sticky rather than fluffy rice. How the rice casserole sat over or was exposed to the flame or embers (more vertically rather than being spread out, or covered with plantain leaves or with a lid, and so on) was another factor.

Preferences, dislikes, and taboos dictated by attitudes regarding the consumption of animal meat also affected the composition of the casserole. The preferred meat was pork, but the parts of the pig that were added to the dish reflected both the material circumstances of those eating it and factors of a more social-psychological nature. In the case of rice and pork dishes, the culinary practices of the elite excluded the use of the animal's extremities, such as the trotters and the head, or the tail and the ears, consigning these to the underclass. Rice with a ridge, that is, rice with a pig's head topping it, is a good example of this division, since, on the one hand, it is represented during the nineteenth century in the context of peasant celebrations,[32] but, on the other, it does not appear in a single cookbook. Animals—rabbits, for example—associated with human qualities might likewise be excluded, as would creatures that people simply feared for one reason or another, such as land crabs that had eaten *manzanillo* (a tree whose fruit and white filmy liquid are poisonous) or fish and shellfish infected with *ciguatera* (a poisonous toxin found in dinoflagellate algae).

RICE FOR PARTIES AND GUESTS

If the most common way of eating rice was in the form of white rice, the preparation of rice casseroles was the favored way to cook and eat rice when guests were invited or when several people gathered in someone's home to enjoy a meal together. On these occasions, meal portions were larger, and one took advantage of foods that were in season or used leftovers from earlier dishes. This distinction is important, all the more so if one considers that it was not until about six decades ago that the majority of Puerto Rican kitchens had more than two burners on their stoves, or a sufficient number of vessels in which to cook several dishes at the same time. When the kitchen was so equipped, guests were able to enjoy not just a delicious rice casserole but other dishes that figured prominently in Puerto Rican gastronomy: a selection of boiled tubers or corn or plantain fritters. Table 1.1 lists some of the recipes for rice casseroles appearing in cookbooks published between 1859 and 1950.

TABLE 1.1 Rice Casseroles in Puerto Rican Cookbooks, 1859–1950

Publication	Year	Recipes
El cocinero	1859	the Valencian way – the Turkish way – with hen or chicken – with pork meat – with clams – with turtle – with beans – with okra – with chickpeas
Home Making	1914	with chicken – with pigeon peas – with salted codfish
Puerto Rican Cookbook	1949	with pork and sausage – with chicken – paella valenciana – with land crabs – with fish – with rice pasteles
Cocine a gusto	1950	with vegetables – with beans and garden legumes – with okra – with tomato and cheese – with tender corn and cheese – with pork – apastelado – with red beans and coconut milk – with pork tripe and Vienna sausages – with chicken – with hen – topped with tomato sauce and cheese – Spanish paella – with fish – with canned sardines – with shrimp – with salted codfish – with fish and garden legumes

Of course, while the person cooking the rice casserole might want to use one of these recipes, its preparation was necessarily affected both by the general agro-ecology of the region and by what was available in the market. Of major importance, too, were the economic circumstances of the comientes (diners sitting down to a meal) and the actual resources at their disposal. The rice casserole was not an everyday dish. Much of the time, in preindustrial Puerto Rico, those eating it could not easily lay their hands on many of its ingredients; and whereas today some of these—such as beans or pigeon peas—are available year-round, they only appeared seasonally in earlier decades. Similarly, a recipe that called for including trotters or special types of sausage could only be followed if a pig was slaughtered.

In both the nineteenth century and the early twentieth, novelists in the costumbrista tradition employed food as a leitmotif. As part of the local diet, arroces compuestos helped mark the element of sociability contained in the act of eating and cooking by appearing in the context of community festivals and celebrations and of visits between friends and acquaintances. "Arroz con carne was heaped about," wrote Manuel Alonso in his sketch of local marriage customs, "Un casamiento Jíbaro."[33] "Rice with a ridge," or rice with a pig's head on it, is served for dinner in Ramón Méndez Quiñones's story "El cuento del matrimonio."[34] In early twentieth century cooking classes given in Puerto Rico's public schools, the preparation of rice with chicken was imbued with a distinctly festive meaning: "This is one of the most popular dishes on the island," proclaimed Grace J. Ferguson, the supervisor of home economics for Puerto Rico's public schools and the author of the recipe that was used in the classes. She went on to recommend that pupils celebrate eating it by having "a little party at the close of school."[35]

Some simple lines of verse in Alonso's "Fiesta del Utuao," about the meal that awaited him at a relative's house, reinforce the teacher's message: "The food that my cousin / had prepared for us / a dish of rice with meat / and another of stewed rice."[36] To dress up visits made by friends or to receive family members, one prepared rice with chicken or hen, or cooked a rich, gumbo-like rice dish called *asopao*. "You go to the store and get a little something. And see here, we're going to kill a young hen, I want to make an asopao for him," was how the old servant of José Dolores, the illegitimate son of a coffee planter in the municipality of Lares, celebrated his master's long-awaited return.[37]

Until well into the twentieth century, some rice casseroles, which are now a fixture on the table, could only be eaten during particular times of the year. Such was the case with rice and pigeon peas, a dish that is now indelibly associated with the Christmas season. In Puerto Rico, its absence during meals on Christmas Eve, New Year's, and the holiday of the Three Kings is considered an unmistakable breach of Christmas culinary tradition. But a fact unknown to many is that in past eras, before agroindustry had made each month like the others in terms of the availability of popular foods, the harvesting of pigeon peas obeyed natural agricultural cycles and coincided with the calendar of Christmas festivities.

Another dish served at Christmas was *pastel de arroz*, a kind of rice pie, to accompany helpings of roast pork. It began as rice cooked in water, to which salt and lard were added. After the rice was boiled, it was mashed into a paste and placed onto plantain leaves colored with achiote. The mixture was stuffed with pork that had been seasoned and cut into little cubes, and—depending on the preferences and resources of the person preparing the dish—could also be garnished with almonds, raisins, cooked garbanzos, olives, and hot chili peppers. It was then wrapped in the plantain leaves and boiled in salted water.[38] The preparation of this dish, like that of *pastel de plátano*, was heavily indebted to traditional African ways of cooking rice and—as we will see—to using leaves for wrapping and steam-cooking different starchy tubers, like the yam, in salted water.

So constant and ordinary is rice in the daily diet today that it is difficult to imagine how special this dish was in earlier times, and not simply because the preparation and cooking of the pastel required considerable time and know-how. The experienced cook had always been able to tell if the pastel was made and wrapped up properly: if so, it would hold completely together while being boiled. Instead, what made the dish so special and kept it from being made week in and week out was the unpredictability, or difficulty, of obtaining all of the ingredients that went into the filling—the pork, the pieces of fatback from under the pig's skin, raisins, almonds, and the like; these were not readily at hand in many kitchens. It made better sense to use rice in simpler ways. That a recipe for pastel de arroz is found in only one of the six cookbooks published between 1859 and 1954 points up the vital importance of an oral tradition in keeping knowledge of the dish alive and widespread.

"BROTHY" RICE DISHES AND "MOIST SWEETMEATS"

Rice was also used as an ingredient in the preparation of soups, of varying consistency, and of sweet confections. Incorporating rice into the former was one way to give them more bulk, as in the case of "rice soups," made with portions of meat and sprinklings of sofrito,[39] or of the thick, brothy rice dishes—known to everyone—called asopao, invariably made with chicken, salted codfish, and pigeon peas.

One of the more specialized ways of preparing some of these dishes, born of the prominent place that sugar occupied in the country's agriculture, was to first soak the rice in liquids that had been seasoned and perfumed with sugar, and to then cook it over very low heat. These preparations, more than any others, were the touchstone of a woman's abilities in the kitchen. They offered women, above all those who cooked day in and day out, the greatest possibility of gaining recognition within the local community and of proving and distinguishing themselves in terms of prescribed male-female gender roles.

In contrast to other rice dishes that appeared on a daily basis, these moist, sweet rice confections (arroces húmedos dulces) were often presented to neighbors and relatives to mark holidays and religious celebrations. Their coloring, texture, aroma, and degree of sweetness, and the various ways of perfecting these qualities, were batted back and forth in conversation, and women of a more mature age used them to point out the successes or failures of younger women for whom cooking and the kitchen were at the center of daily life, the trademark—along with child rearing—of their role in society. They also came into play in matters of the heart, presented either as the sign and symbol of one's love and affection or as a gift to mollify hurt feelings. On one level, then, arroces dulces, like the majority of popular sweets and pastries, were public or social constructions, tasty and appealing food that "gave one pause for thought" or "sparked conversation."

One of the most frequently served sweetmeats in the homes of the well-to-do in mid-nineteenth Puerto Rico was rice pudding, or custard (budín de arroz). This dish, traced back to the region of Andalusia in Spain, blended cooked rice with sugared milk suffused with the aroma of cloves, cinnamon, lemon rind, and nutmeg. After the mixture had been allowed to cool down, beaten eggs, orange blossom, and anise were added to it, and it was put into the oven in a special bowl.[40]

With its pasty consistency, and after being soaked in coconut or almond milk infused with different spices (cinnamon, anise, or cloves), dried fruits (raisins), orange blossom, ginger, and sugar, and then cooked on very low heat, the rice meal was the basis for the sweet, perfumed confections deeply popular even today during Christmas festivities on the island. These treats, bearing the stamp of earlier Mediterranean, Andalusian, and North African recipes, were also frequently prepared for days on the religious calendar that required abstention from meat. They went under a variety of colorful names, and costumbrista literature as well as cookbooks and other gastronomic writings are replete with references to them and to their particular ingredients.

One of the most traditional versions was that known as manjar blanco criollo. According to the recipe that appears in El cocinero puertorriqueño, this delicacy was made with rice meal soaked in a half pitcher of leche buena (fresh cow's milk), sweetened with half a pound of refined sugar and two spoonfuls of orange blossom.[41] The specification of leche buena, rather than the humbler coconut or goat's milk, and of refined sugar, rather than moscabada or melao (a rich syrup from sugarcane), reflects not only material and economic distinctions but a more primordial identification as well, an identification with the brightness and luster of the color white, which in the minds of some was viewed as a symbol of prestige. The use of rice meal, however, implied that the sweet would not be made that often, since rice in its granular form had so many common uses. The dish—which has come to occupy a venerable place in Puerto Rican gastronomy—is quite likely adapted from the classic manjar blanco of the Mediterranean region, the recipe for which had appeared in European cooking guides since the Middle Ages. The preparation of manjar blanco called for using rice, sugar, cinnamon, milk, almonds, and fish or chicken broth.[42]

It is possible that the author of El cocinero was familiar with one of the old editions of Ruperto de Nola's Libro de cocina, which describes manjar blanco, or that the inspiration for its Puerto Rican variant came from one of the many cooking manuals published in France between 1714 and 1799. The opinion of specialists is that the generic use of the name "manjar blanco" in many European cookbooks is deceptive. People are led to believe that the European and Puerto Rican recipes are one and the same, when in fact there are considerable differences in how this sweet is actually prepared.[43] Whatever its genealogy, manjar blanco criollo disappeared from Puerto Rican cookbooks during the first two decades of the twentieth century. It turned up again in 1948, when Eliza Dooley—a North American—classified it as a dish intended exclusively for Christmas time.[44]

Another confection very similar to manjar blanco was that known as "majarete de harina de arroz" (rice meal pudding or custard).[45] This preparation called for the addition of pork fat, to give more consistency to the mixture. It was flavored with lemon rind or with the leaves of new shoots from an orange tree.[46] One of the most popular versions of majarete was made with cornmeal.

Arroz con coco (coconut rice) was made with rice grains, and because it required the use of a device for milling, not every cook had the resources to make it. Several steps were needed to extract the milk from the coconut as well as the ball of coconut inside the shell, steps which modern agroindustry, and conveniences like tinned coconut milk, have made obsolete. All the same, in kitchens where tradition still reigns, above all in the coastal municipalities of northeastern Puerto Rico, such as in Loíza, Canóvanas, and Río Grande, the same procedures that were followed centuries ago are still followed: dry the coconut, peel away the outer shell, break the nut, extract the meat of the coconut, chop it into little pieces, boil these in water, and—as last steps—press them to get the "coconut milk," which is afterward added to the rice.

As with other sweetmeats, arroz con coco recipes vary from one kitchen to another depending on personal taste, economic circumstances, and the creative inclinations of the person preparing it. For example, some might opt for brown sugar over white; others might fold in shavings of the coconut meat, use ginger as a flavoring, or perfume the coconut milk with aromatic cloves. The use of brown sugar imparts the dark color to the confection that, for the most snobbish and jaundiced of those sitting around the table, marks it as having been prepared by someone of limited means. In the kitchens of the better off, the dish is dressed up with raisins, typically found around Easter in urban markets and groceries, along with candies, dragées, dates, nuts, and hazelnuts—all of which feature importantly in Spanish commerce on the island.

By and large, arroz con coco was prepared during the Christmas season. In similar fashion to manjar blanco, it is evidently linked to the celebration of holidays and the presentation of gifts, as well as to the desire, among those most faithful to the liturgical calendar, to abstain from eating meat, since it has no meat in it nor is pork fat used in its preparation.

Throughout the twentieth century, arroz con coco was also known as *arroz con dulce*. It is this dish, more than any other, that has kept alive the mestizo culinary tradition of arroces húmedos dulces, although its taste must undoubtedly have changed once canned, concentrated coconut milk began to be used.

Still another moist rice dish, called *arroz con perico*, seems to have been made in the nineteenth century. This version was seasoned with sugar and perfumed with ginger.[47]

The use of two different forms of rice (ground versus granular), two types of sugar (white versus brown), two types of milk (coconut versus cow's milk), and the presence or not of such extra touches as raisins and coconut shavings point up that there were dual ways of preparing rice sweetmeats—one for the well-to-do and one for the poor; one that pertained to more urbanized environments, the other to coastal and rural regions and to a population more African in origin. Today, almost no one notices the differences that in past centuries must have advertised, in clear, stark terms, such distinctions of social and economic class. Nevertheless, if it is true that almost no one takes much notice at present, it is also true that some of these lines are still drawn and discerned.

By the same token, the ready availability of arroces húmedos dulces today, as facilitated by the operations of the food industry, make it difficult if not impossible to evoke the power that these dishes previously had to define differences in the social hierarchy. In a patriarchal society of sharp social divisions, in which the task of cooking fell principally on women from the lower classes (black, mulatto, or poor white cooks) and the serving of food in both domestic and community contexts generally bestowed first honors on the man, a cook's abilities and creativity in the kitchen gained her attention and respectability.

The cook's need to follow a complicated series of steps, true especially in the preparation of arroz con coco, demanded a special understanding that brought out the qualities that the men at the table, or those who occupied a higher rung in society, admired in cooks. Thus it was (and the practice continues today) that many a confection carried the name of the person who first prepared it (e.g., the majarete of Dolores, Vicenta's arroz con coco, Colasa's manjar blanco), and the possibility that some other kitchen might produce it, in exactly the same way, was dismissed out of hand, because the secret of the recipe was closely guarded by its author. While this situation might obtain with other types of dishes, it occurred much more frequently with rice delicacies and other sweetmeats.

With respect to social norms and rules of conduct, the arroces dulces not only symbolized graciousness and deference but also served as aids for maneuvering in a masculine world: the effort they represented was both a visible token of friendship and an instrument of courtship. Presented at the end of a meal, eagerly awaited, soft and moist in texture, the sweet dessert was full of undertones.

As the twentieth century approached, another moist rice dish appeared. Marketed and sold as *arroz con leche* (rice milk), it became a staple in infants' diets.[48] Its central place as one of the foods given to newborns was such that the most popular song sung by mothers and wet nurses to get the attention of their babies at feeding time, particularly in the homes of the well-to-do, was entitled "Arroz con leche."[49]

Still another form of cooking rice was to fry it. After moistening it in milk or lard and seasoning it one way or another—for example, with sugar and cinnamon, or with salt and cheese—the cook, using her hands, made little rice meal *bolitas* (round in shape) or *tortitas* (small cakes) which were then fried in lard. This dish was the basis for the *buñuelos de arroz* (rice fritters) that have appeared in cookbooks since the nineteenth century and are still sold on street carts in the municipalities of Humacao and Caguas. They were initially known by the name granitos (because cooks molded them into a shape that resembled a grain of rice) and included cheese as an ingredient. In Caguas, they are called almojábanas (fritters or crullers) and are made in the shape of a ball.

Eating Rice: The Development of Expectations, Simplification of the Diet, and Food Insecurity, 1850–1940

That a rich and varied set of rice dishes was emerging on the island, knowledge of which was transmitted via different channels (word of mouth, cookbooks, housewives' personal recipes, and through what Claude Fischler calls "mothers' cuisine"[50]), does not mean that everyone in Puerto Rico cooked and ate them, occasionally or even at all. On the contrary, the dishes and confections that appear in cookbooks, including the most recent beginning in the decade of the 1950s, could not be prepared with the ease and comfort that they are today.

The possibility of eating rice in the creative ways outlined thus far simply did not exist for some groups in a society so sharply differentiated along class and economic lines. Yet given this reality, why was there an expectation, passed from one generation to the next, that rice would be ever abundant, central to one's diet, and flavorful as well? Why did this expectation still maintain its grip (as it continues to do even now) at the end of the 1970s?[51]

There are three underlying factors that intersect to create these broadly shared expectations. The first is that of "habit," or of the rules and conventions governing certain segments of the population (soldiers, plantation slaves, prisoners, hospital patients) whose restricted, unvarying choice in the food they were given made rice the key component in their diet.[52] The second constitutes a subset of the first: when options were limited, as they were, the preference was for food with a high fat content, which enhanced flavor and made meals tastier.[53] The third lay in the "received wisdom" that rice was the key food in guaranteeing that a meal would be nutritional and filling. This attitude would harden as the shrinking of options that occurred between the end of the nineteenth century and the first quarter of the twentieth produced a simpler diet and a growing insecurity about the availability of food. To a greater or lesser degree, these three factors have shaped the ways in which rice is cooked and eaten in Puerto Rico to the present.

Moreover, it is the third one—the belief that rice was the heart of the meal—that has exerted the strongest influence on determining how rice is prepared and eaten. Even today, at banquets where rice is plentiful, it is customary to hear the time-honored refrain: "So, if we stop, nothing's to be lost since we've already eaten?" Although on the surface it may sound like an invitation to indulgence, a very different meaning is concealed underneath, one out of which the popular saying itself was born, that is, a call to seize the moment, to capitalize on the present abundance, which before—for a great many—had been constantly eclipsed by an insecurity about food.

SIMPLIFYING THE DIET

In the face of present plenitude, it is often forgotten that in past eras choices about what and how much to eat were closely tied to agricultural contingencies and, as we will see, to the priorities and contingencies governing the market for imported food. These factors could quickly alter the dietary expectations of groups that produced a substantial part of their own food, if not all of it. In Puerto Rico's nutritional history, a plague, or a hurricane, or the shifting priorities of monocultural latifundia had the greatest impact on changing food and dietary practice.

In the case of rice, the adoption of large-scale agriculture in zones long dedicated to rice (sugarcane cultivation commencing at the beginning of the nineteenth century is one example) reduced its footprint in wet, low-lying coastal areas, spurring campesinos to plant the cereal at higher altitudes, which resulted in the production of a "dry rice." Since these uplands could not be irrigated or flooded to the same extent, lacked the necessary exposure to the sun, and were tended by campesinos who possessed little understanding of their quirks and characteristics, the varieties of rice became intermixed, undergoing a slow but steady process of degeneration that in time produced yields of lower-quality rice.[54]

It is worth emphasizing that in 1859, in the very year that saw the first publication of El cocinero puertorriqueño—with all its enticing recipes for rice dishes and confections, recipes aimed fundamentally at an urban public— 5,345,984 pounds of imported rice entered the country.[55] This figure is all the more striking because it approached the quantity of rice, 8,049,800 pounds, produced in Puerto Rico around 1831.[56]

Could it be that the amount of rice produced in small, single-family plots began to prove insufficient for a population on the rise that contained a growing number of young people? The answer, quite possibly, is yes. Is it also that rice fields lost ground against the force and momentum of sugar plantations, and that communities which had previously cultivated rice were now destined to take up agricultural work that had nothing to do with the planting of rice for local consumption? That, too, is possible. As an added factor, were plantings of "dry rice" affected by the cultivation of coffee in areas of higher elevation?

Whatever the principal underlying cause, starting in the middle of the nineteenth century, rice faded as a crop of choice on the part of farmers and campesinos, its cultivation taking up less and less land relative to other foodstuffs.[57] Even for the poorest campesinos, the dry rice they grew began to be used more as an exchange crop than as food for their tables.[58] As this change was under way, polished, short-grain rice— grown in English and German colonies in Asia— began to appear in ever greater quantities in Puerto Rican markets.[59] The decrease in local rice cultivation, on the one hand, coupled with the growing volume of imported polished, short-grain rice, on the other, helps explain two fundamental transitions in the culinary history of the country: a sharp change with respect to the type of rice people preferred to eat and a solidification of the place of rice within a diet that was growing more limited in scope, becoming simpler, owing to the noncultivation of basic foodstuffs. This second factor meant that diets were deprived of well-nigh all variety, or at least of a minimal amount of nutritional components. Among the poorest elements of the rural population, daily food intake began to be limited to small portions of certain foods rich in nutrients—salted cod, fatback, dried beef, animal extremities steeped in brine, and dried imported legumes—as accompaniments to increasingly larger amounts of rice.

Through this process of dietary shrinkage and simplification, the population would find itself depending more on the market for imported polished rice than on the whole grain rice of its island agriculture. Thus, while the amount of imported rice was estimated at 77 million pounds near the end of the nineteenth century, local rice production covering the same period was calculated at 4,500,000 pounds, or more than a million pounds less than the corresponding figure for 1827 (5,357,000), when the population was much smaller.[60] This situation became more sharply defined in the first decades of the twentieth century, with the development of largescale sugar estates and the further industrialization of rice growing in the United States.[61]

TABLE 1.2
The Importation of Rice to Puerto Rico (in Millions of Pounds)

Year	Quantity
1859	5,345,984
1869	7,961,362
1879	24,128,975
1895	44,199,499
1896	70,614,957
1897	77,994,122

Source: CIH, BM

During this stage of the simplification of the Puerto Rican diet, rice's role as a basic, central food was intensified not because of its capacity for multiple harvests, or because it conserved well, or—as people had come to realize in the seventeenth and eighteenth centuries—because it blended well with other food. Rather, its central place in the diet reflected its growing status as the most reliable food.

As a point of interest, in 1891, as part of his once-a-week food purchases, a farmer in the community of Utuado (located in the mountainous region of central-western Puerto Rico) acquired between four and six pounds of rice.[62] This quantity translated into an estimated total of 13.7 ounces of rice consumed daily and contrasts sharply with an estimate of the amount of rice consumed on a weekly basis in 1937. Among two hundred families living in the region of sugarcane plantations it was 18.1 pounds per family (or some 2.58 pounds per family per day); among two hundred families in the coffee-growing zone it was 17.6 pounds per family (2.51 pounds per day); and in the tobacco-growing zone it was 20.2 pounds per family (2.88 pounds per day).[63] Some years earlier (in 1930), the Department of Education had found, in a sample study of thirty rural families (subdivided by low, medium, and high-income levels), that each family ate rice ten times per week.[64] In 1937–38, the annual consumption of cereals, including rice, wheat flour, and cornmeal, was estimated at 20 percent of total food consumption in the island, 15 percent of which corresponded to rice.[65] In the mid-1940s, 42.3 percent of the Puerto Rican population ate rice twice daily.[66]

These examples do not validate the notion, contrary to the conclusion drawn in most of the studies of Puerto Rican food and diet carried out in the first decades of the twentieth century, that rice was consumed in great quantities because—and exclusively because—it was the "preferred choice." Nor do they establish, in themselves, that as the Puerto Rican diet was being scaled down and simplified, the habit of eating rice and the expectations that accompanied it would necessarily make this the preferred food. The examples also point toward a "budgetary, physiological" reason for rice's popularity. It became the least expensive option for satisfying hunger. Since such high-energy foods as fresh meat or poultry were generally unavailable or beyond a family's reach, a meal of rice and legumes was a good alternative—not as rich or energy providing but still substantial and filling. Food insecurity and the simplification of the diet, however, would eventually exact their price.

As the process of dietary simplification gathered force in Puerto Rico between the end of the nineteenth century and the first decades of the twentieth, the central role of rice played out in other ways. One of these was related to the hard-core belief—on the part of the population that depended most heavily on rice—that the cereal was the key element in turning simple food into a "meal," into a sustaining and satisfying experience, something comparable to the place of *fan* (rice/grain) in Chinese culinary tradition.[67]

The attribution of this special quality to rice caused it, during episodes of food insecurity, such as occurred in the aftermath (1928–30) of the San Felipe hurricane and during the Great Depression, to be expressed in unanticipated ways and through acts of violence. In the first instance, for example, farmers ate the seeds distributed by the Department of Agriculture to increase output on the island; in the second, they ransacked neighborhood corner groceries, to the point of threatening the supplies of rice furnished by the import market.[68]

Later, during the Second World War, the same cycle repeated itself when food rationing was instituted (1942–45). The impulse to secure this key food for one's family again inspired demands that turned violent and led to the ransacking of grocery stores. Such incidents followed a government announcement that the amount of rice entering Puerto Rico would decline from 268.5 million pounds in 1940–41 to 198 million pounds annually and that a system of fixed quotas would be established, limiting each person to a weekly allotment of one and a half pounds of rice.

Thus, when the rumor circulated in Ponce in November 1942 that a ship carrying a full load of rice had anchored in the port, the city's residents poured into the streets in search of the precious grain: "The frame of mind of the people may be accurately gauged from a story that appeared in the Puerto Rico World Journal on 13 November, 1942, when word had gone round that a shipment of rice had arrived in the town of Ponce. The story ran: 'At Ponce, early yesterday morning long files of people lined up at the entrance of stores facing the public square to try to buy one pound of rice each, and they did not disperse until it was proved to them that the rice had not yet been distributed. There was considerable fighting and shoving, and police intervention was necessary.'"[69]

The conviction that rice was the essential source of sustenance, and that without it one could not survive, was addressed by Edward J. Bash, the Caribbean director of the War Food Administration: "Rice continues to be the number one problem here in Puerto Rico. Daytime thoughts, night time dreams, newspapers, the radio, conversations, everything seems to hinge on this fact. Until the supply of rice is adequate, it will probably be best to remember that Puerto Rico, translated into English, is RICE."[70]

Starting in the early twentieth century, as the simplification of the diet gained ground, Puerto Ricans made rice into a "symbol of protected food." To have rice was to have a meal, sustenance, the hope of satisfaction. This conviction, and the certainty that informed it, was displaced onto postwar generations; for them, too, rice was the symbol that kept the specter of hunger away.

It is thus not surprising that many years later, in 1973, when food conditions in Puerto Rico were much more stable and the supply of food more varied, the population again stampeded into the streets in search of rice. The precipitating factor this time was that the major importers had chosen to idle their freighters on the California docks as a tactic to try to force the Puerto Rican government to grant them a subsidy.[71] If there were sufficient supplies available for the consumption of meat (calculated at 124 million pounds), as well as healthy supplies of wheat flour and other cereals, which had been scarce at the beginning of the century,[72] why in this context, so radically different from that which obtained in the years 1942–46, did people still feel compelled to act in the old way, taking to the streets to assure themselves of rice and rice alone? In the 1970s demands for rice security were heard time and again. The role of "fan," which the population ascribed and assigned to rice in contexts of food scarcity and insecurity, was still operative in people's minds and imaginations when they sat down at the table to eat it.

AGAINST POLISHED RICE:
"CONVERTED" AND "FORTIFIED" VARIETIES
As we have seen, the notion about the "necessity" of rice was grounded in the universal belief that without it, a meal was not really a meal. The importance ascribed to it, however, was also tied to a concern about nutrition originating in the teachings of food chemistry and nutritional science. Two developments in particular brought this concern into focus. The first entailed the effort, championed at the beginning of the 1940s by several women nutritional experts based at the University of Puerto Rico, to redirect the population's preference away from polished rice; the second—stemming from the failure of this effort to change popular tastes—lay in

the adoption of a regulation that all rice imported into Puerto Rico must be "fortified." A review of these developments illustrates just how slowly change occurred in the domains of food and diet, and in the "food culture of rice" especially.

Between 1918 and 1951, the limited nutritional benefits of polished versus whole grain rice became increasingly known to nutritionists, public health officials, scientists, and others, as did the associated problem that populations whose diets included little other food were at risk of developing chronic vitamin deficiencies. In those years, while rice-based dishes and sweetmeats continued not only to be consumed (especially by the more educated and advantaged among the citizenry) but to embody Puerto Rican gastronomy par excellence, a diet that concentrated heavily and monotonously on rice (for example, an everyday meal of white rice with the sole accompaniment of beans) began to be seen as the model of an inadequate diet conducive of malnutrition.[73]

These concerns would have to contend both with the reality of a more simplified diet and with a host of attitudes and conventions, forming and reforming since the end of the nineteenth century, regarding the consumption of polished, short-grain rice in opposition to the far more nutritive whole rice that Puerto Ricans had previously grown and eaten. For those most dependent on rice, the polished, short-grain variety offered some practical and visual-aesthetic advantages—long dreamed of by certain social groups—over whole rice: the elimination of the time-consuming tasks of hulling and sifting, and the acquisition of a shiny, soft, and finished grain. In his trenchant reaction to the project of revitalizing the cultivation of local rice by farmers of family plots, a Puerto Rican agronomist put his finger on the essence of this opposition: "The biggest problem affecting our country's rice among its potential consumers lies in the inadequacy of its preparation. No one wants to purchase rice that has been split and cracked by the blows of a pestle."[74]

The opposition, however, ran counter to the new, enlightened nutritional knowledge and was thus largely ignored. Preoccupied to a fault by the wholesale decline in local rice production and swayed by the limited nutritional value of polished rice in a context in which the average consumption per person approached almost one pound daily, nutritionists opted for "converted" rice.[75]

In 1943, driven by both commercial interests and the concern for better health, a campaign was begun to promote the consumption of what was called "converted" rice, better known today as "parboiled" rice.[76] Born of nutritional angst as well as of the ingenuity of the agroindustry in its quest to lower costs, parboiled rice was more nourishing because, in its preparation, the elimination of the bran came after grains had been soaked and steam-cooked. As a result, the B complex vitamins, especially B1, or thiamine, and niacin, were retained inside the grain.[77]

"Converted" rice, however, had to measure up against tastes and outlooks that had coalesced around polished, short-grain rice, and for this very reason, it failed as a substitute. When parboiled rice was brought to the table, it displayed a yellowish color that people found altogether unsatisfying. Unlike polished rice, after being cooked it acquired an opaque appearance that clashed with the look and appeal of the commodity most rooted in the gastronomy of Puerto Rican rice: white rice. It also failed to work for a number of highly traditional preparations, such as the arroces dulces and arroces húmedos, or for the soupy rice dishes such as asopao, because it would not absorb the broth at the right moment when cooked. Equally unsatisfactory, when cooked by itself, it did not come out of the cauldron with the crusty pega'o, as everyone wanted and expected, and its texture turned out too "gummy" for the Puerto Rican palate.[78] In short, converted rice would have to await the arrival of different times and circumstances before it could win acceptance.

In light of these negative results, a debate ensued in 1951 about the possibility of making an enriched rice available by legislating its adoption, as had been done for wheat flour ten years earlier. Through the efforts of the indefatigable nutritionist Lydia Roberts,[79] and the Committee on Nutrition that she had founded at the University of Puerto Rico in 1943, legislation was passed mandating the enrichment of all the rice imported into Puerto Rico for consumption.[80]

The new regulation was a tacit admission that there would be no reversion to the production of whole rice in Puerto Rico, given the deep-seated preference for the polished variety. The underlying concerns about nutrition remained, however, and so the guiding principle behind this reform was a serious acknowledgment of the vitamin deficiency problem resulting from the diet's narrowing and simplification. This acknowledgment was strengthened by the findings of several investigations into diseases triggered by malnutrition.[81] It was evident that among the segments of the population most dependent on rice, the greatest vitamin deficiency was that of B1, or thiamine. Consequently, researchers at the University of

Puerto Rico's School of Tropical Medicine began to study the nutritional value of different types of rice and to publish the results. In addition to dramatizing the problem created by the lack of nutrients in polished rice, this initiative fostered the ideal environment in which to marshal arguments that the rice of the future should be converted rice, or at the very least, local "criollo" rice. When translated into the number of milligrams of vitamin B1 obtained through consuming a portion of edible rice, the figures proved revealing: polished white rice, 0.30mg; converted rice, 1.2mg; whole criollo rice, 1.35mg; and enriched rice, 2.0mg.[82]

The superiority of the rice once grown in Puerto Rico was also evident to a less technical-scientific community participating in the national discussion about diet and nutrition. Yet the reality was that farmers were not about to gamble on reviving the cultivation of whole rice when the level of imported polished rice was so high, nor was the population at large, given its irreversible preference for the latter, about to accept converted rice. People were even less disposed to revert to a hard rice, one having a coarse, opaque grain; and they would equally resist changing styles of cooking and sensations of the palate to which a diet of polished rice had long accustomed them. If it was not possible to overcome the headwinds of importation or of established taste, the logical solution was to make available a short-grain, polished rice that was enriched, or fortified.

According to the description given by Roberts in her pamphlet *Mejor arroz, mejor salud*—which spurred passage of the 1951 legislation that helped convince people that a better rice was not some experimental variety different from polished rice—"fortified" rice was made by adding a pound of mixture known in English as "pre-mix" to every hundred pounds of polished rice. After the combination, rich in thiamine, niacin, and iron, was added to the rice, it was covered with an edible viscous substance. With this technique, the nutrients in the pre-mix adhered to the grains of rice and subsequently passed into the water in which the rice was boiled—the standard method employed by Puerto Ricans when they initially cooked rice.

For all the good intentions behind the science and the nutritional guidelines and promptings, certain food and dietary practices deeply rooted in the population militated against any attempt to institute a progressive nutritional policy.

As noted earlier, in preparing rice to be cooked, it was customary—and had been so since the early nineteenth century—to rinse it twice. This practice continued in the twentieth century, even with the mass-produced polished rice that came from the United States. It was by this means that domestic cooks and housewives got rid of the residual particles that inevitably remained after husking (even when industrial methods of husking were employed). In addition, there was a belief—strongly held by people—that rinsing the rice ultimately made it whiter. Thus the time-honored practice of washing the rice before cooking it undermined the newly formulated nutritional policy with regard to enriched rice. In the years following passage of the legislation, the Committee on Nutrition had to design a forceful educational campaign to explain the harmful effects of washing enriched rice and likewise discredit the belief that the mixture added to the rice contained harmful residues and that it adversely affected the look, feel, and taste of favorite dishes.[83]

So, if the population did not renounce its high consumption of polished rice, or suddenly cease its practice of rinsing rice before cooking it, how could the nutritional problem—first precipitated by the narrowing of the diet—be addressed? As we shall see in greater detail in the chapter devoted to meat, starting in the 1940s, canned meat products began to appear more frequently in the country's markets and to play a larger role in the food strategies pursued by the state, such that the lack of vitamins which the practice of washing rice might cause was counteracted by the availability of foodstuffs that, though much desired, had up to this point not been an option for the general population. The various canned preparations of rice with meat that appear in the 1951 cookbook *Cocine a gusto* bear eloquent testimony to this development.

In subsequent years, moreover, enriched wheat, powdered milk, meal programs introduced in school dining halls, and the availability of frozen meat all contributed in important ways to the normalization of the diet. The population would recover through other foodstuffs what it lost by continuing to wash rice.

These supplements were invaluable, because rice continued to be the main food in people's daily diets, with white rice retaining its place as the preferred variety. The "custom" or attachment that took hold in the nineteenth century, the transmission and passing down of culinary notions and conventions via "mothers' cuisine," the simplification of the diet that occurred during the early twentieth century, and the pressures exerted by the foreign importation market all conspired to turn rice into our daily fare, a status it continues to enjoy today.

Rice as Daily Fare: Some Contemporary Observations

Between 1960 and 1980, the planting of arroz criollo came to an end in Puerto Rico. In 1969 the Mayagüez branch of the Agricultural Experiment Station tried to stimulate and increase local production through an experimental project that employed a new strain of seed.[84] Later, in 1973, the impasse caused by the interests of the large rice importers, on one side, against the government's tariff policies, on the other, inspired a legislative initiative aimed at making rice cultivation a governmental priority.[85] By the end of the 1980s, however, the political indifference displayed toward imposing effective regulation of the import business, the loyalty that consumers had built up for certain imported brands (e.g., Valencia or Red Seal), and the erratic agricultural policies adopted after 1976 ruined any chances this effort might have had to succeed.[86] Not even the attempt to package locally grown rice in terms that appealed to Puerto Ricans' sense of a distinct national-cultural identity, by labeling it Arroz Comet: *De Aquí Como el Coquí* (Comet Rice: Like the Coquí, It's From Here), could overcome the force of entrenched taste and custom. The tiny tree frog known as *coquí* might have symbolized Puerto Ricans' identification with their island and its singular history and traditions as powerfully as any other image or object, but the association was not compelling enough to persuade them to replace white polished rice with arroz criollo.

The statistics for the overall annual per capita consumption of rice—polished, converted, and whole—disclose frequent rises and dips starting in the first years of the 1970s. In 1975, the per capita consumption was 142 pounds, whereas in 1980 it dropped steeply, to 79.8 pounds. By 1987 it had partially recovered, increasing to 99.5 pounds, only to drop again, in 1992, to 70.8. Five years later, in 1997, it had jumped back up to 122.2 pounds. Between 1999, 2000, and 2003, there were similar fluctuations.[87] Throughout, polished rice—which in the Department of Agriculture's statistical compilations was calculated separately from "converted," "whole," "mixed," and "broken" rice—continued to rank as the rice preferred by Puerto Ricans, whether in its long, short, or medium varieties.

Importation figures, from which the amounts of overall consumption are derived, reveal similar fluctuations. What is more, this side of the ledger recorded a considerable decrease after 1975, when the total figure reached 419 million pounds. In 1980, it had declined by roughly a third, to 267 million pounds. In 1990, it was 295 million, dropping in 1995 to 203 million,

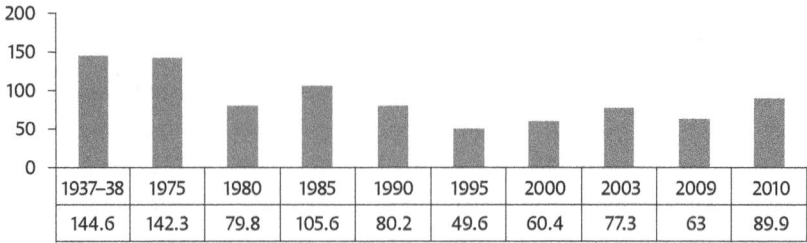

	1937–38	1975	1980	1985	1990	1995	2000	2003	2009	2010
	144.6	142.3	79.8	105.6	80.2	49.6	60.4	77.3	63	89.9

FIGURE 1.1 Annual per capita consumption in pounds of all types of rice, using 1937 as a base

Source: Estado Libre Asociado de Puerto Rico, Departamento de Agricultura, Oficina de Estadísticas Agrícolas, *Consumo de arroz en Puerto Rico (arroz total) 1975–2010*, folder 1759b1.

and in 2000 it rose modestly, to 230 million. This latter-most figure is lower than that recorded a half century earlier, in 1948–49, when it stood at 280 million pounds.[88] The trend line for imported rice as a whole is thus gradually downward.

Does this mean that, in general, the consumption of rice in Puerto Rico has also exhibited a decline? All indications are that it has. With respect to the consumption of all types of rice, including "whole," "converted," "mixed," and "polished," figures compiled by the Department of Agriculture show a slight decline in the last three decades of the twentieth century. The figure for 1975 was a high-water mark that has not been reached since.

This detail is important because it is the spearhead of a phenomenon characteristically noted in developed countries, whereby foodstuffs that are considered scarce or whose high rate of consumption reflects their status as the food that people believe they must eat—as in the case of rice in Puerto Rico—have begun to lose their primacy in the selection of food.[89] It is important, too, because it suggests that certain complementary foods that will sometimes take the place of rice might be emerging, slowly but surely, to replace it as the basic components of the everyday meal.[90] Despite the nearly limitless capacity of the North American rice-growing interests to exploit a deep-rooted preference, the consumption of rice in Puerto Rico has begun to shrink.

In addition to the gradual reduction in the sheer amount of rice consumed, it is clear that the island's "rice culture" has also changed, by absorbing other ways of cooking and eating rice practiced elsewhere in the world and through the popularization of some dishes that follow, to a greater or lesser degree, traditional recipes from abroad. There has also been a move toward using vegetable oils in the preparation of rice dishes, despite the long-standing preference in the Puerto Rican culinary tradition for lard, and a more notable—though still minimal—focus on "whole" and "converted" rice, prompted by various ethical and medical ideas about taking proper care of one's body by eating a healthier diet.[91]

Moreover, in recent years there has been a change of preference in favor of medium-grain and long-grain polished rice, in place of short-grain rice, which has fallen in popularity to third place. Statistics gathered in 1997 showed an overwhelming preference—85.2 percent—for medium-grain rice; "large polished" came in at 10 percent, and short-grain at only 4.8 percent.[92] The lower price of the medium grain versus that for the other two undoubtedly helps account for these percentages, as does agroindustry's strategy of combining different types of rice—or of rice that has been bruised in the hulling—and selling them as "medium" grain at much lower prices. On this point, trade statistics for the fiscal year 1999 indicate that 28 million pounds of rice classified as "milled mixtures" entered Puerto Rico.[93]

It is also noteworthy that, despite the strong pressure still wielded by the United States—and by the state of Texas in particular—on rice consumption in Puerto Rico, the various rice dishes eaten every day on the island are not prepared exclusively with rice imported from the United States. At present, rice is also exported to Puerto Rico from the Republic of China (53 million pounds in 2000), Egypt (11 million pounds in 1999), and Argentina (260,884 pounds)—all of the medium-grain variety.[94]

All in all, to have eaten a bona fide meal in Puerto Rico, as it is understood by Puerto Ricans themselves, still means eating rice every day in a form that gratifies the senses. The greater variety of food in contemporary Puerto Rico notwithstanding, a complete meal is one that includes a side of rice, or some specific rice dish, be it broth-based like asopao, a great favorite on rainy days or on the cool, slightly stormy early mornings of the Christmas season; or a casserole like stewed rice; or "white" rice, garnished with the crusty scrapings called pega'o. These last two dishes preferably come accompanied with the food taken up in the next chapter: beans.

2 | Beans

> ... its plant is always covered with flowers and pods
> containing beans, which are pleasing to the taste, dark
> red in color, not very attractive looking, although the
> natives do not hesitate to enjoy them.
>
> —IÑIGO ABAD Y LASIERRA, *Historia geográfica,
> civil y natural de la isla de San Juan Bautista*, 1788

In 1999, in the midst of all the millenarian prophecies foretelling the end of the world, the Medalla brewery released a television commercial playing on the idea that we can never really be certain of what lies in store for us tomorrow. The commercial, set in some indeterminate future time, featured a young professional hurrying to have his main meal of the day—lunch. Walking through a dark passageway, the young man comes to a vending machine selling drinks and snacks, puts in some coins, presses a button, and receives three capsules from the machine, each one representing a particular food. He picks them up, peers at them more closely—the light is very dim—and suddenly gives way to anger. And the reason for this reaction? Medalla beer was not among the three capsules. Instead, they contained *flan de coco* (a caramelized coconut custard), rice, and beans—three of the foods and confections to which Puerto Ricans are most endeared.

The commercial and its story line convey certain messages that I intend to clarify in this chapter. The most transparent is that a large segment of Puerto Rico's male population, men between the ages of twenty-five and fifty, are in the habit of drinking beer with their lunch. On the other hand, the meaning that attaches to the capsules—the rice, beans, and flan de coco—is not quite as apparent to the viewer, since the immediate message, logically enough, focuses on the lack of beer.

In terms of marketing strategy, however, what is compelling about the commercial is how it tries to create in consumers the impression that drinking Medalla is a foregone conclusion by identifying it with two items of food that Puerto Ricans can scarcely imagine not eating at least once every day—rice and beans. If rice and beans are considered an essential part of lunch, then so, too, is a glass of Medalla beer.

Another interesting element of the commercial is the presence of what might be called "the palate's memory"—that bond which unites food and dishes with vital experiences and remembrances—projected in the commercial as an imagined future. Although the commercial conjures up an uncertain tomorrow, it is one in which Puerto Ricans will still be eating "rice and beans," albeit out of capsules dispensed from vending machines. Why is it that the food in the lunches people eat in the future are foretold as rice and beans, and not something else? Do the marketing futurologists believe that people's memory of what they ate, of the food with which they have identified most closely, will not change, even if the context changes? The answers to these questions presuppose a power exerted by particular combinations of food or, put another way, by a relationship of reciprocal expectations. In simplest terms, there are no beans without rice, and there is certainly no rice without beans. Within this interdependent historical pairing, however, how was the role of beans configured?

In considering this question, the conquest and colonization of San Juan (1508–32) marks a useful starting point, focusing first on the legumes that the Taíno population on the island had long planted and consumed (*Phaseolus vulgaris*)—or on what the Spanish called *fríjoles* and Puerto Ricans commonly refer to as *habichuelas*.[1]

In covering the past and present role of beans in the spectrum of Puerto Rican food, I plan to address several other points: the possible role played by the African population in furthering the adoption of beans as a food crop, the qualities they possess that have made them desirable, the relationship between the preparation of bean dishes and the basic seasoning mix in Puerto Rican cooking known as *sofrito*, and, finally, the movement of beans—understood as both merchandise and food—through the ins and outs of the market, agroindustry, and dietary habits and practice. On this basis, I shall try to answer the question: Why is there a preference for "red" or "kidney" beans over the other varieties?

As in the analysis of rice, the treatment of beans spans an extensive time period, ranging from the sixteenth century to the twenty-first.

The Taíno Beans

Like many of the foods that still form part of the diet eaten at home by Puerto Ricans every day, some varieties of the *Phaseolus vulgaris* species were widely cultivated as food by the indigenous populations of the Caribbean before the arrival of the Spanish. During the initial phase (1492–1524) of imperial expansion across both the islands of the Caribbean and the Meso-american land mass, Spanish chroniclers took to calling these legumes *fésoles* or *fríjoles*. In his *Historia general y natural de las Indias*, Oviedo used beans found in the region of Aragón as a reference point to orient readers to his description of their New World counterparts.[2] Later in his text he noted that "on this island and many others, and even more on the mainland, the Indians had this bean from the fésoles . . . ; and on the lands along that coast and others there are numerous types of fésoles besides the most common, there is the yellow bean and others that are spotted. Another legume they have resembles broad beans, but is much bigger, and somewhat bitter, they eat them raw; the Indians generally sow their fields with each and every one of them."[3]

In time, the indigenous beans that writers like Oviedo called fríjoles came to be called habichuelas, perhaps because of its similarity to the term *favichiela*, which the medieval-period *mozárabes* had assigned to the bean pod of an edible legume that was smaller than the *fabes* (fava beans) of the Iberian Peninsula. The introduction in the colonies of the Castilian term *judihuela*, a derivative of the Mozarabic term, may also have aided in this process.[4]

Although in his description of the abundance and great variety of New World beans Oviedo focused more on Central America, this does not mean that they were any less present in the Caribbean or less important than other foodstuffs as a component of the Taíno diet.

On the contrary, in the period 1508–21, when the drive by Spaniards to find and extract gold was at its height and hundreds of Taíno families were subject to harsh exploitation and mistreatment, beans (like corn and cassava) were indispensable to the Indians.[5]

The conquering Spaniards were well aware of this fact. Much of the food that they provided the Indian workers forced into excavating gold from the rivers came in the form of beans shipped from the neighboring islands of Mona and Hispaniola.[6] From their earlier experiences on other Caribbean islands, the Spanish had learned that the local beans had a number of virtues: they sprouted easily, lasted relatively long before degrading, and ranked as a staple in the Indians' diet. This last factor took on added importance in light of all the new, unfamiliar foods to which the Spaniards were exposing them. The mobilization of a high percentage of the male Taíno population on the island to extract gold, and the concomitant need to feed them, not only accounts for why beans were imported in such quantity from other islands; it also helps explain why the production of foodstuffs declined to the point of stagnation.[7]

Between 1512 and 1513 alone, 6,480 pounds of beans were imported onto the island from Hispaniola.[8] Their storage and distribution were even turned into a business operation (as similarly took place with corn, cassava, and sweet potatoes), controlled in many cases by administrators of the Royal Treasury, whose purpose was to provide food to Indians who had been placed in the service of the king. Any food left over was then sold to conquistadores who had been granted Indian laborers.[9] The native beans became a complement to a standard, unchanging diet that the conquistadores—using as cooks a portion of the Taína women who had not been detailed to the mining work[10]—fed to the indigenous workforce during the most callous, bloodstained phase of the colonization of San Juan.

Lentils, broad beans, and to a greater extent garbanzos were also imported from Spain to the island during this initial phase of conquest and settlement, and in much larger quantities than those contained in the shipments of native beans from Hispaniola. For example, in 1516, 12,240 pounds of garbanzos, 3,400 of them carried on a single ship, entered San Juan.[11]

It would be naive, however, to think that in this period the legumes brought over from Spain were destined, in practice, to augment the food available to the Taíno workers, and it is equally unlikely that they were systematically planted as a food crop. In a context marked by both food insecurity and the fear of experimenting with new foods, the conquistadores did everything possible to assure themselves that they—not the indigenous population—would have adequate quantities of dry legumes, as well as supplies of other foodstuffs shipped from Spain.[12] So long as the Indians were forced to abandon their fields and work outside of agriculture, and the depredations of conquest shrunk their numbers and sapped their morale, the cultivation of beans stagnated. Moreover, because it was the indigenous population, Indian women in particular, who knew when, how, and where to grow and gather them, and because it was the Indians who best understood the value of beans as food, this process of stagnation widened and deepened. The reappearance of the Taíno bean as a common crop and food would have to await different circumstances.

The African Bean

As noted earlier, in the decades that followed the gold mining phase, a substantial number of Africans, of different ethnicities, were transported to the island (as distinct from the Spanish-speaking Ladino Africans who were part of the first wave of Spanish conquest and colonization). It is estimated that by 1531 the island counted some 2,264 African slaves among its population, a number that would increase sharply as the colony gravitated toward an economy centered on the production of sugarcane.[13]

All indications are that the different groups of African slaves, in their capacity as a labor force, played a decisive role (much as they did in spreading rice cultivation) in revitalizing the production of native foodstuffs—beans, corn, and tubers—whose systematic cultivation had been abandoned in the aftermath of the conquest. How was the bean brought back as a crop? What factors intermingled to explain its resurgence? While the participation of African slaves was critical, the contribution of the indigenous population in transmitting specialized agricultural knowledge should not be discounted.

Within the social structure of the colony, the Africans, in their condition both as slaves proper and as runaways, found themselves, in the years after the conquest, in closer contact with the surviving indigenous population than with the Europeans. This situation must have facilitated the exchange of botanical and agricultural insights and experiences particular to each group. With respect to the reemergence of beans, the Indians knew the best places in which to grow them, the best times of the year for planting them, and the revitalizing effect that they had on the soil.

For their part, the Africans quite likely contributed by introducing a legume native to their coastal regions. In parallel fashion to what occurred with the rice species *Oryza glaberrima*, various African groups from the areas comprising present-day Ghana, Angola, Botswana, Ivory Coast, and Equatorial Guinea gathered, planted, and consumed a type of legume long before Europeans explored and colonized the islands of the Caribbean.[14] In fact, shortly before the end of the tenth century a legume was included in the *Kitab al-Azizi*, a geographical dictionary compiled by the

Arab scholar al-Mullabi, as one of the plants grown between the seasons for wheat and millet in Audaghast, a settlement in the southeast of present-day Mauritania. Subsequently, Arab expeditionary forces, such as that led by al-Qazwini e Ibn Battuta, traveling through areas of West Africa (specifically in regions south of present-day Ghana) during the Middle Ages also reported a legume that was gathered in the wild as well as cultivated as a basic food crop in more agriculturally developed areas.[15] Battuta, in fact, observed that women in the markets sold flour made from legumes. Near the middle of the fifteenth century, the Portuguese explorer Luis Ca da Mosto also mentioned a legume that was planted along the coast of West Africa.[16]

The African legume cited by these travelers and explorers may be the species that botanists call *Vigna unguiculata*.[17] Small in size, the "vignas" have come to be known in Puerto Rico as *fríjoles de carita* (black-eyed peas), or as *bizcos* (cross-eyed) in some parts of the island's interior. The vigna seems to have been domesticated around 3,000 years before the Christian era in those regions of West Africa that are now part of Mali and Mauritania.[18]

In all likelihood, the Africans experienced little difficulty in discovering the legumes that the Taínos gathered, cultivated, and consumed. Their keen ability to identify and judge the prospective nutritional benefits in plants, stemming from their long tradition of gathering and cultivating foodstuffs, must have equipped them to do likewise with the native bean, which continued to germinate on its own around the small plots abandoned and left untended during the early years of conquest. Similarly, they would have encountered little difficulty in replanting the vigna, which was familiar to them and which they themselves possibly introduced to the island.

Thanks to the intermixing of Africans and Indians, racially and culturally, both the *Phaseolus* and the vigna flourished in urban settlements, which began to expand in number and size starting at the end of the sixteenth century, as well as in the small holdings of mestizo and cimarrón (escaped-slave) settlers who had fled the cities. Around 1627, as set down in the ordinances passed by the town council of San Juan to regulate the supply of foodstuffs reaching the capital, all of the legumes cultivated on agricultural land outside the city were grouped under the generic name "beans."[19] It is possible that this grouping included the *Vigna unguiculata* as well as the varieties of *Phaseolus*, especially when one considers that, along with rice and yams, beans were firmly associated with African agriculture and cuisine.

Against this background, then, the blending of insights and information about food and agricultural techniques between the native and African populations must have been decisive in restoring the *Phaseolus vulgaris* and in disseminating the vigna within the island's agriculture. The long-standing predilection of the Spanish for lentils and garbanzos was important, too, in helping establish the pervasive taste for legumes, in particular those of the *Phaseolus* variety,—that is, beans—in all sectors of island society. What botanical, bromatological, and nutritional qualities did the *Phaseolus* beans have that prompted people to continue cultivating them and that, over time, made them a basic, highly popular, and worthwhile food to eat?

Good to Eat . . . and Good for Planting

A quarter of a century ago, Marvin Harris argued that human beings fail to consume all of the things that are potentially nutritive for them.[20] In addition, he proposed that the acceptance or rejection of certain foods, such as dog meat in some Asian cultures, or horse meat in Italy and France, must take root only after an extended period of evolution and development. Although not denying the symbolic and religious role assigned to particular foodstuffs in different societies, Harris believes that this manner of comportment—acting on decisions about what is and is not fit to eat—is practical in origin, a result of the interaction of social, physical, and ecological factors, rather than the outcome of an opposition between nature (the qualities or characteristics of edible resources) and culture (ways of thinking about food), as Lévi-Strauss proposed. For Harris, such opposition occurs after a period of testing, when the question of whether a specific food is or is not good to eat has already been resolved.

Although Harris's idea about the development of food preferences and dislikes focuses more on meat products, it also enables us to understand the preference for beans—and other types of food—among the indigenous population, as well as their adoption and popularity as a basic food in the diet in periods following the conquest and colonization of the island. Applying Harris's schema, the taste for beans grew out of their ready adaptability to the agro-ecological environment, with the result that early on the island's indigenous inhabitants discovered both the ease of cultivating them and their sensory and nutritional qualities.

In the opinion of botanists, the domestication and evolution of *Phaseolus vulgaris* took place in an area running from Mesoamerica to the Andes. It thrived equally in a dry subtropical environment and in the humid tropical environment characteristic of the Caribbean region.[21] Aware of its botanical and nutritional value, successive groups of migrating agriculturalists spread the beans first into northern South America and then into the Antilles. The *Phaseolus* was recognized as a good food to eat as soon as the first wave of Indians reached the Caribbean.

In all likelihood, however, this recognition alone could not have created the preference for beans. The fondness for them, and the realization that they were good to eat, must have gained strength from the observation—on the part of both the Indians and Africans and the mestizo population that emerged later—that the legumes not only enriched the soil in which they were planted but also benefited the plants that were cultivated around them.[22] *Phaseolus* beans are capable of improving soils low in nitrogen, even to the extent of providing nitrogen to enrich the process of photosynthesis in plants cultivated next to them.

Although the Indians, Spanish farmers, and mestizo campesinos never understood how to explain this relationship scientifically, today it is known that it happens through the actions of a bacterium, belonging to the genus *Rhizobium*, that lives in the nodules of the roots of legumes. The bacteria exist in reciprocity with the plant, drawing in nitrogen from the atmosphere for the benefit of both the host plant and the surrounding plants.[23] That is why historical references to campesino crops and cultivated land around their huts spotlight the legumes that are close to either other food crops or to crops with a higher market value, such as tobacco and corn.[24] As new generations of farmers and campesino smallholders became aware of this fruitful relationship, the preferential liking for the *Phaseolus vulgaris* beans was extended and reinforced.

This species, and more particularly the two varieties best known by Puerto Ricans—the red and the white—begin germinating quite soon, in well-drained soils a mere thirty-three days after seeding.[25] Although the white variety germinates after the red, it customarily produces a more abundant yield.

Allowing for all of the changes that have affected the ecology of the island since the 1950s, and considering that today it is only farmers living in the island's interior who know what it is to plant, harvest, and eat fresh beans, the *Phaseolus* can still be cultivated twice annually: in the winter, after the period of heavy rainfall (December and January), and in spring (March and April). In the fresh-air conditions of higher-elevation land, the seeds can be planted at the end of spring and during the first months of summer. Barring the occurrence of some natural disaster, this schedule produces beans for the table during a good part of the year, and both farmers and campesino smallholders can count on a well-ordered agricultural cycle given the recurrent periods of planting, germination, maturation, and harvesting. For example, beans planted in December and January (when another legume, the protein-rich *gandul*, or pigeon pea, is harvested) are ready to eat at the onset of spring, during Easter, and in the first weeks of summer. Those planted in spring and summer are similarly ready as fall approaches. Any excess can be dried and preserved to last until the next December-January cycle, when the gandul is again harvested.

In sum, beans became a desirable food owing to several factors: their short period of germination, the considerable and exceptionally abundant yields, respectively, of the red and white varieties, and the possibility of realizing two harvests per year. As long ago as the eighteenth century, the Benedictine monk Iñigo Abad y Lasierra found the red bean under cultivation in the majority of communities that he visited. From his "physiocratic" perspective, he concluded that although the peasant farmers failed to put much effort into cultivating beans systematically, "nevertheless . . . the worker's labors get as good results as they do with rice. As long as the weeds, which grow luxuriantly in this soil, do not overtake them, its plant is always covered with flowers and pods containing beans that are pleasing to the taste, dark red in color, not very attractive looking, although the natives do not hesitate to enjoy them."[26]

The intrinsic agronomic qualities of beans rendered them more of a subsistence crop for campesinos than a food destined for commercial production. Hence, while the *Catastro de fincas rústicas* (census of farmlands) for the decade of the 1880s has them planted in the majority of rural plots and gardens, throughout the nineteenth century their impact on agricultural statistics as a whole was insignificant.[27] Around the year 1832, 1,134,600 pounds of beans were harvested, and at the end of the century, when the cultivation of basic foodstuffs had already begun to enter a period of decline, one and a half million pounds of beans were still being produced in Puerto Rico.[28]

As noted above, however, their productiveness accrued more to the home than to cash crops. The best part of the yield was expressly reserved for domestic use, a practice observed by the Agricultural Experiment Station in 1903. A report by the station lamented the poor quality of legumes that reached city markets: "The bulk of these legumes are inferior in quality. One of the reasons for this fact is that they represent what is left over from the produce of home gardens [located] within a radius of several miles from the city."[29]

In 1907, the manner in which the *Phaseolus* bean varieties germinated simply as a matter of course in both campesino plots and in the wild caught the attention of a North American botanist, Janet Russell Perkins. In studying the range of legume flora in Puerto Rico, Russell Perkins realized that there were "innumerable varieties" of *Phaseolus vulgaris*, both cultivated and uncultivated.[30] On wild lands she also found a bean that the campesinos called *cimarrón*, and another to which they applied the same name—an allusion, on their part, to the natural way in which they flowered and grew in the uncultivated mountainous highlands, and suggestive also of how maroon slaves were forced to live, "undomesticated," on the margins of society to regain their freedom. In her ramblings across the countryside, she also observed the *Vigna unguiculata*, the bean introduced to the Caribbean from Africa, jotting down that it was under cultivation in the municipalities of Yabucoa and Mayagüez. Russell Perkins's observations, made early in the twentieth century, thus underscore that it was on the small plots of a rural, mestizo, campesino population where practical wisdom about the qualities that made beans a favored and nutritive food to eat continued to register and get reinforced, as it had since the sixteenth century. Indeed, four centuries had passed since Oviedo had described *fésoles* as central to the agriculture and diet of the native population. The North American scientist found something not dissimilar, except that now the island's population was almost entirely mestizo. In concluding her treatment of the varieties of *Phaseolus*, Russell Perkins observed: "Of this species there are innumerable varieties. The green pods are used as a vegetable in the form of 'string' or 'snap' beans. The mature seeds, of which there are a number of different colors, are, on account of the abundance of legumin and starch, very nutritious. . . . They are consumed in large quantities, [and] cooked in various ways."

Beans and Sofrito: The Result of a Bricolage

The key role played by the *Phaseolus vulgaris* beans in the islanders' agriculture and diet from the early sixteenth century on does not diminish the importance of other legumes. The *Phaesoslus lunnatus* variety, known in

Puerto Rico as the *habichuela blanca*, or white bean, and in many other places as the lima bean, also played an important role, as did the African bean, or *Vigna unguiculata*. Around the close of the eighteenth century, another legume, the gandul, (*Cajanus cajans*) began to occupy a central place in the agriculture and general diet of the island. There were two others that never succeeded as a crop but that over time, imported from abroad, also won acceptance as basic to the diet: lentils and garbanzos.

Broadly speaking, however, the role of the *Phaesolus* in domestic horticulture would be decisive in establishing a strong predilection for beans in the island's cuisine and popular taste. In turn, that leaning would be joined with the preparation of a *fondo de cocina* (a seasoning base or mix) used in cooking legumes to produce a distinct taste referred to in Puerto Rico as *sazón* (seasoning). The seasoning mix also appears in other cuisines of the Caribbean under the name "sofrito."

In Puerto Rico, as in many other islands of the Caribbean, there has never been a single, standard way of cooking stewed beans. To a person, everyone has wanted a particular taste, insisting, time and again, that his or her results are the best. Preparation of the dish requires that one know about a series of steps: why "dry beans" are used; why "rainwater" is employed for the stew; why the cook always maintains the dish on a *hervor de sonrisa* (gentle boil); why it must be allowed to simmer; why "small pig's feet" are added; why, to get the right thickness in the soup, black-skinned, not yellowish, pumpkin is added when one starts—not finishes—the cooking.

As a rule, the goal in preparing beans in Puerto Rican cooking is to alter their texture, soften them, to produce a semi-thick, soupy dish, something akin to pottage or vegetable soup.[31] One must be careful, however, not to go too far, because the intent is not to sip it, or spoon it up as a liquid, but, rather, to serve it next to or mix it with—above all—white rice.

Furthermore, the aim is not simply to render the beans palatable and digestible. The cook also has in mind a certain ideal blend of flavor, aroma, and color, which is produced by adding the sofrito to the dish while it is being cooked and when it is ready to come off the stove. Although this seasoning has been and is still used with other stewed and braised dishes and other rice preparations, it is most closely associated with the consumption of beans. Indeed, when one contemplates sofrito today, the image that it immediately evokes is that of beans. Without sofrito, sensory, physiological, and even erotic expectations go unfulfilled. For example, for some men, a young woman who makes use of a good sofrito to produce a stew of "good" beans immediately calls up the image of a woman "luscious" and ardent in her sexual performance.

The making of sofrito has become more or less formulaic, with its ingredients now the same from one kitchen to another. This seasoning mix is perhaps the best example of a bricolage-style cuisine, a cuisine created out of the diverse foods, memories, and survival strategies of populations that, throughout a long period of time, have stamped on the insular Caribbean in general and Puerto Rican society in particular their distinctive character.[32]

With a bricolage as a model, the ingredients of sofrito include wild coriander (*Eryingium foetidum*), also referred to as *recao*; sweet pepper (*Capsicum chinense*); capsicum; green pepper (*Capsicum annum*), also referred to as *pimiento de cocinar*; annatto (*Bixa orellana*); and tomato (*Lycopersicum esculentum*). Other than the tomato, these were known to and used by the indigenous population and formed part of the flora of the Caribbean before the arrival of Europeans and Africans. The remaining ingredients—all of them "adopted"—are: garlic, onions, cilantro, vinegar, capers, cumin, and either lard or oil. Because they were not produced in the region, vinegar, capers, and oil always distinguished the sofrito of the rich from the sofrito of the poor.

As the culinary history of Puerto Rico unfolded, these ingredients were not all present at the same time, as is true today in home preparations of sofrito, or in the store-bought versions produced by large companies. Quite possibly the complete sofrito came together bit by bit, as the result of countless attempts at creating a basic cooking mixture that would preserve meat in a tropical climate.[33] The use that is made of it today, as a seasoning for stews, came later.

The healing properties of certain plants, such as chili peppers, garlic, and onions,[34] as confirmed through the personal experiences of many islanders who used them medicinally, very likely also contributed to the development of a common recipe for sofrito, as did the use of wild herbs and spices. The incorporation of herbs and spices, however, was more problematic, because it reflected the diverse medical, religious, and culinary practices of a multiethnic, multiracial society and the stigmas and proscriptions about the use of particular food items to which it gave rise.[35]

Each group that came to constitute the mosaic of Puerto Rican society made regular use of at least one if not more of the items that eventually blended together to form the sofrito as it is known today. To preserve, marinate, and flavor their food, the indigenous people of the Caribbean used several types of chili peppers, spices, sweet ingredients, and even leaves.[36] The record suggests that they also used coriander (recao).[37] As both food and condiments, onions and garlic were central to the cuisines of Castile, Extremadura, and Andalusia. In addition, Andalusian cooking had absorbed from North Africa the use of coriander and cumin, which later—according to individual taste and circumstance—were used in making sofrito.[38] Onions, chives, and garlic leeks were known to some ethnic groups in West Africa. In addition, these people used the leaves of various plants to season their food and also employed (as they still do) palm oil (Elaeis guineensis) to give it seasoning and color, making a sauce for this purpose that they call ata.[39]

The use of achiote (Bixa orellana) in rice and stews to add color and seasoning, which eventually became common in Puerto Rican cooking, is in all likelihood tied to this centuries-old African tradition, as well as to the equally venerable practice, in Mediterranean cuisine, of using saffron for color and seasoning. The preparation of sofrito was also influenced by the practice, common in Murcia and Extremadura, of cooking with dried, ground sweet red peppers, called pimentón.[40] As a measure of this influence, 64,253 pounds of Spanish pimentón were imported into Puerto Rico in 1879.[41] Capers, a constant in the Mediterranean diet, first made their appearance on the island during the initial years of Spanish settlement, as part of the food brought into the colony on ships leaving Seville. They subsequently became a luxury item sold in city markets around the Caribbean. Arab-Andalusian stewed legume dishes had long incorporated fats as an ingredient, and—as we have seen—palm oil was commonly used in African cooking.

As for the order of adoption of the various ingredients comprising sofrito, it is likely that chili peppers, achiote, and cilantro came first, followed by garlic, onions, fat, and pimentón. There are references in eighteenth-century sources mentioning that cilantro was used exclusively for cooking purposes.[42]

The last ingredient to appear was the tomato. Interestingly, although they grow easily in Puerto Rican soil, tomatoes are barely mentioned in the literature before 1859, though some years later the idea of making sofrito without them had become unthinkable. Their slower introduction into Puerto Rican cooking may reflect the longer period of time it took for tomatoes to be widely accepted in the European diet.[43] Capers followed a similar trajectory, and since they were not produced in the region, those using them in cooking had to depend on the foreign import market.

In short, the creation of sofrito illustrates one of the great virtues of " Puerto Rican–Caribbean" cooking—its rich inventiveness. Recalling part of Sidney Mintz's analytical framework, it is a living example of the potential of human beings to experiment, compare, sift choices, work out preferences, and effect combinations.[44] Quite possibly it was slave cooks— male and female—who with time were responsible for turning different versions of this mixture into a basic seasoning, especially if one considers, like Mintz, that among the entire population, it was African slaves who were tied most closely to trends in agricultural production and changes in the range of foodstuffs. They did the spade work that produced the food that was consumed by those who, in time, wrote the cookbooks.

In the meanwhile, recipes were transmitted by word of mouth and by imitation and borrowing, such that each kitchen and each Caribbean population worked out its own methods and techniques. Sofrito, with its sister versions in the cooking done on other Caribbean islands, is one of Puerto Rico's most appealing contributions to world gastronomy.

The Oldest Sofrito

That the cookbooks compiled from the mid-nineteenth century through the first two decades of the twentieth lack even a single recipe for sofrito is surprising, though they do note the use of a *fondo*, or *fond de cuisine*, with garlic, tomatoes, onions, and sweet chili peppers as its customary core ingredients, for seasoning. Likewise, visitors to the island, such as Margherita Hamm, observed that Puerto Rican food contained a "prodigality of spices and condiments."[45] In cookbooks, the fondo never stood by itself as a recipe. Whether used with rice, or a stew of some kind, or some other meal, it was always part of the preparation of a dish.[46] Its presence in the kitchen and in food tended to be seen as natural, inevitable. The fondo was so fundamental to people's cooking, and so unlikely not to be part of the daily meal, that one of its ingredients—cilantro—came to be called "recao," a corruption of the noun *recado*, meaning "message" or "errand." At the beginning of the twentieth century, according to the lexicologist Augusto Malaret, this usage signified the action of sending servants to the market to purchase the provisions that were needed and used every day in the kitchen.[47]

Consequently, as long as knowledge about sofrito and its preparation continued as it did to be passed on from one cook and household to another, through conversation and imitation, it was not considered necessary to publish a formal recipe for it. It was in the third decade of the twentieth century, when the notion of *puertorriqueñidad* (the essence of what it meant to be Puerto Rican) was being redefined, that a written recipe for sofrito appeared for the first time.

Elsie Mae Wilsey and Carmen Janer Vilá, both of whom taught in the School of Home Economics at the University of Puerto Rico, published the recipe for it in 1931. The cooking manual in which it appeared, however, dealt with the most novel ways of preparing tannier, not beans, illustrating that—in the Puerto Rican culinary context of the early twentieth century—sofrito had come to be used as a seasoning for a wider range of foods and had acquired a character and autonomy of its own within a more developed and well-defined style of cooking. No longer was it just the fruit of intuition, of simple survival strategies, or of what a cook could contrive out of the resources at hand. The scene had changed. People now approached a meal with a different set of expectations about how it should taste, and these could not be satisfied without sofrito. By this time, to cook without it was to cook food that was flavorless, flat, lacking in character. The unfailing addition of sofrito to a dish, day after day, was what distinguished Puerto Rican cuisine from the cuisines of other countries. The aromas and flavors it lent to food is what led visitors like Hamm to conclude that Puerto Rican cooking had a personality all its own: "Puerto Rican cookery is at first a disappointment to an American visitor. The use of olive oil instead of butter, the liberality displayed toward onions, shallots, garlic, and chilies, the prodigality of spices and condiments . . . are in the beginning novel and oftentimes unpleasant."[48]

Wilsey's and Janer Vilá's manual also made special reference to sofrito.[49] The oldest written recipe for what had served as a base to season beans, stews, and other commonly cooked dishes was straightforward:

> ¼ cup of ham, ¼ cup of fatback, 2 spoonfuls of lard colored and seasoned with annatto seeds, 2 teaspoons of salt, 1 spoonful of capers, ½ cup of onions, ½ cup of tomatoes, ¼ clove of garlic, ½ cup of capsicum, 1 spoonful of herbs—wild marjoram, coriander, parsley.
>
> Chop and measure out the ham, fatback, onions, tomatoes, and capsicum. Sauté the ham and fatback. Add the remaining ingredients and cook for five minutes.
>
> Use in soups and stews.[50]

During the 1950s, two cookbooks, *Cocine a gusto* and *Cocina criolla*, would be the sources from which other cookbooks devoted to Puerto Rican food and cooking, including those published in the United States for North Americans and "nuyoricans" (Puerto Ricans living in New York), took the recipe for sofrito and disseminated it more widely.[51] Once it appeared in these two cookbooks, sofrito began to enjoy a new image—it was now a major symbol of the island's culinary identity, associated most strongly with stewed bean dishes.[52] Henceforth, in cookbooks on Puerto Rican cooking published up to 1990, it would be highly unusual not to encounter a recipe for making sofrito.

In a word, the arrival of foreign populations on the island and the evolution of a new, heterogeneous society, the experimentation with novel foodstuffs, the desire to preserve them, the creation of a trail of memories about food and cooking, and the wish to endow dishes with taste, aroma, and color were the building blocks of the basic seasoning mix that today stamps the island's cuisine as criollo or Puerto Rican, all the more so when one sits down to a plate of stewed beans.

In contemporary Puerto Rico, not everyone cooks or eats beans on a daily basis, but the somewhat vinegary overtone and pungent olfactory sensation that sofrito produces—above all when the coriander, sweet chili peppers, and garlic come into contact with the hot, sizzling fat—signals unmistakably that stewed beans are on today's menu at home, or in the restaurant or neighborhood eatery. What is more, in the popular imagination about food and its preparation, the slightly bitter aroma given off by sofrito is tied most closely to the *colorás*, or red beans. Why is there a preference for them, as opposed to "pink," "black," or even "white" beans?

The Red Bean: From "Fresh" to "Dried"

In parallel fashion to rice, legumes acquired a central place in the daily diet of Puerto Ricans as early as the sixteenth century.[53] The island's first published cookbook, the 1859 *El cocinero puertorriqueño*, contained recipes for black and red beans and pigeon and black-eyed peas, as well as for judías, lentils, garbanzos, and *arvejas* (snap and other varieties of peas). In this same period, the volume of legumes purchased monthly for preparation in the kitchen of San Juan's Carmelite nunnery, seventy to one hundred pounds, gives some indication of the importance of beans as a basic food.[54] This total, which included garbanzos, and red, black, and other beans, translates into a daily consumption, by approximately two dozen individuals, of between 2.6 and 3.3 pounds.[55] As we will see, the steady ramping up in the volume of imported dry beans during the second half of the nineteenth century illuminates two trends in the Puerto Rican diet: its simplification and its definitive embrace of this nutritional food.

In essence, what in Puerto Rico is called the "red bean," or is still called—somewhat enigmatically—the *marca diablo* (devil's brand) in the most hidebound kitchens, belongs (just like its pink, white, and black cousins) to the *Leguminosae* or *Fabaseae* family. And like them, it has been grouped in the *Papilionideae* subfamily under the species *Phaseolus vulgaris*. At the beginning of the twentieth century, agroindustry dubbed it the "kidney" bean. Puerto Ricans, on the other hand, called it colorá, because of the pronounced dark red coloration of its skin. For them, as for the monk Iñigo Abad y Lasierra writing at the end of the eighth century, this aspect of the bean was more prominent than its kidneylike shape.

As suggested earlier, the biological properties of the *Phaseolus* beans helped carry them to the fore in Puerto Rican cooking. Their rising importance is reflected in statistics from the nineteenth century, numbers that, impressive as they may be, cannot convey either the benefit of multi-year harvests for those living on subsistence diets or—again with respect to such diets—the relative ease with which they grew. In 1832, 1,134,600 pounds of *Phaseolus* beans were harvested; in 1891, when the production of basic foodstuffs was apparently declining, the harvest reached 1,500,000 pounds.[56] Furthermore, throughout the nineteenth century, the total volume of beans produced locally was increased by quantities of "dry" *Phaseolus* beans imported from Spain, Germany, and Italy.[57] Subsequently, in the first decades of the twentieth century, and despite a jump in local production (of both fresh and dry), enormous quantities of beans reached the shores of Puerto Rico from the United States.[58]

This dramatic increase in the imports of *Phaseolus* beans must have reinforced the habit people already had, as they had with rice, of eating them on a daily basis.

Among all the varieties of *Phaseolus*, the tilt toward red beans was notable. It was already firmly lodged during the 1930s, but it gained even more strength during the decade of the 1950s.

For example, at the start of the 1930s, research uncovered that, during a seven-day period, 150 families cooked red beans on 137 occasions.[59] In

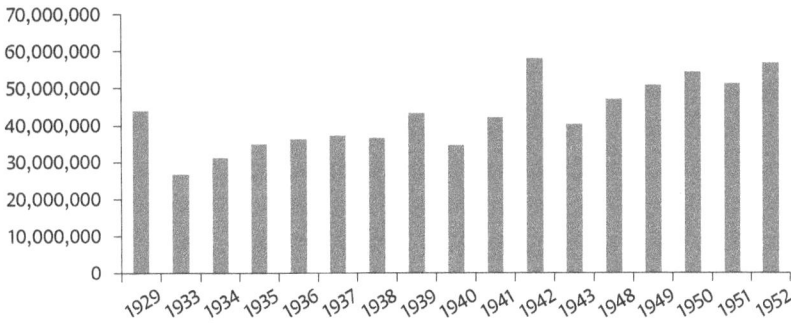

FIGURE 2.1 Imports of dried beans from the United States, 1929–1952
(in millions of pounds)

Source: Estado Libre Asociado de Puerto Rico, Junta de Planificación de Puerto Rico, Negociado de Economía y Estadísticas, Anuario Estadístico, Estadísticas Históricas, 1959.

contrast, white beans and garbanzos were prepared only 29 and 24 times, respectively.

In 1949, the weekly consumption of legumes was estimated at 19 ounces per person, but of this modest total, 97.7 percent corresponded to red beans.[60]

During these years, the sociologist Clarence Senior was unable to discover an explanation for the marked preference for red beans. In the midst of the initial efforts by the state to address the problems occasioned by the simplification of the diet, and having learned that the red bean was less nutritious than others, he posed the question: "What resistances will have to be overcome before soy beans, lima beans, and garbanzos will be preferred to the less economical and less efficient red kidney beans?"[61]

Although none of the studies carried out in this period indicates what type of red bean—whether fresh or dry—was being used by those in sample groups, it is highly plausible that researchers took dry beans as their point of reference.[62] The success of the foreign import market, which expanded its horizons once the Second World War had ended, appears to have fueled these trends by capitalizing on the traditional liking for legumes to increase the supply of the "dry red kidney" bean, imported from California since the early years of the century.[63]

In trying to explain the unbroken preference for red beans, which since the beginning of the century had veered toward the dry variety, it is important to keep this supposition in mind, since it is possible that during the immediate postwar period, the cultivation of red beans (and thus their subsequent availability) had consistently declined, as happened with rice and—as we shall see—as would also occur with corn.

Several developments make this scenario likely. First, following a drop in the importation of dry legumes from the United States during the Depression years (when compared to levels achieved in earlier years), and despite solid legume production (habichuelas, gandules, and fríjoles) inside Puerto Rico (31.4 million pounds in 1937–38 versus 37.1 million pounds of imported dry legumes), after 1940 the importation of dry legumes from the United States not only recovered its previous momentum but, in some years, as shown in figure 2.1, outstripped pre-Depression levels.

Paralleling this recovery, agronomists in Puerto Rico's Agricultural Experiment Station began to study beans to develop better techniques for growing them and to isolate those varieties displaying the greatest resistance to the diseases that frequently broke out in home gardens and smallholder plots. The studies were aimed at trying to sustain local, small-scale production, especially of fresh red beans, which had been a feature of the countryside between 1930 and the middle of the 1940s.[64] The agronomists' research, however, verified that, in contrast to the white variety, the fresh red bean was less resistant to the saltón (Emposaca fabalis), an insect that attacked plants during the summer months in the hot lowlands and, by robbing them of their nutrients, unleashed a virus that made their leaves turn pallid and sickened their stems and seeds. The agronomists' pinpointing of the insects' destructive effect on the fresh red, as opposed to other varieties, is critical in understanding the turn toward dry red beans. The serious degradation of the red bean plants in the months when it was attacked drove home the destructive role played by the saltón.

As already noted, the capacity of the Phaseolus beans to be planted and harvested year-round, complemented by the harvests of pigeon peas, helped stabilize the food supply for those most dependent on them. The appearance of the saltón during summer, however, made that season off limits for growing fresh red beans. Admittedly, the cementing of a preference for dry red beans seems to call for more of an explanation than simply the intrusion of the insect. If one considers that summer—at the beginning of the twentieth century—was universally known as a "dead time" of year, a time that campesinos always associated with seasonal unemployment in sugarcane fields, hence with a fear about hunger, it is possible that the cultivation of fresh red beans, and consequently the fresh red as a staple food, became an afterthought for them and for small-scale farmers generally.

Discouraged by the unstoppable saltón, and fearing the onslaught of hunger in the event they planted only red beans, campesinos and farmers faced two stark choices beginning in the late 1940s: they could either plant white beans, which were resistant to the insect, or—during the "dead time" of year—they could resort to obtaining imported red beans on credit, for these were increasingly available in plantation canteens and small groceries.[65] The second choice was apparently the preferred option for two reasons: thanks to their slow rate of spoilage, dry red beans lasted longer in small grocery stores, and their bromatological and culinary attributes enabled people to face the adverse food conditions of the 1940s with a greater chance of success.

The qualities described below, which people who consumed them discovered in dry red beans, created a favorable environment for them in the marketplace. These attributes appear to be intertwined with several elements inherent in the dry red, but not in other varieties of the same species. While it is true that the red bean (whether fresh or dried) has less protein value than dried peas or dried soy beans, which began to be imported into Puerto Rico at the start of the twentieth century, it has other virtues underlining its popularity.[66] Preeminent among these is its excellent taste, which sets it apart. Were a new survey conducted in Puerto Rico to determine the reason why people prefer dry red beans to others, the response would be the same as always: they are preferred because of their "taste," even though respondents could never offer a referent.

The texture of dry red beans is another spur to its popularity. When dried, the skin of this bean may be hard, but the outer film is softer than on other varieties of *Phaseolus*, such as the black and pink. Furthermore, although it is advisable to soak every variety of dried *Phaseolus* in water before cooking it, the red beans—in contrast to others—wrinkle up quite early in the process. In culinary and physiological terms, this quality is important.

"Soaking" allows the decomposition of the cell walls of the bean to begin, which in turn permits the *Alpha-galactósidos* type of complex sugars, present in all legumes, to be released.[67] As experiments in chemistry have shown, these sugars cannot be decomposed by the human body, because if they are (an action that would be controlled by certain bacteria living in the intestine), gases such as methane, hydrogen, carbon dioxide, and others would be produced.[68] The sensation of flatulence experienced by persons dining on beans is a function of this process of decomposition, and the reason why a prudent approach to eating them has always been recommended.[69]

It is not the matter of flatulence, however, that warrants emphasizing, but, instead, how relatively quickly the skin of the red bean wrinkles up when soaked, which then makes it softer, more pliant, than other beans once the cooking begins. The softer quality of the red bean when it is put into the stew shortens the cooking time, which in the era before electricity entailed a considerable savings in fuel and also brought the food to the table sooner. Thus it was that during the cooking, the level of boiling was checked periodically to see that it was not too high—something never allowed by the most watchful cooks—who saw to it that the beans stayed soft but did not "shred" into little pieces.

Technically, the faster release of indigestible complex sugars in the water that is used for both soaking and stewing makes the red beans more digestible. However, in the more down-to-earth terms of expectations about one's daily fare, the release of sugars helps thicken the water in which the beans are stewed, producing a broth that is not only tasty but can also be used to soften and moisten other foods, above all rice. It is perhaps for this reason that there are still people in Puerto Rico who prefer to be served a caldito (brothy stew) of red beans on top of their white rice.

Yet another advantage enjoyed by red beans is the greater possibility they offer of satisfying a diner's appetite. The kidney bean is longer than other beans, and dry beans double in size during cooking. These attributes translate into a larger volume of food, no small consideration if people are experiencing bouts of hunger and one likely to help solidify the preference for red beans.

From the point of view of the nutritional and agronomic knowledge that was brought to bear, in the mid-twentieth century, on the problem of protein deficiencies in the Puerto Rican diet, the partiality of the population for the colorá was a source of much questioning. In the Department of Education and in the University of Puerto Rico's School of Home Economics, the most progressive voices were those of Lydia Roberts and Esther Zeijo de Zayas, both of whom lobbied for the consumption of more nutritional legumes, such as the soy, garbanzos, and pigeon peas.[70]

Such advocacy notwithstanding, the islanders' preference for the colorá was an unavoidable reality. Nutritional science that focused on the home and small garden plots keenly understood the difficulty of transforming engrained habits and instead recommended that, if there could not be greater intake of more nutritional legumes, then the amount of red beans contained in daily meals should at least be increased. In Zeijo de Zayas's words: "It will be useful, then, to increase the consumption of garbanzos and gandules, above all in families that do not consume a sufficient amount of meat, milk, eggs, and fish. . . . The Puerto Rican woman has to be encouraged to prepare and serve more frequently garbanzos and gandules. It will also be helpful for us to teach them to eat more legumes in combination with rice, and to eat, if possible, 'beans with rice' instead of rice with beans."[71]

The agronomists, ever attuned to discovering a bean capable of meeting their economic criteria, aligned themselves with Puerto Ricans' preference for red beans. Early in the 1950s, they produced a new colorá, one far more robust and resistant than those, brought onto the island from outside, that had previously been tried and tested. To this bean they gave the emblematic name *Borínquen*.[72]

The inroads made by U.S. agroindustrial companies continued to expand, despite an effort by Puerto Rico, in the following years, to exploit the local preference for the colorá. In 1938, the island produced 31,432,488 pounds of legumes (including 15 million in the *Phaseolus* family), and imported 37,046,242 pounds from the United States,[73] whereas in 1975 local production had dropped to scarcely 665,400 pounds.[74] At the same time, the quantity of dry beans imported from the United States, the majority of which were kidney, or colorá beans, reached 50,266,400 pounds. This trend was not reversed.

The Colorá and the Puerto Rican Mental Foodscape

During the end of the 1960s and the early 1970s, through a commercial still remembered by a great many Puerto Ricans, the preference for the "dry red" bean was used as a marketing ploy to sell the Sello Rojo brand of rice. The commercial presented two winsome, cartoonlike characters: the "little Sello Rojo white rice grain" (*granito*, playing the male) and the "little red bean" (*habichuelita*, playing the female) who together symbolized one of the classic combinations in Puerto Rican gastronomy. The commercial featured short love stories in which the two courted each other and were presented as inseparable companions. The subliminal messaging was clever, and after some time, the public found itself less concerned with the surface gloss of the commercial than with the love story of "granito" and "habichuelita," who—in the end—married one another, becoming—like white rice and beans—an everlasting pair.

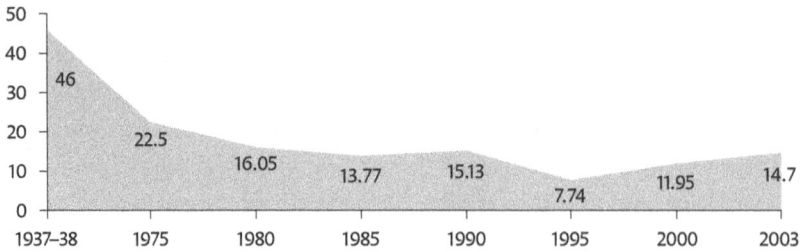

FIGURE 2.2 Total per capita consumption, in pounds, of all legumes dried, fresh, and canned

Sources: Descartes et al., *Food Consumption Studies*; and Departamento de Agricultura, Oficina de Estadísticas, *Consumo de Alimentos, Legumbres*, folder 20-57bb1, 1975-2003. Includes chickpeas, pigeon peas, and others phaseolus varieties.

In Puerto Rico's "culinary imagination," every islander steeped in local dishes knows that any diner whose meal includes a *matrimonio* has chosen an accompaniment of rice and beans, and not just any beans, but the col- orás. Why, at the end of the 1960s, when beans produced by large-scale agroindustry had become freely available, did advertising companies not use the pink or white beans, or black-eyed peas? Very simply, because then and even now, in the twenty-first century, the preference for the red bean reigns supreme in the representation of Puerto Rican food. Thus, for exam- ple, when a new "outlet" for local food recently opened in the San Patricio Shopping Center—where more types of cuisine are available than in any other central part of metropolitan San Juan—it was named The Red Bean.

By the end of the twentieth century and into the first years of the twenty- first, the per capita consumption of legumes in Puerto Rico had declined in comparison to the levels recorded in the early decades of the 1900s. The average annual intake of legumes was estimated to be 46 pounds per per- son, or almost one pound per week (15.2 ounces), in 1938.[75] From 1975 on, the figures reported by the Puerto Rican Department of Agriculture for the total consumption of legumes have generally followed a downward curve, as shown in figure 2.2.

Since the 1970s, the consumption of dry beans (the *Phaseolus* varieties only) has also declined by increments: in 1975, the figure was 16.7 pounds per person annually; in 1985, 11.8 pounds; in 1990, 11.03 pounds; in 1995, 8.5 pounds; in 2000, 8.1 pounds; and in 2003 it bumped up slightly to 9.4 pounds.[76]

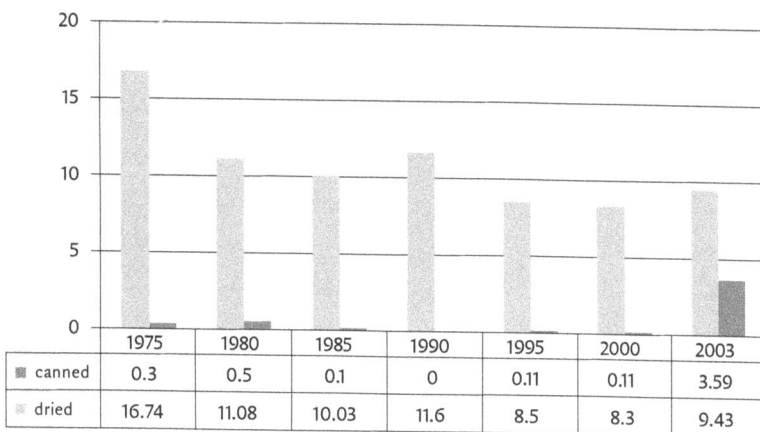

	1975	1980	1985	1990	1995	2000	2003
canned	0.3	0.5	0.1	0	0.11	0.11	3.59
dried	16.74	11.08	10.03	11.6	8.5	8.3	9.43

FIGURE 2.3 Per capita consumption, in pounds, of all dried and canned varieties of phaseolus beans

Source: Departamento de Agricultura, Oficina de Estadísticas Agrícolas, Consumo de Alimentos, Legumbres, canned beans, and dried beans, folder 2057b7, 2057a15.

Is this decline due to a move in favor of "canned" beans? Although the figures for imported canned beans indeed show an increase (for 1975, 143,200 pounds; for 1980, 319,800 pounds; for 1995, 422,900 pounds; and for 2000, 448,000 pounds), they are greatly exceeded by those for "imported" dry beans.[77] As indicated in figure 2.4, the quantity of canned beans consumed is negligible compared to that for dry beans.

In 1937–38, the island's harvest of Phaseolus variety beans alone was estimated at 15 million pounds. Contrast this figure with the miniscule harvest, in 2001, of 1,728,400 pounds of legumes of all types. Of this latter total, some 1,164,400 pounds were attributed to Phaseolus beans.[78] In July 2004, this number was approximately halved, when the Department of Agriculture calculated the 2003 Phaseolus harvest at 596,000 pounds.[79]

The marked decline in consumption implied by these figures may reflect the availability of a wider range of food, resulting in a more variable diet, with a greater intake of proteins than before. Yet there are other factors at play too.

Beans, against all the weight of the traditional love for them, have begun to be seen as requiring too much "cooking time" and so have been replaced—at least to some extent—by semi-prepared "convenience food."[80]

In their favor, canned foods open up shortcuts in the kitchen, yet as every cook knows, to prepare a dish so that it turns out right—even if

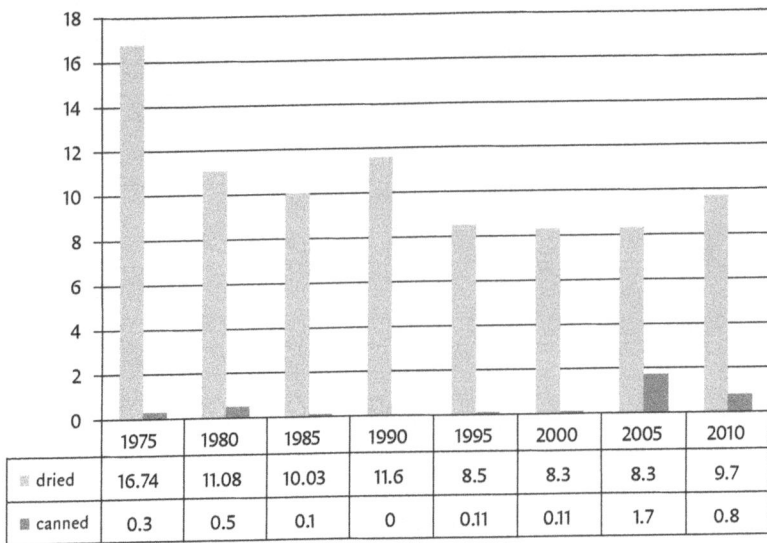

	1975	1980	1985	1990	1995	2000	2005	2010
dried	16.74	11.08	10.03	11.6	8.5	8.3	8.3	9.7
canned	0.3	0.5	0.1	0	0.11	0.11	1.7	0.8

FIGURE 2.4 Per capita consumption, in pounds, of dried and canned beans (phaseolus beans), 1975–2010

Source: Departamento de Agricultura, Oficina de Estadísticas Agrícolas, *Consumo de Legumbres,* 1975–2010, folder 2057A16

canned beans are used—still means paying careful attention to how the ingredients are blended and cooked. That is why dry legumes, which in fact need more cooking time, are more and more becoming a food that one cooks on weekends, or—if eaten during the week—enjoys outside the house.

Beans have also encountered opposition from advocates of better nutrition intent on balancing the need people have to take in food during work hours with the need to treat one's body prudently. Their orientation, which at bottom justifies an ethic of work and discipline, is decidedly "anti-carbohydrates" and favors eating light foods in the meals taken during working hours. Moreover, they have concentrated a good part of their criticisms on beans, given both how heavy and filling they can be and how they can lead to stomach upsets.[81]

Yet through all the modifications wrought by four centuries of cooking and eating, beans—especially when combined with white rice—have become a new and powerful symbol of ethnic and national identity. They have crossed the frontier of being merely a tasty and filling stew and become the subject of cultural-institutional dialogue and the object of people's imaginations about food and cooking. As such, beans are seen as emblematic of the traditional values shared by and familiar to all Puerto Ricans.

The responses that people gave when asked to describe their favorite meal (from the introduction) would seem to validate this association, as would the action taken by the recently inaugurated Department of Education school meal program, which—in eliminating so-called junk food—highlighted rice and beans as basic components of its menu.[82] Even more telling was the response of the singer Olga Tañón when asked how she felt after winning a Grammy award in February 2001: "I feel more rice and beans–like than ever, more Puerto Rican than ever."[83]

Conclusion

Beans (*Phaseolus vulgaris*) were a daily food among the indigenous peoples of the Caribbean before the European incursion. In the years following the first stage of the Spanish conquest, they may have lost some of their importance as a crop, especially when one considers that the native population applied its agricultural energies and knowledge more to corn and yuca, products that in turn won greater acceptance among the Spanish since they could be sources for making bread. In addition, the traffic of goods from the Spanish Peninsula to the colony often included other types of dry legumes.

Subsequently, the arrival of groups of Africans familiar with the cultivation of another legume (*Vigna unguiculata*), followed by the close contact they had, in the social world of the colony, with the native population, enabled them to absorb the body of local knowledge that had accumulated about the *Phaseolus* beans. The Africans' familiarity with the cultivation of the *Vigna unguiculata*, together with their strong aptitude for identifying the nutritional potentialities of plants, helped reinstate the importance of legumes in agriculture, and thus in the islanders' diets as well.

In time, and as successive waves of immigrants to the island introduced novel food, familiarized themselves with the new environment, and salvaged the memories of their own culinary traditions, a more or less standardized way of seasoning and cooking the *Phaseolus* beans gradually took shape.

Moreover, a seasoning base—that came to be called "sofrito"—was also perfected, most likely as the result of people's experimentation during a long period with different spices, condiments, and food items. While sofritos of one sort or another may have been basic to the cooking of people who arrived and settled throughout the Caribbean, the version that emerged in Puerto Rico was unlike any other.

Although it initially varied according to the personal taste and economic wherewithal of those preparing it, the ingredients in the seasoning mix eventually became the same for everyone. And while used, historically, for different stews and rice dishes, sofrito in Puerto Rico would be linked most closely to the preparation and consumption of beans.

Of the multiple varieties of *Phaseolus*, the red bean would in time capture the fancy of most. This preference is much remarked, since it separates Puerto Rico from other Caribbean countries, where—though people are familiar with and eat red beans—they prefer the "black" bean.[84] Such is the case, for example, in Cuba, Venezuela, and Colombia.

In Puerto Rico, the preference for red beans apparently helped solidify the ever-growing prominence of the dry variety of red (kidney) bean, imported from California when the cultivation of food crops declined during the first half of the twentieth century and islanders experienced a narrowing of their diets. The taste of the dry red bean, its greater size, and its capacity to soften more rapidly than other varieties were key factors in securing its primacy among the population at large.

In addition, the constancy of red beans in the daily diet of Puerto Ricans has fueled the creation of a stylized image of "food and nation." Eating red beans marks Puerto Ricans off from Cubans, for example, or from Venezuelans, both of whom prefer the black variety of beans.

Above all, however, to consume any type of beans, invariably in combination with rice, has become a potent and defining image of Caribbean identity. Whoever spots a diner spooning up beans by themselves out of a bowl can surmise that the person is not Caribbean. In the case of Puerto Rico, the combination of beans and rice is unquestioned and therefore defines people's tastes and habits with even greater force.

The food examined in the next chapter, *harina de maíz*, or cornmeal, no longer carries such strong connotations. It has others, however, which call up grim memories filled with derogatory implications.

3 | Cornmeal

During the war years, when rice was often unattainable,
cornmeal was used with beans in place of rice and jokingly
called "the Second Front."

—LYDIA ROBERTS AND ROSA LUIS STEFANI, *Patterns of
Living of Puerto Rican Families*, 1949

In Francisco Oller's emblematic painting, *El velorio* (*The Wake*), the viewer's
gaze tends to be drawn to the human figures in the center of the composition, but if we look above them, near the top of the canvas, we see twenty
or more corncobs hanging from a beam running below the roof. The cobs
are "getting aired," or dried.

In the days before industrialized farming, corn harvested for domestic
consumption was dried inside rural dwellings, hung from posts or walls
and not left out in the open, where it was easy prey for birds, rats, and
foraging pigs.

Although the focal point of Oller's painting appears to be the unfettered
naturalness of simple country folk gazing happily at a roast pig strung
above them, the artist has not included the corncobs simply as decoration.

On the contrary, they carry a specific meaning within Oller's larger de-
piction of rural life, a meaning—in this context—that we can apprehend by
applying the ideas of Carolyn Korsmeyer.[1] According to Korsmeyer, when
food plays a subordinate part in a larger visual narrative—as it does in
El velorio—it typically goes unnoticed or at least fades into the background.
Nonetheless, it still lends its meaning to the painting's wider subject, re-
inforcing the symbolic value of the painting's narrative line.

Thus, Korsmeyer asserts, while food and other mundane objects rank
only as humble elements in grand paintings, they still have vital importance for society and for the context in which they are represented: corn—
as conveyed in Oller's visual language—is a basic, essential food, and so are

the bananas that hang in bunches in the painting, and the rice that appears to be half eaten in the gourd that has toppled onto the floor.

If one looks at the scene in El *velorio* with a view toward picturing what transpires later, the kernels of corn are going to be stripped off the cobs and—when they have dried—ground up, to be turned into cornmeal. After being passed through a sieve, the mashed kernels will swell up with the addition of water, or cow's or coconut milk, leading to the preparation of a *funche* (a thick cornmeal mixture, similar to polenta). Throughout the history of Puerto Rico, no dish made from corn has satisfied the appetite—especially around the tables of less advantaged families—more than funche.

Corn converted into cornmeal, however, and corn eaten specifically in the form of funche, hardly register on the food scene, and in what people eat, in contemporary Puerto Rico. Its popularity was diminished by the image it acquired after the Second World War as a "poor man's food." The availability of other flour mixtures and cereals beginning in 1950, along with the fast-paced globalization of food in recent years, has also contributed to this decline.

Nevertheless, some adults continue to eat the dish for breakfast, as it is easily digested on an empty stomach. The minority of young people who still consume it prefer the version that comes precooked and seasoned under the name *cremita de maíz* (creamed cornmeal), a rather insipid name given to the preparation by the agro-food industry as a way of appealing to people in various age groups.[2] As a result, the young do not call it funche, although the only difference between the two is the rather soupy consistency of the former.

At present, cornmeal in Puerto Rico is primarily used for making corn bread or *sorullitos* (cornmeal fritters resembling a small stick—one type is stuffed with cheese, the other is sweetened and flavored with cinnamon and anise—deep-fried and eaten by hand). It is also used as the base for making *guanimes*—seasoned cornmeal mixed with water (there are two types, sweet or salted) and shaped into tamales that are wrapped in banana leaves and boiled in salted water—a popular item among "foodies" who enjoy guanimes in combination with salted codfish, as a kind of "blast from the past," on weekend excursions out of the capital. The cornmeal used in preparing guanimes is usually mixed with coconut milk, to counteract the saltiness of the codfish. Ultimately, though, cornmeal was most commonly prepared as funche because of its simplicity, ampleness, and bland taste. At one time, such was the importance of funche to the daily diet of

Puerto Ricans that it gave a new verb to the language—the frequently heard *enfucharse*, meaning, according to the linguist Manuel Álvarez Nazario, *enfadarse*, or to become irked or angry.[3] The association came from the hard, rough texture that funche acquires when it turns cold.

The Virtues of Corn

Corn is an annual grass plant, with robust vegetation and deep roots. It prefers a hot climate and humid soil, and a single seed can produce plants that grow more than ten feet high. In fertile land, one stalk of corn will yield between one and three ears. In the sixteenth century, it was estimated that one ear of corn could contain between two and three hundred kernels.[4] A minimum of three hundred was the calculation made in the nineteenth century.[5]

Moreover, corn is nothing if not promiscuous. It has an extremely high potential for fertilization and reproduction, whether through self-pollination or through wind-borne pollen belonging to the same species. It was this attribute that caused Europeans to encounter so many different kinds of corn as they explored the Caribbean and surrounding lands.

In contrast to wheat, which—to prevent the propagation of its pollen—seals up its flowers tightly, the corn plant's male flowers blossom on the panniculus or stamen that forms at the top of the stalk and release their pollen when brushed by the slightest wind. The female organs of the plant are fertilized via this process, since out of the central nodules of the stalk grow "ears," from which emerge innumerable silky strands. These are the female flowers, whose pollen mates easily with the male pollen wafting through the air. The union of the two produces a tube that grows inside the strands until it reaches the ovary. In this way, the male gamete fuses with the female cell, spawning the kernels of corn within the tube, which is called the "cob" or "ear."

Before the days of agroindustry, the cobs, in fertile soil, could be harvested within a period of ninety days.[6] The indigenous peoples of the Caribbean were aware of the exceptional fertility of this plant long before the arrival of the Europeans, a fertility later touted by Oviedo when he wrote about the farm that he maintained in Santo Domingo in the mid-1600s: "This corn germinates in a matter of a few days, and is harvested in four months, and some even earlier, in three months. And there is another seedling which is harvested in three. A planting of one fanega [either a unit of land or of productive capacity—in this case the latter] of corn usually yields six, ten, twenty, thirty, and [up to] fifty or more fanegas, depending on the fertility and condition of the land where it is planted. This year, that took us past 1540, on a country estate of mine, I brought in . . . one hundred and fifty five fanegas, from a single fanega that I planted."[7]

As food, corn can be eaten in two forms: the kernels can be eaten fresh or roasted or boiled with the leaves shucked or not; or—after drying out—they can be made into cornmeal.

According to Oviedo, the Indians commonly ate corn in one of two ways. They either consumed it "as toasted kernels or, if tender, without toasting them, [take it] almost like milk"; or they ate it in the form of bread rolls: "A kind of paste or dough is made, from which they take a little and make a bun [and] wrap it in a leaf from the same plant . . . and cook it [in water] . . . , if they prefer not to cook it, they roast these buns on braziers . . . , and they let the bun harden, and they get it to be like white bread . . . and make the crust . . . and the inside comes out softer than the crust."[8]

The Indians' new masters quickly familiarized themselves with all of these qualities and techniques. Above all, it was the ready conversion of corn into flour that allowed the Spanish to accept it without the qualms they suffered over other indigenous foodstuffs. They could roast it over embers wrapped in the leaves of the cob and, without any need for ovens, have food that bore some similarity to wheat bread. In addition, cornmeal could be toasted and preserved for several days if stored in a cool place. Then, by simply adding water and stirring the mixture, they would have a kind of doughy porridge, sufficiently filling and nutritious to feed them while they tramped through island forests or sailed the waters of the Caribbean.[9]

As the sixteenth century wore on, new groups of people arriving in San Juan soon became cognizant of the value of corn as a crop and foodstuff. In 1579, the municipal council requested that a special ship, independent of the regular fleet, be allowed to deliver a cargo of wheat flour to the capital, "since on many occasions there has not been any flour for making the host [in the celebration of the Mass]," due to the lack of cassava and corn, "which is what we subsist on."[10] Eighteen years later, the colony's governor, Antonio de Mosquera, decided to establish a farm where "corn would be planted and plantains harvested to feed and sustain the blacks who must work on the military fortifications."[11] John Layfield, the chaplain on a fleet of English ships whose officers and crew occupied the island in 1598 before abandoning it after dysentery broke out, summed up the excellent qualities of corn as a food and crop: "Besides cassava they have corn, from which a very fine bread is made, much used by them. . . . There are two kinds . . . , the smallest is not much different from rice; in taste and size: I never saw this one in the fields or uncooked, but I have seen it in the form in which it is eaten, and at first I took it for rice, except that I thought it a little puffier. Those who have eaten it said it tastes like rice. I have seen the other kind as plantings and it is the same or very similar to the grain that we call wheat; it grows with a knotty stalk like a reed with large splayed out leaves; it grows to a height of at least a fathom and a half, and the cob sprouts from its tip."[12]

Because corn was easily cultivated, yielded a crop quite rapidly, conserved well once the kernels were dry, and, as flour, could be made into bread, it had earned a special niche in the agriculture and diet of the island's native inhabitants. For the diverse population of the colony, it was equally important, attaining the status of an everyday food.

Not surprisingly, when the San Juan municipal council issued a set of ordinances at the beginning of the seventeenth century designed to regulate the capital's food supply, corn was counted among the most important foodstuffs, because—like only a handful of others—it could be used to make bread.[13] As the eighteenth century drew to a close, the annual harvest of ears of corn on the island amounted to 1,550,600 pounds.[14]

Corn has still other virtues, one of which is its considerable potential to enhance the energy level of those who eat it. For example, 100 grams of an edible portion of cornmeal—when converted into porridge—can provide 362 kilocalories.[15] When combined with other food that bolsters its nutrients, such as coconut oil, salted cod, jerked beef, or fats derived from the fattier parts of meat, this characteristic is enhanced.

For this reason, at the outset of the nineteenth century, when the era of the slave-based sugar plantation was coming into its own, corn made into funche, and accompanied by salted codfish, herring, mackerel, or jerked beef, represented the core hope of plantation owners: that of instilling maximum energy into their slaves at minimum cost.[16] Cornmeal was also a lifeline for poorer elements among the non-slave population, especially at the beginning of the twentieth century when many Puerto Ricans experienced a narrowing of their diet.[17]

Cornmeal has yet another virtue: its taste, on the whole, is mild, if not bland, enabling it to temper or neutralize the strong flavors present in even small quantities of other foods, such as salted codfish or smoked herring, which were typically added as complements to cornmeal in the simple fare offered to field hands in the countryside or to day laborers in the cities.[18]

Other items, such as sugar, *melao* (sugarcane syrup), pork fat, and coconut oil were used as seasonings with cornmeal, as were such aromatic spices and condiments as anise, cinnamon, and cloves. These ingredients are also used in the preparation of sorullos, nowadays produced on an industrial scale but still eaten as part of a simple breakfast, accompanied by coffee with milk.

Corn possessed a last important attribute, one dating to earlier times. In the campo, it was part of the daily routine of feeding domestic fowl and animals. The slenderest dried kernels were scattered about as food for chickens and pigs. The pigs also fattened themselves up on the corncobs that had been stripped of their kernels and on the dried leaves from the ears.

Grinding Corn

Before the advent of agroindustry, the high value of corn as a crop and dietary staple compensated for the burdensome work of converting it from its raw state into an edible food, especially for those who cultivated it for their own domestic use, or who faced obstacles to acquiring it in urban markets, which were kept abundantly supplied with cornmeal flour from the fertile corn belt in southeastern Puerto Rico.[19] The millstones that some restaurants on the island feature as part of their decor are fancied today as picturesque cooking utensils, but such nostalgia for the rustic is simply that; in reality, the job of grinding corn to put food on the table was among the most onerous and complicated of domestic chores, and—like so many others that revolved around the kitchen—fell to the women or female servants of the house.

If circumstances allowed, grinding could be done on tender kernels, which were stripped off of cobs that had not been harvested more than a few weeks earlier. This practice, known as grinding *en crudo* (raw grinding) or *a la antigua* (in the old way), yielded a very nutritive milky paste, but one that did not last long without spoiling. Grinding could also be done *en seco*, that is, using kernels that had been stripped—with a knife or one's fingers—off of fully dried cobs.[20]

But whatever the method, grinding required time and physical exertion, as much or more as that expended in first removing the leaves from the ear (leaving it *desperfollado*) and later stripping off the kernels from the dried cobs, leaving them *desgranado* (with the kernels separated from the cob). In the case of the tenderest corncobs, the process of removing the kernels was called the *guayado*, or—loosely translated—scratching off. Furthermore, to obtain a smoother, cleaner, more aromatic cornmeal, additional steps were required. The kernels had to be soaked in water with salt, anise, and a solution obtained from boiling ashes; then left to dry, after which their outer filmy skin was removed by placing them on a sieve or strainer, or *jibe*, as it was called, and rubbing them gently. Only after these time-consuming procedures were finished could the grinding finally begin.[21]

Majarete and Mundo Nuevo: Sweet Cornmeal Cuisine

For Spaniards who left the peninsula to take up residence in Puerto Rico, and who were attuned to a culinary tradition that emphasized wheat flour, the adjustment to cornmeal cost some effort. Such was the case, for example, for Friar Damián López de Haro, accustomed as he was to delicacies from Toledo, cakes from Seville, and the food served at a bishop's table.[22] As a result, it is hardly surprising that some works published before the end of the eighteenth century make scant if any reference to the taste and culinary qualities of cornmeal.

Starting in the sixteenth century, corn began regularly to figure in the meals eaten by those newly settled on the island, and the culinary practices and traditions they brought with them were enriched by the food and cooking customs of people from the west coast of Africa and the Canary Islands, who over time fanned out toward Puerto Rico.

It is a commonplace that Africans and Canary Islanders used corn as a foodstuff long before Europeans.[23] Both groups formed part of the population growth that took place in Puerto Rico during the eighteenth century,[24] and both applied their fund of gastronomic knowledge in using cornmeal to create confections, different from those in their birthplaces, to which they gave names that came from their native languages. Such was the case, for example, with Angolan *ngfungi*, which later came to be known as *funchi*, or "funche,"[25] as it also was with *gofio*, a term from the Canary Islands.[26]

As time passed, the culinary possibilities of cornmeal were extended and enriched, especially in the preparation of fritters and other fried delicacies and through the use of different aromatic spices like cinnamon and anise, which reflected the Andalusian tradition of confecting sweets. By the nineteenth century, the range of offerings in Puerto Rico included *mundo nuevo*, *tortitas de maíz*, *pudín de maíz seco*, *buñuelos*, the *buñuelo de maíz veracruzano*, and *rosas de maíz*, a type of popcorn characterized by Fernando López Tuero as "blossoms or croutons that boys go for."[27]

Also popular were *alegrías de maíz*—these were simply rosas de maíz that street vendors caramelized, plunging the popcorn into sugar syrup. The pieces were placed on a sheet and cooled. They were then cut and separated, leaving a delicacy with an outer shell of hard, crunchy caramel. Until a few decades ago, alegrías were an inevitable accompaniment to the celebration of a patron saint's day, on which occasion they were given the Gallicized name *crispé*. But now they have been superseded by commercially produced sweets available in markets.

Two other sweet dishes, mundo nuevo and majarete, deserve special mention, although they are rarely made any longer. The ready availability of prepared sweets and pastries, including those supplied by an international bakery goods market, and the sheer amount of work involved in making these two desserts from scratch, have caused their almost complete disappearance from home kitchens.

Majarete is more easily prepared if one uses cornmeal as the base, but the preference, or at least the recommendation, in earlier generations was to strip corn off the cob while it was still soft and tender. For mundo nuevo, even the latest recipe books call for a traditional method of preparation. First, the corncobs should be grated; the kernels are then soaked in milk and finally squeezed out through cheesecloth to obtain the "cornmeal," which serves as the basic ingredient of the dish. Interestingly, even though these recipes appeared in cookbooks published between 1859 and the late 1990s,[28] and knowledge of majarete was passed on in some families from mother to daughter, these recipes are scarcely employed today.

Among the few persons who still make majarete is Sandra Rodríguez, a native of the Collores neighborhood in the municipality of Humacao and the lady who looks after my house. One morning in July 2001, as the two of us were breakfasting on corn muffins, she suddenly expressed aloud: "I have to make majarete for my granddaughter's baptism."[29] In contemporary Puerto Rico, everyone associates majarete with disorder, rowdiness, and confusion. No longer is it seen as one of the delicacies—like *manjar blanco*, *dulce de coco*, *arroz con dulce*, and *frutas en conserva* (fruit preserves)— that for so long people had made, and brought as gifts, to help celebrate festive gatherings and other special occasions.[30]

The preparation of corn-based sweets played the same role in male-female relations and in defining the status and position of women in the family and community as did their rice-based counterparts. These delicacies were the province of women, offering them, whether free or slave, whether simple housewives or cooks by occupation, the opportunity to excel in the eyes of others. In the homes of the more prosperous, majarete or mundo nuevo—consistently well made—enabled the servant class to earn a measure of admiration and prestige from persons of higher social rank. Sweet dishes also helped fix the sensation of pleasurable tastes and flavors in one's memory. In her autobiographical novel, *Bajo el vuelo de los alcatraces*, Pepita Caballero evokes this experience on the part of one of the characters, master José Dolores: "Those afternoon snacks prepared by the old black women in the kitchen—now, once again, he could recollect the aftertaste of guava jelly, majarete, corn bread, and that coconut delight that the black [servant], Natalia, made like no one else."[31]

It was also the custom to prepare these homemade sweets to give them to neighbors who lived nearby and to relatives residing in the vicinity. They were part of the cultural fabric, appreciated by rich and poor alike, though socioeconomic status might distinguish the uses people made of them. Cooked in the most humble kitchens, these delicacies were a way of expressing solidarity and warm feelings on the Three Kings feast or on the occasion of a campesino wedding. When prepared in the kitchens of the more well-to-do, and brought as gifts to mark holiday celebrations, they sparked conversations about who among the ladies of long-established families did the better job of producing them, inspiring comparisons—and furtive jealousy—regarding the relative merits of their cooks.

At bottom, these sweets were individual creations, with a meaning that transcended the stove and its coals, a meaning best grasped by the cooks themselves. Their work was a language with its own grammar. In the prologue to her book, which she dedicates to her black cook, Isabel, Eliza Dooley captures this special quality:

Everything went by rule of thumb. One night there was unusual cake, light, and delicious. When asked for the recipe, "well you creams de butter." "How much?" "Oh, jes' enough to mix up." "But can't you tell me the amount?" "Well, dat depen's on de size of your cake."

"But Isabel, success depends on accuracy." "Oh, go 'long, chile, dis cake depens on me an not you. You take yourself out de kitchen."

It was true she needed no "prescriptions" for she never had to ask what to put in a Dish, but by some sixth culinary sense or subtle reckoning concocted delectable food.[32]

In this way, with the kitchen as their personal domain, cooks managed to reaffirm their own dignity before the lady of the house, who only entered the kitchen to issue orders, sample food, or propose some technical improvement.[33]

Majarete and mundo nuevo also served to broaden the base of culinary knowledge. Legions of anonymous cooks, as well as housewives who employed more than one cook, could devise new versions of these dishes by altering and jotting down opinions about the recipes. Such, at least, seemed to be the purpose behind the blank pages inserted after some recipes, including those for making majarete, in the section entitled "Christmas Dishes" in Dooley's The Puerto Rican Cookbook, which also included recipes for sweet dishes that she had copied from various friends during the 1940s.

To judge from cookbooks, the preparation of majarete seems quite simple and straightforward, as it basically involves mixing cornmeal with milk and sugar, then heating the mixture on a low flame, stirring constantly to prevent lumps forming. The mixture is poured into cake tins and allowed to cool. The last step is to sprinkle it with cinnamon powder. Some cooks will also put the majarete into the oven to brown it. Small differences often creep in, from one kitchen to another, in the procedures and ingredients used for making majarete. For example, the oldest formal recipe (1859) for the sweet recommended using corn grated off of cobs that were near tender, "but [also] good and ripe, so that the kernel begins to harden,"[34] a detail not repeated in Dooley's 1948 cookbook, in which commercially produced ground cornmeal now figured as the basic ingredient.

In addition, the 1859 recipe specifically called for using a refined white sugar and good-quality milk, implying that other types of sugar, such as moscabada (a moist, mellow, dusky sugar), which tended to darken the sweet, were sometimes used, along with other types of milk, such as goat, almond, and coconut.[35] Coconut milk, a central ingredient in the Afro–Puerto Rican cuisine of the island's coastal regions,[36] seems in fact to have been the norm, to judge by the recipes for majarete, including those calling for the use of rice flour, which appeared in later cookbooks. In the preparation of majarete one also had to take care to get the cornmeal base right (the 1859 cookbook recommended stripping kernels from a dozen cobs) and to not burn the dough in the vessel, which often happened to less experienced cooks who forgot periodically to stoke the embers so the heat would be evenly distributed, or to stir the mixture away from the open fire. The same vigilance had to be exercised with majarete cooked in the oven. In roomier, better-equipped kitchens, one had the choice of cooking the dish in the oven or of baking the mixture by using an *infiernillo* (small brazier) that was placed in the oven, and subsequently employing a heated metal paddle or spatula (*pandero*) to gratiné the majarete from above. With this last method, the cornmeal base was cooked *a dos fuegos*, (on double heat, or two temperatures).[37]

In the kitchens of the very poorest, however, majarete was cooked on dampened leaves stripped off corncobs, or on plantain leaves placed among the embers, or it was put on clay griddles over the heat and covered with plantain leaves or an earthenware dish. There are still some versions of majarete—such as those served in modest restaurants in the municipality of Loíza—which are prepared over iron griddles, with the cornmeal wrapped in plantain leaves. The variation in the use of spices and aromatic ingredients—in some cases cinnamon powder, in other cases crushed cloves, in still others grated coconut or lemon shavings—attest to the different ways of preparing the dish and of different preferences in taste and aromas. There are different ways, too, of decorating the sweet. In the nineteenth century, this was sometimes done "with the scrapings taken off the bottom of the vessel in which it was prepared, these usually come out as a burnt layer."[38] Such local variation, however, never altered two long-standing things about majarete: its close connection to the celebration of festive meals and its role as a gift that families brought when socializing with friends or relatives.

Funche

In contrast to majarete, funche never acquired such connotations. It is little mentioned in nineteenth-century *costumbrista* literature, especially in writings that portray the lives and experiences of the more privileged classes.

A *niño*—as young white men from well-off creole families were called—could offer majarete, but not funche, as part of the ritual of courting a young woman.[39] If funche was so offered, in front of other privileged young men, and particularly if from "a huge dish of funche with salted codfish," as Luis Bonafoux Quintero characterizes it in his "El carnaval en las Antillas," it conveyed a meaning that was directly opposed to the feeling of sociability, or sense of courtesy or gallantry, that sweet confections represented in the codes of masculine behavior observed among old, established creole families. Funche was identified as a food consumed by people of color, and it thus bore all the lustful, erotic, sexual overtones attributed by the elites to the black race.[40]

The plantation cooks who prepared it day after day in massive amounts for men, women, and children of like social circumstance had no illusions that the dish would enhance their culinary reputations or lead others to view them more highly. Nor did those eating funche have any expectations that it would be prepared as a separate, or "starter," dish, served by itself during the meal. It is possible, in fact, that the popular saying "hacerle el funche aparte," identified by Álvarez Nazario, derives from these low expectations.[41] According to him, the expression could mean "give special treatment to someone so that he/she does not become annoyed or angered." In a society characterized by class conflict, it could also have had a more conspiratorial meaning: the idea of dragging someone into a shady deal.

In any case, funche was a phenomenon of poor urban kitchens and of campesino huts and the meager rations eaten in slaves' quarters. As soon as it was cooked and placed in a *dita*, it cooled down, acquired a coarse texture, and resembled porridge. These qualities inspired the colloquial term *enfuncha'o*, said of someone who is in a bad mood or who is hard-edged, with a disagreeable personality.[42] The dish also gave rise to other colloquialisms, such as the expression *cara de funche en batea*, used—sometimes with an air of contempt—to describe someone whose facial bone structure is not quite even. A person referred to as *cara de funche* has a squat profile.

Because it acquired a hard, firm texture after being cooked, funche could easily be scooped out of the bowl, where it was generally combined with some salted fish or jerked beef, or rice and beans, or viandas, and eaten by hand. According to the handbook of social etiquette used in the Puerto Rican public schools at the end of the nineteenth century, eating food with one's hands was permissible only when picking up slices or little pieces of bread, or the "corn muffins" that were sometimes eaten in place of wheat bread. Under no circumstances was it acceptable to eat the main dishes of a meal by hand. For that, cutlery was always required.[43] Eating funche was thus associated with the vulgar practices of lower-caste persons who lacked manners and had not a spoon, knife, or fork to their name. So it was decreed by the social classes who faithfully observed the protocol and mannerisms devised to govern the table in the nineteenth century.

The linking of funche to the diets of black Africa probably occurred during the first part of the nineteenth century, when sugar plantations were at their most prosperous.

The first appearance of the word "funche" may date to this time, and it possibly derived from *jundy*, a preparation of stewed, ground guinea corn (*Sorghum bicolor*) made in the Congo,[44] or from *ngfungi*, which in the Kikongo and Kimbundu languages of Angola refer to a form of bread made from cornmeal.[45] It was in the period 1815–50 that the island's sugar plantations reached their full strength with the addition of thousands of slaves (*esclavos* "*bozales*").[46] By then, indeed, since the end of the eighteenth century, corn had replaced traditional food plants and become centrally important for some ethnic groups in regions of the Congo, present-day Benin, and western Nigeria.[47] It had also figured in the diet of the majority of Puerto Rico's black population of West African ancestry for some three centuries.

It was also during these years that plantation managers made two discoveries about corn that helped tie funche firmly to black society in the image that people formed of food and cooking on the island. First, they realized that cornmeal was an inexpensive food, of high nutritional value, that could not only satisfy people's hunger but was abundantly cultivated on the island.[48]

This realization was coupled by their awareness that cornmeal had been a key part of the diets of some of Puerto Rico's blacks since before the nineteenth century, and it came full circle with the promulgation of the slave regulations of 1825, which imposed obligations on slave owners regarding the minimum amount of food they were required to give their slaves. Furnishing them with substantial portions of cornmeal not only provided slaves a filling daily meal; it also meant that those newly arrived from Africa would be eating food to which they were already accustomed. By providing ample quantities of cornmeal, plantation and large estate owners—operating within a society whose gross inequalities necessarily affected what and how much people ate—appeared to have acted magnanimously: giving to another food that he likes. Though couched on occasion in sexist, indeed, bawdy terms—*dale por donde le gusta* (let her have it where she likes it)—such treatment in contemporary Puerto Rico means offering food that is pleasing, plentiful, and comforting to the palate. By giving ngfungi to their slaves, plantation owners managed to deflect or rectify any complaints about meager portions, strange food, or spoiled meals.[49] Although slaves were allowed to maintain small plots of their own on land far away from their workplace, using whatever these yielded to supplement the fixed rations they received in the slave quarters, cornmeal—along with rice, plantains, and tubers—constituted the heart of their daily meal. Converted into funche, it served as the core food, accompanied by minuscule portions of salted meat that served a limited purpose only: to lend flavor and to ensure that the slave population received the necessary minimum of protein and salt.[50] In 1843, in the face of complaints about an inadequate diet voiced by his slave Blas, a plantation owner in Guaynabo tried to defend himself by asserting that, in addition to salted meat—the entrails (mondongo) of cattle prepared on Thursdays and Sundays, and fresh meat served on Wednesdays and Saturdays—his slaves and servants received, every day of the week, exactly one pound of cornmeal "made into funchi."[51] In a society in which, during the nineteenth century, heightened social tensions led to a greater separation between classes, and the possibility of having a minimally varied diet was difficult for many, funche played an outsized role as a food consumed, to a very large degree, by the poorest of the poor, and in particular by slaves and their black or mulatto descendants. This pattern was observed, in 1898, by Henry King Carroll, the U.S. Commissioner to Puerto Rico, in his assessment of cornmeal's commercial prospects.[52]

Funche was also the keystone, the point of reference for the range of corn dishes that constituted much of the diet of the majority of the island's poor.[53] As such, the word was bound up with class distinctions and racial prejudices, as well as with the occurrence of pellagra, a vitamin-deficiency disease caused, in this case, by an excessive dependence on cornmeal in the diet.

Both its high nutritional content and its importance as a mainstream food for large segments of the population influenced the lunch menus adopted in the first decades of the twentieth century for public school dining halls. For example, the 1929 Manual del comedor escolar included two versions of the dish: "cornmeal with milk funche," accompanied by "grated coconut" or "an orange," and funche formed into "balls" that were mixed into stewed okra.[54] The menu called for these dishes to be served twice per month.

Funche also featured prominently in the study of living conditions of Puerto Rican families carried out by the nutritionist Lydia Roberts in 1949.[55] At this time, when Second World War food rationing still loomed in people's memories, references to funche were recast in the terminology of war: it was called "the second front." People especially took to calling funche by this name when it was mixed with the "main front"—the stewed beans that had been substituted for rice.

Nowadays, for Puerto Ricans older than fifty, the recollection of funche is bound up with the image, a perhaps idealized image, of a simple but ample agrarian system, in which smallholders worked hard but satisfied their basic food needs. It is also connected, however, to the reality of daily food deficiencies, something that Roberts's fieldwork during the late 1940s verified empirically.[56] Moreover, since this connection was clearly less apparent with rice, it is quite possible that at certain intervals, when other food was available, funche served as a second option, or as the last, irremediable option during periods in the twentieth century when conditions of hunger swept the country.

It seems, therefore, that funche was tied to people's ability to maintain a basic subsistence diet, a struggle experienced, for example, by the father of Epifania Estrada on his small plot in the municipality of Ceiba during the 1940s: "Then"—recalled Epifania in April 1995—"papa got and harvested a lot of corn, and he had a mill, one of those round mills [grinding stones or millstones], and he ground that corn and mamá made guanimes and funche, . . . she made it with coconut, sometimes she threw in fish, beans, she even made it with pigeon peas."[57]

This recollection is of a bleak yet manageable self-subsistence. Funche, however, also evokes the food handouts furnished by the state to balance the rations of the poorest families, or of landless families. On this score, funche recalls the *mantengo* (maintenance), a euphemism for the food and nutritional assistance programs implemented between 1940 and 1950. As late as 1994, various women in the eastern section of Puerto Rico retained clear memories of the cornmeal that—more than other foodstuffs—formed part of the rations they received through the government's food assistance program.[58] Ramona Denis, for example, replied to the questionnaire (see note 58): "Yes. I latched on to PRERA. I used to make little flour, porridge, and funche cakes, with water and salt."[59] Another respondent, Julia Acosta, had more vivid, extended recollections: "My parents got hold of the prera [*sic*] when I was a little one. These foods were rice, powdered eggs, dry beans, spam, cheese, powdered milk, canned meats, and cornmeal. My mother always made cornmeal funche, cornmeal fritters with cheese, and guanimes."[60]

Secundina Ortiz, a resident of Maunabo, on the southeastern coast of the island, remembered that in addition to millo (sorghum), another cereal was distributed that was used to make porridges consisting of flour and milk, a cereal that struck her as being "like a wispy rice."[61] Similarly, when the interviewers mentioned funche to the owner of the restaurant El Fogón de Víctor, in Humacao, the first thing he remembered was having eaten it every morning for breakfast. As he searched his memory, he recalled that when there was nothing else on which to dine, he also had it as his evening meal, with sugar spread over it, using his fingers to pick up the burnt scrapings off the bottom of the pan.[62]

In the current context, when cornmeal of different types (fine or thick), preseasoned and flavored for instant use, is stocked on hipermercado shelves, and various preparations from other corn-growing regions of the hemisphere are available in frozen packages or are supplied via the international baked goods market, funche has disappeared from a good many kitchens. Its infrequent appearance is probably also attributable to the desire to forget a dish that reawakens memories of times of hunger. All the same, sweet and cheese-filled sorullos—fried in fat—are still to be had. Their appeal, however, is more to those in other age groups.

Funche has thus been forgotten, or relegated to the recesses of the memory, when other premade porridge-like dishes have not. Its name alone evokes a distasteful image, an image of uncomeliness, as Fernando Ortíz implied in analyzing the terminology of Afrocuban cooking. Ortíz noted that when the ending "ngi" is changed to "che," as occurs in the Caribbean with the word "funche," it carries a derogatory meaning, like the endings "icha," "iche," and "uche."[63] It is revealing, too, that funche is largely missing from the menus of restaurants specializing in the style of cooking known as nuevo criollo, which prides itself on employing new techniques, exotic ingredients, and evocative decor to prepare dishes that use the food eaten by past generations of Puerto Ricans. The same is also true with related confections, such as mazamorra, marota, or marifinga, all of which can bring up bleak memories of once-common food.[64]

Funche has also disappeared from the pages of various cookbooks published during the past few decades, cookbooks carrying the appellation "Puerto Rican," or "of yesteryear," or "criolla."[65] One of the few to include it is A Taste of Puerto Rico: Traditional and New Dishes from the Puerto Rican Community, which is written more for aficionados of multiethnic cooking in the New York area than for devotees of the most traditional cooking on the island.[66] The author makes an interesting move, calling funche the "Puerto Rican Polenta," as a way of capitalizing on the high standing that a humble, rural food of Italy has recently come to enjoy among gourmands worldwide to elevate a dish that in Puerto Rico had belonged above all to slave-quarter kitchens, bore the mark of black culture, and denoted economic impoverishment. Like funche, polenta has a long history, having served as a staple in the diet of Italy's Emilia-Romagna region since the end of the eighteenth century.[67]

Denouement?

In contemporary Puerto Rico the consumption of cornmeal, fresh corn, and other corn derivatives has declined considerably. For example, in 1982–83, the Department of Agriculture tabulated the per capita annual consumption of cornmeal at 9.8 pounds,[68] a figure very close to the 9 pounds of cornmeal consumed per capita in the island's urban areas in 1940.[69] At the beginning of the 1940s, however, it was precisely families living in cities and urban zones who consumed the least amount of cornmeal. In broad terms, the total annual consumption of cornmeal, unground corn, and of other corn derivatives was 12.3 pounds per capita in 1983.[70] This figure is less than the amount of cornmeal—cornmeal alone, exclusive of any derivatives—consumed in rural parts of Puerto Rico in 1939–40, which came to 19 pounds per person.

The Department of Agriculture's figures show an uptick, because the figures for the consumption of cornmeal and those for its processed derivatives are added together. But the consumption of cornmeal itself, which was always the most heavily used derivative, has declined during the past three decades: in 1975, annual per capita consumption was 2.31 pounds; in 1985, 2.74 pounds; in 1995, 0.02 pounds; in 2000, 0.19 pounds; and in 2003, 0.22 pounds.[71] Unlike rice, cornmeal and the dishes made with it have dropped sharply in popularity.

At the same time, the packages of cornmeal (white, and the fine or thick yellow varieties) stacked on hipermercado shelves suggest that even now—when scarcely any corn is grown in Puerto Rico[72] and a globalized food market has made other types of flour and cereal available—certain dishes maintain their appeal, though they must contend with still other factors that help reshape people's food preferences (for example, the amount of advertising for sorullos, as the accompaniment to a main dish, is much less than that devoted to French fries). The recipes found on the back of packages of cornmeal provide some indication of the continued fondness for certain preparations that use cornmeal. Moreover, informal observation demonstrates that along the coasts, especially in the Joyuda district of the municipality of Cabo Rojo, sorullos, purchased from street stalls or shops, are still highly popular, as they are in cafeterias that serve a selection of fried sweet goods for breakfast.

However, among the island's younger population, which is a key market for advertising and tends to consume on the basis of peer-group preferences, the majority of these confections and dishes are completely unknown, or at best seem stuffy and out of date. Also working against them, especially in a domestic setting, is the amount of time their preparation requires. And, conversely, shoppers will not find them, as they will other attractively packaged delicacies, conveniently sitting on grocery and supermarket shelves. Majarete, mundo nuevo, crispé, and gofio were, in earlier times, reserved for particular occasions. They have this same character today, though it plays out differently: now they figure almost exclusively, as "folkloric items," at food fests that are advertised as offering typical or traditional fare.

On the other hand, 2001 Department of Agriculture statistics indicate that 20,921,616 pounds of corn chips or similar snack foods were imported from the United States into the Puerto Rican commonwealth in 1999.[73] Although, given the ever stronger practice of "nibbling" (mordisqueo) between meals, both adults and young people undoubtedly still eat some traditional confections, these are simply not perceived as being genuine snack food.[74] Of all the traditional items, sorullo dulce and corn bread would be likely to enjoy the widest acceptance. In the end, however, the market for the retail sale of imported prepared baked goods is very strong. In 1999, 11,618,398 pounds of such goods were imported into Puerto Rico from foreign countries alone.[75] The comparable import figure from the United States was 19 million pounds.[76]

Still and all, for Puerto Ricans born between 1920 and 1950, dishes made with cornmeal—and funche more than others—have a double meaning: they recall times of scarcity and want but on that very basis continue to be seen as food that is simple, healthy, and reliable. These paradigms have not been lost on large agroindustrial concerns, such as Goya Foods and Molinos de Puerto Rico, which not only sell various semi-prepared confections, such as frozen sorullitos and *arepas*, but which market them as a kind of authentic heritage food that keeps the flame of tradition burning.[77]

It is possible that the trajectory of corn-based dishes in Puerto Rico differs fundamentally from that of rice, that unlike recipes for rice dishes, which have evolved to absorb new ingredients and to reflect new styles of cooking, preparations made with corn remain stubbornly the same. Rice unquestionably lends itself more readily to such adaptations, and while some things about cornmeal —its qualities as a processed food and its nutritional composition—have changed in line with agroindustrial advances, its preparation in the kitchen still follows a standard procedure: it gets mixed with water or milk and must then be beaten by hand. The process, which has not changed for centuries, is tedious and time-consuming. In a society in which large segments of the population have less and less patience for labor-intensive routines, a task like beating cornmeal appears anachronistic and self-defeating. On that score it is akin to guanime, whose very name calls for dusting off ancient cookbooks to eat a tidbit that stretches our culinary skills to the limit, or, alternatively, requires that we search out small restaurants tucked away in some remote corner of the island.

As a result, it may be that not too many years hence, recipes that emerged from the Afro–Puerto Rican plantation milieu, from the delicacies made in the family kitchen for festivities and celebrations, and from the creative capacity to produce a lot out of a little, will fade entirely from the domestic scene, their preparation taken over by the processed food industry. Thus obtained, in semi-prepared or precooked form, they will have the character of appetizers and snacks. Not long from now, preparing them at home will have a contrived quaintness to it, like attending an antique food fair.

4 | Codfish

Hey, salted codfish! I know your face though you come disguised.
—Popular saying

Although found in the frigid waters of the north Atlantic, cod became the source of and a principal ingredient in some of the dishes most distinctive to Puerto Rican cuisine, often accompanying or being mixed with other food, such as *chayote* (a pear-shaped, squashlike vegetable) and eggs to make the stew known as *alboronía*, or eggplants or seasoned *viandas* to make salads and other dishes. It was commonly mixed with rice to produce the popular *arroz con bacalao*, or incorporated into a thick soup dish called *sopón*. For all these preparations, however, it was first desalted in water; transformed, as it were, from its dried, salted state—the way in which it arrived on the island—back into a soft, damp, flavorful fish.

When preparing salted cod with *sofrito*, tomatoes, raisins, capers, potatoes, and wine, the cooks for some Basque families took to calling it *a la vizcaína*, though it differed considerably in this form from its Vizcayan namesake. In the kitchens of simpler folk, this dish has always been known, straightforwardly, as "codfish stew." When salted cod is accompanied by onions, capsicum, hardboiled eggs, oil, and vinegar, and sometimes avocado, it goes by the name *serenata*.

To make the Puerto Rican version of what is known in Cádiz and the nearby coastal town of El Puerto de Santa María as *tortillitas de camarones* (crisp shrimp fritters) and on the island—where salted cod has been so prominent—as *bacalaitos*, one first mixes wheat flour and water, to which are then added finely chopped tomatoes, *recao*, sweet chili peppers, small coriander leaves, and some achiote lard—in other words, sofrito.

For all its popularity, however, salted codfish has been consumed in progressively smaller quantities, a decline brought on by advances in the technology of refrigeration and the more rapid distribution of fish and shellfish, both fresh and frozen, as well as by a rise in its cost on world markets. Between 1950–51 and 1973–74, the annual consumption of salted and smoked fish in Puerto Rico declined from 15.9 to 7.23 pounds per capita.[1]

Yet at certain times in the island's food history, the frequency with which salted cod was consumed, in particular by those in the population suffering the greatest undernourishment, became a source of major concern for nutritionists and policy makers. Formulaically associating the food with nutritional ignorance, low-income levels, the lack of adequate measures for preservation, and gastrointestinal diseases, these critics and observers failed to perceive the deeper material, social, and cultural forces underpinning the reliance on salted codfish. Its consumption was driven by two extremes: on the one hand, obedience to the imperatives of the Catholic Church, crowned by numerous periods of abstention from meat on certain days of the week and during various times of the year, as dictated by the liturgical calendar; and on the other, the sheer struggle on the part of the poorest elements of society to amass enough food to survive. A certain type of importation business, which succeeded in cutting off other products from the food market, developed around these two factors. Consequently, the distribution and sale of salted codfish evolved into one of the island's most exclusive and profitable businesses.

The majority of traditional dishes that combine salted cod with other foods and are still consumed to this day were the result of adaptations, readaptations, and experiments made by people—women above all—compelled to abstain from eating certain foods and to patch meals together in a dietary context that was rich in foods from rural gardens but poor in meat products and in the foodstuffs found in urban centers. From a nutritional point of view, between the end of the nineteenth century and the 1950s, salted codfish was the pole around which the intake of proteins revolved, for those eating a simple diet characterized by a preponderance of carbohydrates and a lack of complete proteins. It was this situation, wherein people had only the same few things to eat day after day, month after month, that caused the consumption of salted cod—though dressed up and cooked in different ways—to be seen as something endlessly recurring. And this, furthermore, was the basis on which the saying quoted at the beginning of this chapter—"I know you salted codfish, even though you come disguised"—acquired its meaning.

Although the order of fish to which salted cod belongs, the gadiformes, is extensive, containing more than two hundred species spread across ten families,[2] since the Middle Ages, the commercial cod trade has revolved principally around just four gadiformes: Atlantic cod (*Gadus morhua*), haddock (*Melanogrammus aeglefinus*), pollock (*Pollachius virens*), and hake (*Urophicis chuss*).[3] The four are all found in Puerto Rican supermarkets today, with Atlantic cod being the most expensive, owing to its excellent flavor, soft texture, and low fat content—qualities that are less pronounced in its three close relatives.[4] Cod are omnivorous, indeed so omnivorous as to feed at times on their own offspring. Their insatiable appetite, ichthyologists believe, may be tied to how they swim about with their mouths constantly open, a characteristic which in turn has made them easy prey for fishermen.[5]

Their relatively easy capture also stems from their preference for shallower waters. For example, schools of Atlantic cod—though able to survive in a variety of ocean environments—are rarely found at depths greater than 650 feet, and during the summer months, when they are caught in the greatest number, they stay much closer to the surface, swimming at a depth of only 200 to 300 feet. During the winter months, their preference is for slightly deeper water, a depth of 300 to 400 feet, though females, who spawn during this time of year, can be found in fishing grounds as shallow as 30 or as deep as 350 feet.

Discovered by Basque fishermen as early as during the Middle Ages, cod populate the Atlantic Ocean in a line extending from Newfoundland south to New England. Although their practice had no firm scientific basis, these Basque—along with the Portuguese and English—always fished in shallow waters, waters that came to be known as "banks," extensive low-lying sea beds running along the North American continental shelf. These banks (the largest of which are the Grand Banks of Newfoundland) were rich in the phytoplankton, zooplankton, and other marine life on which the voracious cod fed.

The majority of gadiformes live in waters with temperatures ranging from one to ten degrees centigrade.[6] While a species of tropical cod (*bergmaceros*) still exists, it is not believed to have any significant commercial value.[7] Other species of cod are prized as sporting fish (tomcod), and still others—that inhabit freshwater, such as the burbot,—are valued in some arctic countries for their flesh, though its quality is not as high as that of the Atlantic cod and its three near relatives, all four of which have been the preferred varieties for as long as they have been fished. Several factors account for this marked preference, the first of which is the quality of their flesh. As the whitest and tenderest, the flesh of the Atlantic cod is superior to that of all the others. Whoever has eaten this fish knows that its flesh can be easily flaked off in large sections, which bear a pleasingly light, shiny hue, in contrast to others of the same species, whose flesh is darker, oilier, and less robust.

Next in importance is the low fat content of codfish. In its fresh state, Atlantic cod contains no more than 0.3 percent fat.[8] Only a fraction behind is smoked haddock, with a fat content of 0.4 percent.[9] This particular feature of cod enables it to last longer without spoiling. While it is true that cod contain a high percentage of water (80.5 percent), the water is easily eliminated when the fish gets dried, owing precisely to its low fat content. In earlier times, the drying of cod was done in the open air, by draping the eviscerated fish over rocks and using the cold Nordic winds that blew during winter as a natural drying agent.

A third factor underlying the preference for cod is its high nutritional potential. Although the protein content of Atlantic cod, in its fresh state, amounts to only 18.1 percent, once the fish is subjected to the drying effects of the cold winds and its water content evaporates, some 80 percent of its flesh turns into protein.[10] Furthermore, its fine flavor has also contributed to making it a premier choice among those who eat fish.

A Complementary or a Supplementary Food?

How is it possible, we might well ask, that a fish caught, cured, and salted in waters and lands so far from the Caribbean should succeed in becoming such a major component of the Puerto Rican diet? Clearly, salted cod was, and remains, no less foreign to the ecology of the region than certain other foods. The yam, plantain, rice, breadfruit (*Artocarpus altilis*), and pigeon pea (*Cajanus cajans*), all commonplace today, are similar to salted cod in one respect—they were native to continents and regions far removed from the Caribbean—but fundamentally different in another: in the culinary history of the island, they were destined to play, as Claude Fischler terms it, a "complementary" role.[11] That is, they fell into position as complements, placed beside native foods that played a central role in meals consumed within the society to which they, the complements, had been introduced: for example, the yam and the plantain next to cassava, tannier, and sweet potato, or rice beside corn. When joined with these native foods, they fulfilled a narrow, purely dietary purpose, without causing any displacement or occasioning any substitution.

Not so salted codfish. This dried fish seems to have arrived and found its place on the island not as a "complement," but as a "supplement."[12] In this case, that is, as a food that survived to serve a different function. By and large, as Fischler pointed out, foods that arrive and gain a footing as supplements do so in contexts of thoroughgoing interethnic contact or mixing, such as has taken place in Puerto Rico throughout its history. At an early stage of their insertion, Fischler goes on to say, they take their place next to similar foods—for example, salted cod and herring opposite fresh fish—and eventually displace these or, alternatively, get adopted to fulfill specific, new culinary functions.

Although Fischler underscores that one cannot really adduce with precision any pure cases, the adoption of salted codfish in Puerto Rico may be the exception to the rule. For example, dried cod always had a high "convenience of use" value in sustaining populations subjected to regimented diets, as were plantation slaves or soldiers during much of the period of Spanish colonial rule in Puerto Rico. In addition, because of how inexpensively and lastingly it preserves, coupled with its high protein content, salted cod was an effective food for groups in the population that, as we saw in the case of rice, were hardly in a position to deliberate over the quality and quantity of what they consumed.

The "convenience of use" factor also played out strongly in the role of salted cod, in both a real and symbolic sense, as a substitute for meat on the days when the church's liturgical calendar called for such abstention. Abstaining from meat served, from the initial years of the conquest, as a clear marker of religious and ethnic identity, and the days that required such observance were so great in number (between 140 and 160 per year) as to preclude any possible reliance on the use of fresh fish.[13] Viewed from this dual angle—both as a fish that preserved well and as a vehicle that helped fulfill religious duties—the adoption of salted cod made perfect sense.

In sum, the practical value of salted cod, its convenience of use, was a key factor in furthering its introduction into Old World diets, and especially into those relied on by the poorest urban dwellers, well before the European expansion into the New World, including the island of Puerto

Rico.[14] Before its decisive role as a staple could take hold in the colonial diet, however, salted cod had first to become a high-value commodity in the food market of the Caribbean.

The Slow Process of Adoption

Figuring from the start as a supplement, salted cod began to assume a prominent place on the dietary horizon of the population only during the last years of the eighteenth century, when the ideas of the European Enlightenment were filtering into the Spanish colonial world and Puerto Rico experienced its share of defining events, such as the birth of the proto-nationalist Ramón Power y Giralt, the completion of the painting of Bishop de la Cuerda by the mulatto artist José Campeche, and the inauguration of San Juan's San Cristóbal fort, the largest military fortification constructed by the Spanish in the New World.

More than two centuries earlier, however, in the mid-1600s, salted cod had comprised 60 percent of the fish consumed on the European continent.[15] Yet according to the manifests of ships arriving in San Juan from Seville between 1510 and 1519, the cured fish imported into the colony were not salted cod but, rather, "mackerel" and "sardines."[16] A possible explanation is that sardines and mackerel, at that time the objects of much fishing activity in the waters of the Andalusian Atlantic, were favored as exports by the Andalusian mercantile guilds that provisioned the ships leaving for the Indies from Seville.[17]

Cod, on the other hand, was caught, dried, and salted in and near the waters of the North Atlantic, far from where Spain's "enterprise of the Indies" was first launched. In addition, fishermen hunting Atlantic cod had to follow the prescribed course that it swam along the waters close into the Newfoundland-Labrador coast.[18] Both factors acted as a brake on its widespread introduction into the Caribbean during the first centuries of Spanish colonial rule.

While Basque, Galician, and Portuguese sailors knew about the rich cod fisheries of the Newfoundland banks,[19] their catch was primarily directed toward satisfying the needs of the Catholic populations in the interior of the Iberian Peninsula, in the French Basque country, and in southeastern Europe, rather than of those in the Andalusian south, whose nearby Atlantic and Mediterranean waters teemed with their own fish.[20] Indeed, the charges leveled at colonial administrators, during the early years of the conquest, over their failure to enforce the church's rules on abstaining from meat,[21] and the frequent petitions later made by San Juan's municipal council to ecclesiastical authorities in Spain, requesting that the population be allowed to eat meat on days when it was prohibited,[22] provide insight not only into the imperfect exercise of Catholic penitential practice and the difficulties encountered by the new settler population in preserving fish caught on the island but also into the relative scarcity of any dried fish, including salted cod, in the colony's few markets.

Theoretically, the fish population on and around the island could have filled the colony's needs, since the Caribbean shelf contains numerous species of fish.[23] However, the high fat content of fish in this region,[24] as well as challenges in mastering techniques for curing them with salt, made the preservation of fish in the tropics a difficult task. It was perhaps for this reason that San Juan's municipal councilors ordered that any cured fish sold in the market had to be "lean and not recently salted."[25]

Factors of a geopolitical nature also figured into the delayed adoption of salted cod in Puerto Rico. These were epitomized by the defeat of the Spanish Armada in 1588, following which England claimed for itself the richest fishing grounds found along the coast of Newfoundland.[26] In addition, Spain's annexation of Portugal meant that Portugal lost, as of 1581, the naval protection that England had always afforded her as a fishing power in the Newfoundland region. This loss had a cascading effect; Portugal's narrowed options for fishing the waters of the North Atlantic reduced, in turn, the amount of Portuguese salted cod that could be stored in Seville to await shipment to the Indies. Although Portugal continued to send out fishing boats, its days as one of the leading powers in the Atlantic cod trade had come to an end. Furthermore, if there had been any possibility that Portuguese salted cod might be included with some frequency in cargos sent out to Puerto Rico during the seventeenth century, it was foreclosed with the change in navigational routes adopted, beginning in the early 1600s, by the Spanish fleet in the Caribbean.[27] The scant amount of fish brought onto the island by the few ships that reached Puerto Rico between 1650 and 1700 may have resulted from this change in sea routes.[28]

The spreading use of salted codfish and its definitive adoption seemingly date to the final years of the eighteenth century and the first decades of the nineteenth. The commercial exchange and interaction, both licit and illicit, that undermined and broke Spain's monopolistic grip on trade in the Caribbean and reoriented it in favor of the English after the signing of the

Treaty of Utrecht in 1713, as well as the identification of the Caribbean as an economic zone composed of sugar plantations worked by slaves, transformed the region, as the eighteenth century wore on, into a potentially strong market for the consumption of salted cod, above all on the plantations of the French and English Antilles.[29] For its part, Puerto Rico, which in this same period lay at the center of what has been called a "rich area of commerce," in all likelihood began to receive, legally and illegally, supplies of Anglo-American salted cod in its ports in quantities far in excess of those furnished earlier through the peninsular market.[30] Ultimately, too, the importance that Puerto Rico and Cuba eventually acquired as military outposts and as centers of sugar production also furthered the growth, gradual as it may have been, of the English salted cod trade in the ports of both colonies. Between 1804 and 1816, the volume of salted cod imported into the Caribbean from England jumped from 55,998 to 167,603 *quintales* (in the metric system, one quintal equaled 100 kilograms).[31]

Salted Cod for Soldiers, Salted Cod for Slaves

The greater use of salted codfish as a supplementary food apparently sprang from the military reforms instituted by colonial authorities in 1765. Among other provisions, these stipulated that each veteran soldier quartered in San Juan should receive an allocation of at least one and a half pounds of salted cod on five days out of the month, although it is not clear whether this regulation was adopted for religious or military reasons: whether to help ensure compliance with the church's rules regarding abstinence from meat on the prescribed days,[32] or whether to bolster the diets of soldiers at a time when a greater military readiness was called for. In either case, under normal conditions, the new directive translated into an allocation of no less than eighteen pounds of salted cod per soldier annually.

The transformation of Puerto Rico's economy, during the first decades of the nineteenth century, into one based heavily on the sugar plantation and its system of slave labor, gave further impetus to increasing the availability of salted cod and other cured fish in the island's ports, since they could find a ready market on the sugar estates, whose owners needed to provide a basic, effective diet for their slaves. Today, thanks to advances in nutritional science and work in food chemistry, it is known that under certain conditions of undernourishment, such as those endured by Puerto Rico's plantation slaves, salted cod played a vital physiological-nutritional role: a tiny portion of it enabled the body to recover the phosphorous and mineral salts lost through the dehydration that accompanied long hours of work in the fields. In addition, its high protein content could help mitigate the otherwise insufficient amount of complete proteins contained in the diets of slaves and other laborers.[33]

Throughout the nineteenth century, merchants who sourced and sold dried cod in large quantity—the English in particular—helped turn the Caribbean into a major market for salted cod (often of second-rate quality), and slave owners factored its acquisition into their economic and administrative calculations. A conservative estimate of the amount of salted codfish allocated per slave on a monthly basis at the beginning of the third decade of the nineteenth century is 5.4 pounds.[34] The release, years and decades later, of former slaves and soldiers into civil society, with their established patterns of eating and the scant possibility of changing these, helped lock salted cod into the dietary practices of the population to the very end of the nineteenth century.[35] Just prior to the middle of the nineteenth century, 7,416,502 pounds of salted cod were imported into Puerto Rico—something unheard of before 1765.[36]

During the rest of the nineteenth century, salted cod began to feature in meals eaten by other sectors of the population. Importation figures reflect not only the rise in the slave and military populations occurring between the end of the eighteenth and the first decades of the nineteenth century but also the increase during the nineteenth century of the Puerto Rican population at large, as indicated in figure 4.1.

The gradual reduction in the amount of land dedicated to growing crops for consumption, the inability of local agricultural and livestock production to thrive against the pressure for land (and labor) exerted by large-scale enterprises like sugar and coffee, and the relentless strength of foreign markets to import food into the island all conspired to turn salted cod into a top nutritional, protein-laden option for many. What had started as an inexpensive fish that would satisfy the requirements of Lent and supplement the diets of soldiers and plantation slaves ended as the most logical dietary staple for hundreds of islanders, both rich and poor. At the end of the nineteenth century, the amount of cod caught in the North Atlantic and subsequently cured and imported into Puerto Rico reached 55.3 million pounds. It was so plentiful, in fact, that what had not been consumed was eaten in place of fresh fish as a Lenten food, and in the households of the poor, it took the place of meat, which by the late 1880s was seldom to be

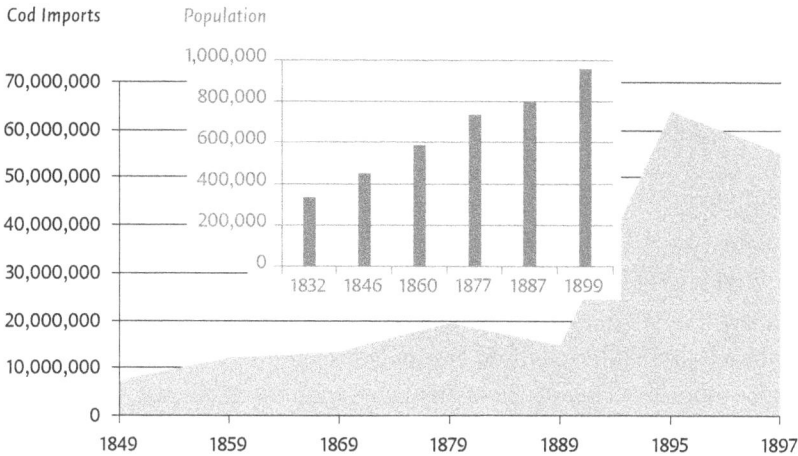

FIGURE 4.1 Population growth and salted cod imports during the nineteenth century

Sources: Centro de Investigaciones Históricas de la Universidad de Puerto Rico, Balanzas mercantiles, Selected Years, 1849–1897; José L. Vázquez Calzada, La población de Puerto Rico y su trayectoria histórica, Universidad de Puerto Rico, Escuela Graduada de Salud Pública.

seen. Around 1897, it was estimated that the supplies of salted cod available on the island were sufficiently large that each person could, on average, consume 55 pounds annually. Perhaps nothing better captures the pivotal nutritional role played by this dried, salted fish than a popular riddle of the day: "¿Qué es la vaca con la o? Bacalao" (What's the cow with the [letter] o? Salted cod).[37]

Not All That Glitters Is Salted Cod

Normally in Puerto Rico, when one thinks of "salted cod," it is with a single kind of fish in mind. Yet a glance at the labels and prices of what is sold in supermarkets as salted codfish is sufficient to realize that, now and in the past, not everything lumped and marketed under that name was, and is, the genuine article. The economic history of the Caribbean, to which Puerto Rico was always closely tied as a sugar-producing colony, has been instrumental in the development of this false notion, which still envelops the use of the fish in Puerto Rican gastronomy.

As far back as the sixteenth century, European fishermen had identified at least four varieties within the cod family. Although belonging to the same family, each was different in respect to the texture of its flesh, its water content, degree of oiliness, flavor, and the manner in which it was dried.

The differences extended, too, to the depths at which and the time of year when they could be caught.[38] Historically, this variation had caused the fishing and curing industry and its brokers to establish a graduated scale of prices. The development of a diverse set of consumer markets was another outcome.[39]

From the seventeenth century onward, for example, Atlantic cod caught in the fisheries close to the island of Newfoundland and dried outside during winter (above all by English and British North American fishermen who lacked a robust sea salt industry) fetched the highest price, because the method by which it was dried and salted allowed it to keep its excellent flavor—one of the qualities that distinguished it from the other varieties—and extracted the maximum water content from its flesh. This treatment not only saved space and weight on ships and boats but also made the product more durable. Atlantic salted cod was sold in the fish markets of Northern Spain (Bilbao and Santander) and in Mediterranean ports for the tables of the more prosperous.[40] It was also brought to the ports of La Rochelle, in France, and to those at the mouth of the Douro and Miño Rivers in Portugal. Meanwhile, the lower-grade salted cod arriving in these ports (such as pollock and hake, which had higher water and oil content and, as a rule, got dried on the vessels themselves) was targeted to less well-off populations in the interior of the peninsula and throughout the rest of Europe.[41]

In the Caribbean, paralleling the growth of a plantation-slave labor economy in the French and British Antilles, cod fishermen from the British isles and North America—who were the biggest suppliers by far of salted fish in this region—discovered that the Caribbean market was not as discriminating or demanding as the European one. Insofar as these fishermen supplied fish from the cod family, they realized that they could without much difficulty confine it to what got classified as second grade in the process of curing and salting. When properly dried and salted, cod can be delectable. But in the process of preserving the cod, fishermen were wont to make a number of missteps: many fish were slit open badly, or dried carelessly in the summer, or under- or over-salted, or mishandled in some other way.[42] In addition to being experienced at their craft, these cod fishermen were shrewd businessmen. As time passed, they realized that salted cod could be sold in the Caribbean as *pieza de mantenimiento* (scrappage), along with other fish of lesser quality, such as mackerel, herring, and whiting, or small hake. Indeed, in the cod nomenclature of that time, inferior-grade salted cod was called "Jamaican fare" (*vianda jamaiquina*), while the high-grade variety, caught in the spring and dried during the winter, was called "spring fare" (*vianda de primavera*).[43] All of the second-class salted cod and other salted fish were paid for in the form of molasses from the Antilles, loaded on ship, and taken back, eventually reaching distilleries in New England, where it was used in the production of rum.

In the nineteenth century, when Puerto Rico had attained the status of a major sugar-producing colony, the principal importers instituted rankings of grade and quality similar to those employed in the French and English colonies. In turn, Puerto Rican custom houses adopted a scale for rating imported salted fish according to both its quality and its place of origin. Throughout the century, the *Balanzas Mercantiles* reflect the different prices set for the salted cod from Scotland and elsewhere (the Nova Scotian was the most expensive), other salted fish, and hake. Similarly, fish such as sardines, anchovies, herring, mackerel, and salmon differed in price from salted cod, since they often came canned and preserved in oil. When the possibilities of enriching one's diet were limited, as was the case in nineteenth-century Puerto Rico, the availability of inexpensive salted fish, all varieties of which were accepted as "salted cod" by the mass of the population, allowed proteins and mineral salts to be more widely distributed among various sectors, including poor campesinos, less economically secure urban workers, and the country's wealthier families. Some 45,311,535 pounds of salted cod and mackerel were imported into Puerto Rico in the fiscal year 1897, the market for which was dominated by Great Britain (with 22,092,000 pounds), followed by the United States (2,149,000 pounds) and Norway (638,000 pounds).[44]

Salted Cod and the Periphery

No citizen of Puerto Rico today would be surprised to find, in the buffet section of cafes and restaurants, a platter brimming with *bacalao guisado* (codfish stew) or *serenata de bacalao* (codfish salad), whether the fish was Atlantic cod or not. Indeed, one could easily gain the impression, when leafing through Puerto Rican cookbooks—including those published before 1960—that salted codfish and its near relatives were abundantly available on the island and that everyone in the population could enjoy preparing them in a number of sophisticated ways, dressing up the most delicate varieties with saffron, nutmeg, raisins, capers, olives, white wine, almonds, eggs, hazelnuts, and more. That salted cod scarcely deserved the lowly reputation that once dogged it would be a further impression.

Yet the reality was otherwise. Salted cod was not a common sight on the tables of many Puerto Ricans, nor—by the same token—did many people have the opportunity to prepare it as a rich, savory dish, even though it cost relatively little. Nor did the majority of people procure the better-quality salted cod, or cook it with the seasonings and spices called for by the more elaborate recipes. Furthermore, as a food that lost much of its body while being cooked, salted cod—when it reached the dining table, especially in poor households—was a fraction of its original size. Thus, if it is true that at one point it came to be a food that was relatively abundant for certain segments of the population, as in the case of slaves, who on average consumed sixty pounds per annum,[45] it is also true that, with time, salted cod became what Mintz calls a fringe, or "peripheral food."

According to Mintz, in societies characterized by systems of subsistence agriculture—and, one could add, by economies built around the export of a single crop or commodity—the food consumed by the majority falls into a "matrix" organized along the coordinates of "center-periphery-legume." Within the matrix, the "center" is composed of cereals and tubers that supply complex carbohydrates. The "periphery" is composed of meat, fats, spices, and condiments, which—more than being a source of protein—enhance taste and flavor. The "legumes" are composed of beans and all kinds of green, leafy vegetables.[46] In the case of Puerto Rico, it is possible that the matrix took shape when meat ceased to play a prominent part in diets starting in the first decade of the nineteenth century.[47] With reference to salted cod, its importance in the matrix as a peripheral food would have increased as it was imported in larger and larger quantity and as both dried and jerked beef and pork giblets became ever more costly, as imported foods, in comparison to salted cod.

Perhaps for this reason, by the close of the nineteenth century, salted cod not only featured prominently in essays and other writings dealing with the diet of campesinos and the working poor but was cast as well in an unfavorable light. The dreariness of their diet, its deadening monotony, was lamented and criticized, as though these groups, trapped as they were by meager incomes and endemic poverty, were somehow free to choose among a wide variety of food and to eat more creatively. Salted codfish thus stands out, in these writings, as the quintessential peripheral food of the poor. "Do you know what makes up the diet of the campesino? Well, pay close heed: four or five ounces of salted cod, usually without any oil, and eight ounces of cornmeal, or—absent the latter—four plantains," declared the newspaper La Razón in 1871.

Salvador Brau was the only commentator to acknowledge that an inferior daily wage severely restricted the portion of salted cod that could accompany an already sparse meal: "Frugal more out of pure necessity than from any sense of virtue, they satisfy their appetite with hardly any food: a piece of dried pollock, a bun or cake of cooked or roasted corn, three or four malangas (dasheen, Colocassia esculenta), and a cup, most often just a coconut shell, of coffee sweetened with honey." Another journalist, José Pérez Moris, observed in El Boletín Mercantil that the poor "are not used to having any food other than sweet potatoes and salted cod."[48]

Francisco del Valle Atiles, Puerto Rico's best-known hygienist-physician, and a man who did more than anyone to set forth a model diet for the island's campesino population, likewise recognized the peripheral role of salted cod and other cured fish, "frequently found in a sorry state of preservation," over meat, even as he expanded the number of edible substances that, in his opinion, were regularly consumed by the poor.[49] Valle Atiles appreciated the importance of salt, which dried codfish contained in great quantity, for the physical welfare of human beings. Thus, in his 1887 Cartilla de higiene (Booklet on Hygiene), salt-containing condiments were defined, for the benefit of school teachers, as "stimulating gastric activity" and as "necessary for nutrition."[50] But Valle Atiles stopped there; he was unable—given his level of scientific knowledge—to propose that salt was as necessary to the body as water. Rather, he saw its use in terms of "[the] need to preserve food substances or . . . to prevent the spoiling of food that we wish to preserve."[51]

The discovery that sodium and potassium were essential minerals in maintaining and regulating the amount of water in the body did not occur until the end of the nineteenth century. Because of its high salt content, dried cod—like mackerel and herring, which were also categorized as cured fish—became a "reconstituting peripheral [food]" that kicked into action following physical exertions that caused the body to dehydrate. In addition, of course—as Valle Atiles and the poor who consumed it on a regular basis well appreciated—it enhanced the flavor of food. Unquestionably, then, salted cod established itself as a peripheral food in the last quarter of the nineteenth century.

Moreover, between 1900 and 1940, during the period of the "simplification of the diet," this process gained greater traction. The way in which salted cod acted as a peripheral food is, admittedly, not easily discerned through textual references, since the fish is always defined or represented as an everyday food. Its peripheral function is better understood in numerical terms.

During the first four decades of the twentieth century, there were two periods during which the importation of salted cod into Puerto Rico dropped significantly, leaving people with less opportunity to consume it. The first occurred between 1900 and 1910, the second between 1934 and 1938. In the first case, statistics demonstrate that a strong contraction first set in during the late 1890s and persisted until 1910. Indeed, the amount of salted cod available between 1900 and 1910 fell to pre-1895 levels, when it was already entrenched as a peripheral dietary item. This first decline resulted from policies implemented by Canada and the United States to protect their respective cod fisheries and trade.

In 1897, Canadian authorities began to take measures to regulate U.S. participation—especially by Maine's fishing fleets—in catching and processing codfish within the fishing banks of Newfoundland, Labrador, and Quebec.[52] These initiatives, which remained in force until 1918, rebounded adversely on the supply of salted cod imported into Puerto Rico during the first years of U.S. control over the island, since the United States responded by adopting similar protectionist measures (which in fact it had begun instituting as early as 1890 at the insistence of Maine's congressional delegation) on all fish caught in waters lying along the British territories in the northwestern Atlantic. The American response picked up momentum as soon as Puerto Rico was incorporated as a colony of the United States and U.S. laws regarding coastal navigation and trade went into force following the passage of the Foraker Act in 1900.[53] Imports of salted cod from Canada, which by the end of the nineteenth century had exported the lion's share of the fish into Puerto Rico, disappeared from the picture entirely.[54] As a result, the amount of salted cod imported onto the island between 1900 and 1910 (1901, 12 million pounds; 1905, 18 million pounds; and 1910, 25 million pounds) fell dramatically from the total imported into Puerto Rico from a group of nine countries during the last years of the nineteenth century.[55]

Moreover, any recovery in the supply of both salted cod and other salted fish furnished by the United States to Puerto Rico would have to contend with another development: the ice-cooled fish that had first appeared not too many years before with advances in mechanical refrigeration were no longer a novelty; there was now a stronger preference on the part of consumers for fresh fish, rather than desiring salted and preserved. Consequently, between 1900 and 1910, only 1 percent of all the fish caught by fishermen working the ports of New England subsequently turned up in the market as salted codfish.[56]

This development was bound to work a hardship on the diets of the poor in Puerto Rico, since U.S. exports of salted cod to the island were already minimal before 1900 and a revival and reorganization of the market to satisfy Puerto Rican demand would necessarily take time. As such, the years from 1910 through 1919 demonstrate that the per capita availability of salted cod—salted cod alone, exclusive of any similar fish—was not equal to what it had been via imports from Canada in 1897, which had hovered at some 23.1 pounds per person annually. The market recovered only in 1926, when between 27 and 28 pounds of imported cod and other salted fish were available on a per capita basis in Puerto Rico.

Moving in reverse, however, the market contracted even more sharply in the ten years from 1929 to 1938. As can be observed in figures 4.2 and 4.3, beginning in 1927, a reduction in the volume of imported salted cod caused a gradual, corresponding drop in the amount of it consumed per capita.

In 1929, in fact, the year's consumption of salted cod per person was only 17 pounds, or more than 5 pounds less than the equivalent figure for 1910 (22.4 pounds). In the six years between 1929 and 1935, those Puerto Ricans who depended most on this cured fish—the rural and urban poor—were forced to make do with considerably less of it. In contrast to rice, whose import numbers increased, or to the availability of different tubers (31,432,488 pounds of which came from local agricultural production[57]), the figures for salted cod show a sudden reduction of imports, similar to that which afflicted corn, bringing them down to levels not recorded since the last years of the First World War. This trend persisted well-nigh unaltered until 1937–38, when the amount of salted cod available per capita in Puerto Rico was still no greater than 16 pounds.

At the close of the decade, the trend line remained essentially unchanged, although the figures for per capita consumption and availability appear, curiously, to be at odds with each other. The islanders' annual consumption, in broad terms, equaled 18 pounds per person,[58] which exceeded by 2 pounds the amount of salted cod reported as available.[59] The

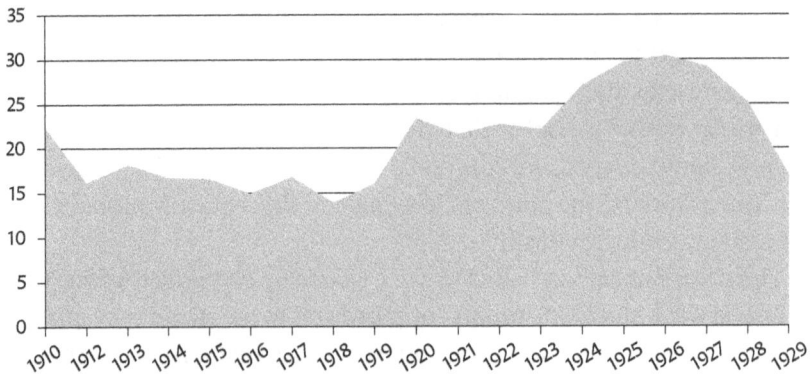

FIGURE 4.2 Yearly availability per capita, in pounds, of salted cod imports

Sources: "Food Imports into Porto Rico from the United States and Foreign Countries," in Victor S. Clark et al., *Porto Rico and Its Problems*, Washington, D.C., 1930; Cámara de Comercio de Puerto Rico, *Boletín Oficial de la Cámara de Comercio de Puerto Rico* 10, no. 6 (September 1934): 22; Government of Puerto Rico, Department of Agriculture and Commerce, *Annual Book on Statistics*, 1924–1943; Junta de Planificación, *Anuario Estadístico*, 1956. The figures include salted cod, salted haddock, and haddock in brine.

actual meaning of either figure, though, is that the nutritional aspect of salted cod—one of the essential functions of peripheral foods, according to Mintz—had ceased to exist for Puerto Ricans. In this period, then, its role in the diet was purely "to enhance flavor."

In 1937–38, nutritionists, dieticians, and others calculated that the highest intake of "calories by the pound" from purchased sources of complete proteins (meat and fish) broke down as follows (after allowing for wastage and loss in the process of cooking): from fresh pork, 874 calories; fresh beef, 652; salted codfish, 300; chicken, 289; and fresh fish, 205. On average, the cost per pound of these was: fresh pork, 19.9 cents; fresh beef, 19.2 cents; chicken, 25 cents; fish, 10.9 cents, and salted cod, 8.5 cents.[60] Depending on the region, these prices would all vary, up or down—but by no more than a single *centavo*.[61]

Thus for these types of meat and fish, salted cod was the most logical choice in terms of cost. Yet the technical specialists made two related observations. A majority of the population was inclined to buy food that was less expensive, such as rice and viandas, as a way of bulking up their diets, and they chose to obtain their protein—to the extent they possessed such awareness—from legumes, not from salted cod. Studies, in fact, disclosed very low levels of consumption per person of salted cod: in San Juan, 0.18 pounds per week and in 22 other communities on the island, an average of

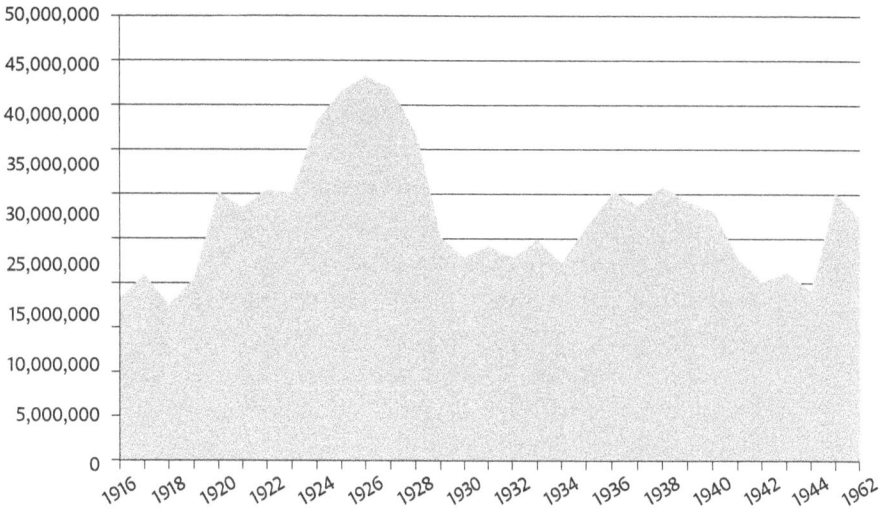

50,000,000
45,000,000
40,000,000
35,000,000
30,000,000
25,000,000
15,000,000
10,000,000
5,000,000
0

1916 1918 1920 1922 1924 1926 1928 1930 1932 1934 1936 1938 1940 1942 1944 1962

FIGURE 4.3 Imports of salted cod, in millions of pounds, 1916–1962

Sources: Clark, Food Imports into Porto Rico from the United States and Foreign Countries, Washington, D.C., 1930; Cámara de Comercio de Puerto Rico, Boletín Oficial de la Cámara de Comercio de Puerto Rico 10, no. 6 (September 1934), 22; Government of Puerto Rico, Department of Agriculture and Commerce, Annual Book on Statistics, 1924–1943; and Junta de Planificación, Anuario estadístico, 1956. Numbers include salted cod and salted haddock as well as haddock contained in brine.

0.31 pounds per week. These figures were extrapolated to reach, annually, 9 pounds per person in San Juan and 16 pounds per person in the other 22 communities. Within rural zones, the annual consumption among a group of 439 families was estimated at 19 pounds per person,[62] or the same figure as had obtained, under normal circumstances, for a veteran soldier in the eighteenth century (18.5 pounds).

The dietary dynamic at the end of the 1930s, however, was markedly different: people were then living under conditions of diminished protein intake, and the larger society faced strong demographic pressures, which was not the case in the late eighteenth century. From all appearances, salted cod in Puerto Rico had entered a new phase in its history: if at one time it was a "supplement" (1765–1880), and later (1880–1930) a "peripheral food" that furnished proteins and enhanced taste, it had now adopted the organoleptic function of a "condiment."

This new role was identified some ten years later, in 1949, by Lydia Roberts, when the problems of malnutrition and food insecurity were increasingly seen to stem from underlying economic structures and conditions of dependency, capable, in their own way, of creating a political situation fraught with risk.[63] In the face of this reality, Roberts summarized the new role played by this cold-water fish:

> Codfish has long been known as a staple in the Puerto Rican diet, and it now appears that it is the most commonly used protein food. Over half (57.7%) of all families customarily purchase codfish once a week, and 16.5 per cent oftener than this. Thus approximately three-fourths (74.2%) of all families may be said to use codfish as a regular part of their dietaries. Others (15.5%) also purchase it, but not with weekly regularity, and 10.3 per cent seldom or never use it.
>
> *Per capita consumption.* The regular purchase of codfish does not necessarily mean that any considerable quantities are eaten. The average weekly consumption for all families is 5.7 ounces, or about 0.8 ounces a day. The average is less in families with incomes below $500,—5.1 ounces for rural and 5.3 for urban families—and still less, 4 ounces, in urban families in the "$2,000 and over" category . . .
>
> To assume that these averages are representative of the consumption of all families in a given category would, of course, be erroneous. . . . In terms of daily averages, 66.8 per cent of all families have less than one ounce per person daily, on the average, and 33 per cent less than one-half ounce or none at all. . . .
>
> What contribution does codfish in these amounts make to the dietaries? One ounce of codfish furnishes about 5 grams of protein, or about one-fifteenth of the day's protein requirement. . . . In the lowest income bracket where codfish is the main and often the only animal protein food used, 70.2 per cent of the families get less than 5, and 37.1 per cent less than 2.5 grams of protein per person daily from this source. It is thus evident that for these families the chief contribution of codfish is that it adds some flavor to an otherwise bland diet.[64]

In 1954, when the process of modernization in Puerto Rico was at its height, medical science recognized the direct association between nutritional diseases and the amount of salt that the poorest islanders were accustomed to eating on a daily basis, once salted cod had become a "condiment": "El Dr. Pons believes it likely that the large amounts of salted cod fish eaten by the chronically poor in our country contribute to augmenting the number of sick people who display nutritional edema."[65] From that point forward, after one and a half centuries of tradition, the significance of salted cod as a supplementary and peripheral food, and as a dietary item equated largely with the poor, began—slowly but visibly—to be reversed.

The Salted Cod of Wealthier Puerto Ricans

If salted cod served a basic physiological and taste-enhancing function for families of piece-workers and the poor, it took on a very different coloration among families of the well-to-do, whether they were native to the island or just living on it temporarily. Depending on individual budgets and tastes and whether recipes had been handed down, the cooks employed by wealthy Puerto Ricans re-created and mastered various ways of preparing salted codfish. Their success, and the elaborateness of the dishes, hinged on using a number of other items: oil in which to marinate the fish, spices for seasoning it, wines to give it flavor, and nuts to give it more body.

The cookbook El *cocinero puertorriqueño* contained numerous recipes for salted cod, all of which called for incorporating ingredients that, owing to their cost or to their unavailability in nonurban markets, not every kitchen could stock or acquire: fine spices, saffron (used in three out of eleven recipes), nutmeg, cloves, white wine, toasted hazelnuts, wheat flour, and eggs. Even hollandaise sauce—not easy to prepare—was recommended.[66] In some kitchens, the most expensive variety of salted codfish, which came from Scotland, was used.[67]

At the beginning of the twentieth century, when lessons about cooking and the kitchen were added to the home economics curriculum by North American teachers, young women in the Puerto Rican public school system were taught the recipes for salted codfish dishes that the newly arrived female educators had learned from cooks of well-to-do families on the island.[68] Recipes such as "salted cod a la vizcaína," "salted cod in cream sauce," and "salted codfish balls" were presented as models of a distinct yet simple and healthy way of preparing the fish. More elaborate recipes recommended the use of ingredients not typically found in many kitchens, such as olives, capers, and raisins in the case of one version of salted cod a la vizcaína. To make salted cod in cream sauce it was necessary to use butter, milk, and wheat flour, all of which—being expensive—were affordable only to middle and upper-class households. And even if campesino families might have obtained some of them as by-products of their husbandry— milk, butter, or eggs, for example—they were more valuable as items to be sold or exchanged than as ingredients to be used in cooking.

In any case, by making their students aware that salted cod could be used in a variety of ways—something already known and practiced in the kitchens of the well-to-do during the nineteenth century—these pioneer home economics teachers broadened the options for cooking and preparing it; the fish—as their students learned—could be presented in more aesthetically pleasing ways; it need not appear only in funche, or as pieces of fried salted cod, or as codfish salad. As postwar (1950–60) agroindustrial advances made headway in reforming the island's economy, and as the programs of direct food assistance began to put high-protein canned meats, fish, and other food on the tables of the poor, a larger segment of the Puerto Rican population could now broaden its use of salted cod to prepare it in more interesting and satisfying ways.

Ultimately, however, the island's fancier, more elaborate salted cod cuisine has always maintained a strong association with the simpler, utilitarian ways in which the fish was traditionally prepared: with rice in a sopón; served up salted with breadfruit and yautías; and submerged in a seasoned flour mix to make the codfish fritters that people make a beeline for in the street stalls or cafés in Piñones. Thus, to a certain degree, the salted cod dishes enjoyed today bear the traces of the physiological, taste-enhancing function that the fish once performed for the poorest elements of the rural and urban population.

Salted Cod Today

During the two decades from 1950 to 1970, Puerto Rican society experienced, unequally across the population, material and cultural transformations that modified the historical role played by salted cod in people's diets. As a result of the campaign undertaken after the Second World War to industrialize its economy, Puerto Rico began to share directly in the recent advances made by the U.S. agroindustry, two of which were particularly significant in reshaping dietary patterns and practices: improved techniques, perfected during the war, for canning and preserving protein-rich products; and scientific research and development, again a by-product of the war, leading to the improved design and manufacturing of such home appliances as refrigerators and freezers. In the first instance, many kinds of food previously considered and treated as luxuries, such as shellfish and canned fish, together with refrigerated or frozen meat and poultry, were now available and accessible to a wider public. In the second, greater possibilities now existed for preserving certain foods, such as "fresh meat," which the population had long desired, even dreamed of, but which—unlike salted cod—spoiled rapidly.

Hand in hand with these developments, the most recent findings published by nutritional scientists, coupled with new messaging emanating from the food-marketing industry, likewise helped alter the dietary landscape, alter it in a way that privileged the virtues of protein-rich meat products in opposition to salted cod.[69] Similarly, a new establishment—the supermarket—began to make its appearance in cities as of 1955. Impressive outlets such as Pueblo, Todos, Superama, and Grand Union opened their doors, employing advertising and sales techniques that had no precedent in the Puerto Rican food market.[70] New products, priced very reasonably, began to line their shelves. All of these changes were felt and absorbed by a population that little more than a decade earlier had lived through food insecurity, rationing, and persistent shortages. In this environment, which popularized hitherto unknown agroindustrial food products and opened new gastronomic horizons, it was only to be expected that the image of salted cod as a poor man's food would be reinforced, stirring up memories—perhaps more strongly than did funche—of times past when people went to bed hungry.[71] The decrease in the consumption of salted cod, to 11.9 pounds per person annually in 1950–51, 10.1 pounds around 1960, and 5.42 pounds in 1973–74, is directly attributable to this association.[72] In contrast, as we saw earlier, the average per capita consumption of salted cod in 1937–38 was estimated at 18 pounds.[73]

Department of Agriculture and Planning Commission statistics create a confusing picture of trends in the importation and consumption of salted cod in Puerto Rico between 1980 and 1995. First, in the inventories covering 1980 and subsequent years, salted cod, its close relatives, and (other) "salted fish" appear individually, as their own categories, in contrast to how they appear both in the Planning Commission's 1956 statistical report and in the study carried out by the commission in 1978.[74] In the latter two sources, there is only one category—salted and smoked fish—which includes imports of salted cod, its near relatives, and varieties of other salted fish. Second, the data for the period 1980–95, while usefully breaking importation and consumption into separate categories, are still not finalized. For this reason, any conclusions drawn must be hypothetical.

As just noted, the most recent figures distinguish salted cod from its other family members (hake, pollock, and haddock), as well as from other salted fish, revealing that a tiny reduction occurred in the consumption of salted cod during the last years of the 1990s. This decline appears to have been preceded by an increase in consumption from the 1980s into the 1990s, an increase that runs counter to what might have logically been thought to occur following the "democratization" of food between 1960 and 1970. A preliminary estimate for 1995, for example, puts the annual per capita consumption of salted cod at approximately 18.5 pounds. Nonetheless, the trend up to the year 2001 indicates a reduction in the consumption of salted cod: in 1996, the amount consumed per capita stood at 8.1 pounds; in 1997, 8.6 pounds; in 1998, 7.5 pounds; in 1999, 4.4 pounds; in 2000, 5.7 pounds; and in 2001, 5.8 pounds.[75]

This reduction, however, involves salted cod alone; it does not apply to hake, pollock, or haddock, nor to salted fish generally. The imports of all of these have increased; and all, to be sure, were always available on the local market and played an important role in diets alongside salted cod. Today, though, they have become more abundant. Their greater availability has been spurred by the severe drop in the cod population of the North Atlantic, caused by the fierce struggle among eight countries that historically competed for the fish without—until recently—setting firm quotas or establishing exclusion zones or defined periods for working the fisheries.[76] The massive depletion of cod has helped to push up its price; with fewer fishermen and smaller catches, the cod-fishing industry necessarily faces higher unit costs.

Not surprisingly, the increased cost of Atlantic cod has played out at the retail end, by promoting the purchase of "dried fish" or "fish preserved in salt," with consumers now favoring the fish closely related to cod, since these have a much higher water content, which makes them less desirable in gastronomic terms but more attractive in terms of market cost.[77] Following this track, the substitute fish have gained an ever greater share of the market as practical, affordable alternatives to Atlantic cod. Figure 4.4 shows the gross import statistics for cod, for its near relatives, and for salted fish as compiled by the Planning Commission during the last years of the twentieth century and the first years of the current one.[78]

The upward trend in the importation of dried and salted fish and of the near relatives of salted cod merits examination, for it suggests that—owing to the high price of cod, hake, pollock, and haddock have become synonymous, in the Puerto Rican mind, with "salted codfish." Anyone peering at the compartments in supermarkets that contain salted fish can experience

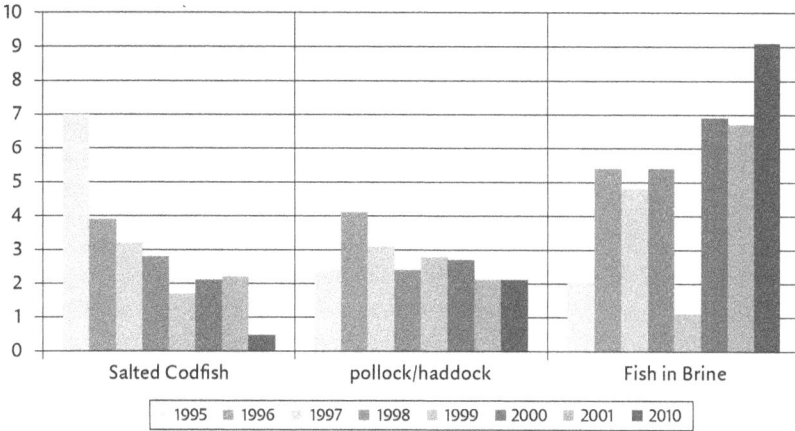

FIGURE 4.4 Approximation, in millions of pounds, of salted cod, salted pollock/haddock, and fish in brine imports

Sources: Junta de Planificación, Programa de Planificación Económica y Social, Oficina de Análisis Económico, Shipments of Merchandise from the United States to Puerto Rico by Commodity, 1996-2010. I am grateful to José Mulero González and William Cruz, agronomists for Puerto Rico's Department of Agriculture and Planning Commission respectively, for granting me access to their agencies' databases. The figures are approximate because they include total imports into Puerto Rico without subtracting reexportations to the Virgin Islands and other Lesser Antilles markets.

this conflation firsthand. The packages are labeled "salted cod," and while the fish have a taste that is reminiscent of salted cod, they are simply not the same. This marketing tactic has reshaped gastronomic attitudes and practice, such that many Puerto Rican restaurants pass off haddock, pollock, and all manner of salted fish as though it were salted cod.

In one sense, if both salted fish and the near relatives of cod are accepted as salted cod by most Puerto Ricans, and they purchase these other fish to make dishes that, to their way of thinking, are being made "with salted cod" (e.g., serenata, codfish stew, salted cod a la vizcaína, salted cod with rice, codfish soup, and codfish fritters), then there really has not been any deep-seated change. At bottom, the surge in the importation of closely allied fish corresponds to the long-standing tradition, among the populace, of consuming salted fish, whether cod or something else. One can therefore postulate that no visible reduction has actually occurred, contrary to what might have been expected in light of the image that salted cod acquired as a staple of the very poor. If different varieties of salted cod and three other fish in its family are considered the same as salted cod, then today, proportionately, people eat as much or more salted cod as they did previously.

It is true that, when it comes to planning Lenten meals, salted cod and its near relatives face competition from shellfish, frozen mollusks, and such processed replacements as "king crab." Yet salted cod, of whatever variety, is still strongly associated in the popular mind with the rituals and celebrations of Easter Holy Week, as it is with the abstentions practiced by those still observant of the old liturgical calendar. As a result, some closely related fish are standard items on the menus of restaurants and cafés every Wednesday and Friday. Nor, for its part, has the demonstrable improvement in living standards tempered, at least so far as the decade of the 1990s was concerned, the desire for salted fish, a desire that—as we have seen—carried a stigma of poverty originating with salted cod.

The importation of other seafood and other prepared fish and shellfish dishes has also increased, as has the consumption of these same products during recent decades. In 1985, 787,899 pounds of shrimp—fresh, frozen, and canned—were imported into Puerto Rico. By 1993–94, this figure had nearly doubled, reaching 1,443,757 pounds, an increase that reprised the onetime ascent of salted cod.[79] And in fiscal year 2001, a total of 4,557,000 pounds of frozen shrimp were imported from the United States alone.[80] Other seafood duplicated this dramatic increase in the same timescale: from 1985 to 1993–94, the importation of lobster jumped from 36,329 pounds to 420,571; in the case of crab, the corresponding figures were 75,873 and 243,315; similar increases were recorded for squid and other shellfish.

Salted cod, like rice, is a prominent part of what today is known as "Puerto Rican cuisine." As such, it stems from the continuous interaction and blending of foodstuffs that existed in the Caribbean prior to the sixteenth century and those that were brought from without and successfully adapted to local conditions. Yet Puerto Rico, throughout a long period of time, was also a land of decidedly monotonous, unvarying food and culinary practices, practices shaped and consolidated by an import market that exploited a society whose dietary habits and structures evolved against the backdrop of a long-lasting plantation economy. Under these circumstances, salted cod became closely interwoven with the repetitious labors of everyday life, as the market hardly countenanced the importation of other products that might complement it. On this ground, salted cod became familiar fare, an item of food that the majority expected they would eat, and eat regularly. It would not be until after the Second World

War that salted cod's horizon would be brightened by the addition of new, complementary foods.

In the midst of this slow-moving stream of history, punctuated by the island's relative isolation, notions and opinions about food were formed and shared, uniform ways of preparing it devised and passed on, and names given to a succession of dishes. Eventually, out of the new dynamic of recent decades, dishes made with salted cod or with the varieties of fish closely related to it were thought of and designated as "traditional," and they have served as a symbol of Puerto Rican identity.

This supposed heritage, however, does not mean that these dishes were always here, on the island, or that everyone experienced them in the same way and under similar conditions. Nor does it mean that new versions and understandings of salted cod, including even its disappearance from the repertoire of Puerto Rican cuisine, are not possible. Yet precisely because the path of change traced over time by this fish has been so long and so slow, it has kept its prominence and its adherents in the gastronomy of the island, or, again with a nod toward history, perhaps it is better characterized as having adopted the double face of Janus, looking back to the past to know the present and to set out in the direction of the future.

Despite the considerable changes on the food scene made possible, in part, by the availability of other types of fish and other foodstuffs, a tangible reverence for salted cod still exists. A full range of dishes made with it is still etched strongly in people's memories. Thus few Puerto Ricans register any surprise when, on a Friday or Sunday, they patronize one of the island's "self-service" eateries and typically find a bowl of serenata among its offerings; and many of them—"yuppies" from San Juan above all—cannot wait to taste crisp fried salted codfish in the seaside town of Piñones. It is not too much to claim that the full culinary and cultural dimensions of this fish in Puerto Rico still await discovery.

5 | Viandas

Vianda: The sustenance and food of rational men:
So it has been said, from the Latin meaning of Vivanda,
because it helps [men] to live and strengthens life.
—*Diccionario de autoridades*, 1737

In contemporary Puerto Rico, no one thinks twice when *viandas* appear as an everyday item on the menus of restaurants serving local fare. Today, however—unlike several decades ago—viandas appear not as the center of a meal but as a side dish, what in Spain is called *guarnición*, or in Italy *contorni*. If we look closely at the menu of one of these restaurants, we will see that viandas are included in the section where diners expect to find an answer to their question, "So, what does this dish come with?" It is a perfectly reasonable question (and Puerto Ricans will ask it with a certain vehemence if the answer is not already apparent from the menu), but one that goes no further than the menu in our hands. Far more interesting, in a broad cultural sense, is that few if any of the people dining in these restaurants could explain why these particular accompaniments are called viandas.

In the lexicon of Puerto Rican gastronomy, the term "vianda" is applied indiscriminately to starchy root vegetables, rhizomes, and fruits, among which cassava, tannier, sweet potato, yam, plantain, dasheen, green bananas, and breadfruit are all prominent. As accompaniments to a meal, several of these will often be served together, or in a combination of at least two or three. As a rule, they are brought to the table after being boiled in salted water. Puerto Ricans, in fact, have taken to calling them *viandas sancochás* (parboiled viandas), in an apparent allusion to the archaic verb *salcochar*—to cook something by boiling it in salted water.

Previously, however, viandas were a central part of meals for a substantial segment of the population. As with cornmeal and rice, they helped the poorest Puerto Ricans leave the table satisfied, by increasing the volume of what they ate. For the more well-to-do, they functioned much as they do today, as simple accompaniments to more varied dishes.

Yet whether essential or marginal to the diet, viandas possessed certain characteristics that made them universally valuable: they could reproduce and grow in different types of soil, withstand radical shifts in weather conditions, and they lent themselves to being cooked in a variety of ways. Even more pivotal, however, was their ubiquity—they could be relied on as a secure item of food, readily accessible and quickly obtained. In a preindustrial society marked by both monoculture and isolation from wider markets, should famine strike, they were always available. It is on this count that the term "vianda," as applied to a broad range of starchy foodstuffs, acquired its full meaning.

In essence, there were two channels through which Puerto Ricans might obtain enough food products to eat abundantly or at least with some degree of variety: through the island's own agriculture—in which viandas played a vital role—or, as is the case today, by relying on the importation of certain basic foods. The flow of the import market, as affected by tariff policies, importers' self-interests, the vagaries of diplomacy, and the structure of the internal market, helped determine whether people enjoyed an abundance of food or struggled to survive.

Even when vulnerable to other contingencies, and though not devoted exclusively to the cultivation of viandas, the agriculture practiced in home gardens proved a richer vein. Their fruitful botanical properties, ability to germinate easily, compatibility with local ecological and climatic conditions, and capacity to add volume to meals, made these starchy foodstuffs so central to the diet that they took on the meaning of "vianda" in its etymological sense.

Just as in the French language the term *viande* came to mean meat because meat was readily obtained in the forests and formed the core of a basic diet, so in the Spanish of Puerto Rico "vianda" came to mean cassava, tannier, and their likenesses, including plantains and unripened bananas. All of these became the food that enabled people to live when other foodstuffs were scarce, and during periodic food crises when conditions became truly dire and the specter of hunger haunted the population, tubers and their cousins invariably became the fail-safe or most secure option. Lydia Roberts observed this pattern in 1949, during the time she spent studying the dietary practices of Puerto Ricans after the severe rationing of food and the nutritional deficiencies brought on by the Second World War: "Viandas is a term used to cover a group of root or starchy vegetables, such as *yuca*, *yautía*, *malanga*, *ñame*, as likewise the starchy fruits, plantain, and breadfruit (*panapén*). These are widely used in Puerto Rico and in low income homes they may make up the bulk of the diet, either alone or in combination with rice and beans. Viandas are, indeed, the 'saving grace' of low income dietaries."[1]

Cassava: A Root Made into Bread

During the initial years of conquest and colonization, Spaniards were drawn more to cassava than to other tubers, in part because it could be used to produce a long-lasting kind of bun or bread. It was soon apparent to them that whether they succeeded or failed in mounting expeditions in this new land and in fighting and subjugating the native population depended on having food that would not ruin quickly. For that to happen they had to adjust expectations and change some entrenched preferences, one of which was a fondness for bread made with wheat flour. Several factors aided the process. On the long voyages from Seville to the Caribbean, wheat flour—like much other food—spoiled very easily. In addition, those who patiently awaited its arrival were at the mercy of a capricious calendar, and when ships did have wheat flour to unload, it went no further than the ports and their close environs, never making it into the interior of the island. Furthermore, the cereal decayed in the humid tropical climate, ruining as easily amid the jungles as did gunpowder. The conquistadores and their soldiers also realized that it was all but impossible to track through dense forest foliage carrying portable ovens for making bread.

Thus the most logical option, or alternative, was to adapt to eating a starchy flour that the indigenous population of the Caribbean derived from the root of a bush—cassava—which they called yuca (*Manihot esculenta* and *Manihot utilussima*).[2] The Taíno followed a complicated, step-by-step process to obtain this flour: they peeled off the rind with sea shells, shredded the flesh with rough-edged stones, expelled the liquid contained in the fibers—some of which was poisonous—dried the fibers, shaped them into buns or little cakes, either by hand or in clay molds, and, as the last step, cooked them over a fire on clay griddles.[3] The end result was cassava, a type of bread that seemed extremely coarse to those accustomed to wheat bread, but it had the virtue of preserving quite well—up to three years. Put to various culinary uses, cassava was the principal food in the diet of the native population, and, in the aftermath of the conquest, it also became part of the diet of the emergent mestizo society.

Cassava: From Essential Bread to Secondary Complement:
The Sixteenth to the Twentieth Century

In 1647, long after the newly arrived Spaniards had been exposed to cassava, the creole canon Diego de Torres Vargas related, in his noted report to the Dominican friar and historian Gil González Dávila, an anecdote about the miracle of Saint Patrick and about how San Juan's faithful and the city's manual laborers began to venerate him and celebrate his good works in an annual feast day.

Since the time of Bishop Alonso Manso, according to Torres, the devotion to Saint Patrick was a formal event on the religious calendar. The background to the anecdote was how vigorously the cassava plants grew, in the 1647 season, on farms located all around the capital. To the great good fortune of both the city's inhabitants and workers in the nearby countryside, the plant began to flourish once again six years after a plague had devastated it, killing the harvests of what seems to have been, to a person, the most favored starchy food. The legend recounted in Torres's fragment drives home the importance that cassava had in the diet:

> In the time of this Bishop [Alonso Manso], ants destroyed the cassava plant, which is what ordinary bread, called cassava [*casabe* in Arawak], is made from; through the fortunate intercession of Saint Saturnino the plague was stopped; afterwards there was another worm that ate the cassava plant, and in another stroke of good fortune, San Patricio interceded, and even more, as it seemed to the Bishop and the Cabildo Eclesiástico, because this saint was little known and of extraordinary power, he repeated this good fortune three times, his intercession the same each time, so that taking it as a most remarkable miracle, they embraced the saint as the protector of cassava and both Cabildos proclaimed a feast-day celebration, in the city, with a Mass, sermon, and procession, which

to this day continues to be faithfully observed, nor has there been (except during times of storms) any notable lack of cassava, and, although the celebration has, as always, been held, the enthusiasm has cooled somewhat, so that this year, 1641, *the worm began once more to eat the cassava, but by throwing ourselves into celebration with three processions, it later stopped and the cassava has returned to growing vigorously,* it is the daily bread in these parts, looked upon with much fondness by the workers, *causing them to understand that the Saints do not become angry but do exact obligations.*[4]

Whether one believes in miracles or not, the canon's story is richly suggestive of the reliance placed both on the cassava plant and on its derivative, the cassava bread or casabe, during the initial years of colonization, especially by the settler population. Amid the many failed experiments to grow crops such as wheat in the tropics, the bread made from the cassava plant became so central to the daily diet that when the first shortages of it occurred, they were interpreted as "states of emergency," similar to those that arose in Europe when bread was lacking, heralding times of anxiety and crisis understood as *penuria panis, exiguitas panis,* and *inopia panis.*[5]

As a further indication of the importance of this plant and the bread made from it, after colonization of the island had taken root, certain words in the Arawak language associated with the preparation of cassava were absorbed into Spanish. Thus, for example, the names given by Fernández de Oviedo to various utensils and by-products used in making cassava (*guariquitén, burén, catibía*) reappear, unaltered, in the description of the cassava factory contained in the sugar plantation owned by the Puerto Rican privateer Miguel Henríquez (1676–1749). Henríquez's account was passed down in the book about his life and exploits written by Ángel López Cantos.[6]

With time, however, as ethnic and racial intermixing became more pronounced and as new materials were introduced to make the utensils used in preparing cassava, the process of lexical absorption and change also worked in reverse, causing some Arawak words associated with the preparation of cassava to fall out of use. Such happened, for example, with the word *cibucán,* as the tube-shaped basket that was used to squeeze the liquid out of the cassava plant was called. Nonetheless, a number of indigenous words survived. For example, guariquitén, as the place where all operations to produce cassava took place; catibía, as the coarse residue that remained after the tuber's rind had been scraped away and its liquid squeezed out was known; or burén, the name for the griddle on which the cassava cakes were cooked.[7] Some of these words are still in use in certain districts of the municipality of Loíza.

The successful cultivation of the cassava plant was also aided by the fund of agricultural and culinary knowledge transmitted by mestizo descendants and by the Africans who were either transported to San Juan as slaves throughout the seventeenth and eighteenth centuries or who arrived in the colony after fleeing neighboring islands. As a result of the transatlantic exchange of foodstuffs that accompanied the European expansion into Africa and the New World, cassava was first carried into Africa by the Portuguese, who brought the tuber from Brazil to feed enslaved Africans on their journey across the Middle Passage. In doing so, Portuguese slavers spread the plant along the upper Guinea coast at the end of the sixteenth century. Although its cultivation spread more slowly in West Africa, by the end of the seventeenth century cassava had become the core food for some ethnic groups in the region, and by the early nineteenth century it was being extensively cultivated.[8] As such, cassava came full circle, returning to the New World to enhance the agricultural and culinary groundings that it had attained both before and after the colonization process.

Although distinctions are commonly made between two varieties of cassava—the wild or bitter, and the sweet, (the former required detoxification before consumption)—it also possessed certain natural qualities that promoted its lasting position in the island's agriculture and helped make it a perennial staple in the diet until the first quarter of the twentieth century. The plant could thrive in soils that had few nutrients,[9] notably in the dry, poor, sandy soil of the coast, a virtue pointed out by the French naturalist and chemist Renato de Grosourdy, who toured the municipality of Guayama in the nineteenth century.[10] Cassava was also highly resistant to drought, tolerated crops being planted near it even in its first year of growth, and germinated easily under a full, hot sun. And while cassava's maturation period was quite long—some eight or nine months after being planted at the start of the rainy season, which in Puerto Rico usually begins around October—those growing the tuber had two options: they could either harvest the roots or keep them intact, safely underground. With the latter option, the roots continued to grow, in which case the harvest was not only larger but could take place at the most advantageous time of year, in the summer months, when there was generally little if any rain.[11] This feature made the consumption of cassava a year-round possibility.

All the qualities that made cassava the logical substitute for "ordinary" bread in turn gave it a privileged position in relation to the other native starchy foodstuffs that made up the diet of the settler population.

In the early seventeenth century, for example, San Juan's municipal officials considered it to be more than a *menudencia*, or something of limited if not trifling importance. In the regulations issued by the city's municipal council in 1627, cassava was not grouped with the yam, nor was it classed as just another tuber or starch.[12] Indeed, in the hierarchy of regulated foods, its derivative—cassava bread—was ranked in second place, behind wheat bread and ahead of meat.[13]

In this same vein, as San Juan in the last quarter of the eighteenth century evolved into a *ciudad garganta* (gullet city) and the countryside was cast as the source of food for the capital, cassava became the central crop on farmland and on work sites recently parceled out by civil authorities. Under a set of reforms issued in 1770 by the colony's governor, Miguel de Muesas, this pattern was underscored and reinforced: "All who hold and own farms and work sites, need to plant a quantity of cassava on them, as arbitrated by each area's local administrative official, where the land they hold is suitable for this product; where it is not they are to give it over to plantains, corn, sweet potatoes."[14]

By the early sixteenth century, cassava, consumed as a type of bread, had—out of sheer necessity—become part of the daily diet of the conquistadores, including their political and administrative leaders, and their descendants acquired the habit of eating it as well. Nonetheless, it is apparent that among newly arrived Spaniards, the more educated and cultured in particular, cassava was one of the local foods that inspired the greatest qualms. The references made to it in some histories and memoirs are rather circumspect. For the authors of these works, cassava is categorized as "other people's bread," a food that never appealed to their taste.

What they disliked about cassava were those qualities that caused it to resemble bread considered inferior or second rate in the food culture of Europe, in opposition to wheat bread: its coarse texture once it was cooked ("the roots are grated, and they come out like sawdust"), a texture experienced on the tongue as well as in handling it; and its insipidness—"something bland, without flavor"; "If it isn't softened with other foods, it is very rough, and has no taste when eaten"—and how at times its coarseness prevented it from being easily moistened, unlike wheat bread "in milk and sugar-cane syrup, it barely even moistens in wine, as wheat bread does";

"Some consider it an excellent food, but since common folk eat it hard and thick, it's like you are chewing on wood chips; it's tolerable if you moisten it. It's a base food, grates on one, and offers little sustenance"; "Although they make it in different ways, I can't get it through my teeth try as I might, and it's the cream of the crop that I brought to the table." These were a few of the verdicts rendered against cassava by Spaniards newly arrived in the colony, though—in its defense—its ability to thicken up soups and fill one's stomach was also acknowledged.[15]

If, on the one hand, the cultivation of cassava continued to be important, above all by peasants who tended small plots along coastal areas, on the other, its value as a product from which bread could be made steadily eroded in the nineteenth century in the households of the well-to-do.[16] In fact, the ability to distinguish between "bitter cassava" and "sweet cassava," or the poisonous versus the edible variety, may have been lost to the buyers of products sold in urban markets or to the domestic help who purchased the food eaten by wealthier families. The warning that accompanies El cocinero's introduction to its recipes for preparing cassava—that care should be taken so that any cassava selected "not be the poisonous kind"—seems to confirm the fact.[17] The trend away from cassava in certain sectors of society was also evident in an exhibition and trade fair held in Ponce in 1882, when farmers showed little interest in featuring it as an edible food that could also serve as the basis for making bread. Their lack of interest was all the more glaring given that prizes were awarded in the category of starchy flours and that new technologies for the industrial processing of tubers were on display.[18]

The absence of recipes for cassava in the two earliest manuals on Puerto Rican cuisine and cooking to appear in the twentieth century, The Porto Rican Cookbook (1909) and Home Making (1914), also influenced and reflected decisions to devote less land to cultivating this tuber. It is true that they were both compiled and written by North Americans, whose understanding of the uses of cassava may have been less keen than that of a native islander. Yet the absence of any recipe for making cassava in Home Making, which was produced to teach cooking and kitchen skills to thousands of female students in Puerto Rico's public schools, is clearly indicative of the decline of cassava and, by extension, of its consumption as well. Cassava, which for nearly four centuries had caught the eye of persons visiting the island and served as the most common type of bread, the ever-present substitute for wheat bread, was less and less to be seen.

At the end of the 1920s, the home economist Elsie Mae Wilsey breathed a bit of new life into cassava by including it in the educational pamphlets she compiled on new ways to cook and prepare viandas.[19] The underlying trend, however, was not reversed. By the early 1930s, the popularity of cassava declined further in comparison to other tubers, in particular to the sweet potato and tannier.[20] Subsequently, in 1937, agronomists realized that a sharp drop had occurred in the production of cassava, which they ascribed, in the first instance, to a lack of care in the selection of seeds. They also pointed, however, to an apparent erosion in the ability of people to differentiate, as they had customarily done in the past, between poisonous and edible cassava: "This tuber was used by the indigenous population long before the coming of white men, but in recent years the selection and planting of this crop has been made so carelessly that many people refuse to use the plant for fear of the poisonous varieties."[21]

Cassava's share of land under cultivation had declined noticeably. Between 1937 and 1938, only 6,846 *cuerdas* of land were devoted to growing it (versus 17,569 cuerdas and 36,947 cuerdas for tannier and sweet potatoes, respectively),[22] with 12 million pounds harvested for domestic consumption. In contrast, 34 million pounds of tannier and 73 million pounds of sweet potatoes were available for consumption during this same period.[23] Both the price of cassava and the amount of it that was consumed demonstrate that it was less valued than other tubers by Puerto Rican families.

Interestingly, two English-language culinary guides, the 1926 cooking manual *Tropical Foods*, compiled by Wilsey, and the 1948 recipe collection *The Puerto Rican Cookbook*, compiled by Eliza Dooley, pay homage to the cassava plant, and both contain recipes for "cassava bread," as well as for more humble creations—cassava "boiled in salted water" and "mashed," and either "steam-cooked" or "fried." Wilsey and Dooley also resurrected recipes based on "cassava flour," which had quite possibly been lost to most cooks who still used the tuber. An example in this category is tapioca, or what Dooley called "cassareep," the difference being that the latter was seasoned with fresh coriander and peppers. Cassareep was recommended for tenderizing meat and for seasoning and thickening soups. Other dishes found in the two publications were "*budín de yuca*," "*guanimes de yuca*," "*alfajor*," and "*panuchos*." These were designed as desserts, either to be consumed at home or sold in markets and at roadside crossings, above all by women of African descent.

Although a handful of recipes for cassava appear in cookbooks published during the 1950s, the changes that affected both city and countryside in Puerto Rico between 1950 and 1960 continued to shrink the tuber's profile. Against the larger trend, however, it was still planted—as a kind of wild crop—in some sandy coastal areas, especially along the belt of land that runs between the municipalities of Loíza and Río Grande, in the north-eastern corner of the island. Agro-ecologically, this area had always been suitable for cultivating cassava, and its inhabitants used the tuber as a core food in much of their daily diet. In Loíza, at the beginning of the 1960s, there was still broad knowledge of how to prepare cassava on a communal burén, how to make "cassava empanadas filled with land crabs," and how to make other sweet meats, such as *rusiau*, and *tortilla*. For the most part, however, these were treated less as food for the home table than as items to be sold.[24]

This commercial motive is what underlies the sporadic preparation of cassava recipes today, especially in the communities of Piñones, Vacía Talega, and Loíza. It is to these locales and their picturesque (as deemed by many), ramshackle *friquitines* made of pieces of salvaged materials that "yuppies" from San Juan are drawn, ostensibly in search of their African roots but secretly eager—as the Puerto Rican novelist Edgardo Rodríguez Juliá says—to shed the image of the "trendy yuppie."[25] At bottom, what they really seek is to evoke memories of a coastal cuisine that has all but vanished, since—in today's world—these ways of preparing cassava have largely become a simulacrum of a once vibrant food culture.

Doña Benicia Carrasquillo, a resident of the Medianía Baja district of Loíza, is among the limited number of people who still make the sweet known as tortilla.[26] In this sweet confection, the catibía, that is, the finest of the floury residue that is left after the cassava has been grated, is placed on the griddle and quickly removed. It is then put in a container, broken up by hand, and has shavings of dry coconut flesh, coconut milk, salt, anise, and cinnamon mixed into it. Pieces of the moistened dough are then made into little balls and placed on banana leaves that have been smeared with coconut milk. The last step is to cover these with more leaves and flatten them, so that each side can be heated on the griddle. Tortilla and other such sweets were once a regular part of the full spectrum of cassava recipes and preparations. For the great majority of Puerto Ricans, and in the culinary continuum, however, they have become passé or, at best, lost any trace of quotidian importance. Since the middle of the nineteenth century, the yam, tannier, and sweet potato have relegated cassava to the margins.

Tannier

Cassava's onetime prominence, as we have seen, was due to its capital importance in the food system, for it could serve as the source for making bread.[27] Before the conquest, however, there were other root vegetables, notably tannier (*Xanthosoma sagitifolium*) and sweet potatoes (*Ipomeas batatas*), which were central to the diet of the indigenous peoples of the Caribbean. Once again, it is Oviedo, writing in the mid-1500s, who has left some of the earliest, most informative descriptions: "Yahutía [tannier], called 'dihautía' by some, is one of the commonest plants that the Indians grow with particular care and diligence. From it they eat the root and the leaves, which are like large cabbages. The roots are the best part, they have shaggy beards that they remove, peeling them off, they cook them to good effect. The leaves, too, are healthy to eat, and taste much better to the Indians, who are drawn to them, than to Christians, for whom they are anything but a treat they might wish for; [the Christians] shy away from them, eating them not because they want to but only as a last resort, if they can find nothing else."[28] To judge from Oviedo's account, the colonists seem to have preferred cassava and sweet potatoes to tannier. Although he reports that tanniers "are good," his somewhat terse description of them suggests a less than enthusiastic response on the part of the Spanish, in contrast to the account he gave of their positive reaction to cassava and corn. As for the plant's leaves, these—according to Oviedo—the colonists unequivocally disliked ingesting, whereas they were apparently a common item of food among the indigenous population. The contrasting reaction to eating the leaves reveals the tensions that arose between the two communities about the division of food; it was only the threat of wasting away from hunger that made the colonists consume and gradually develop a taste for them.

Like corn and beans, tannier received only passing reference in the accounts and memoirs written by visitors to the island, and it was largely ignored in the development of agricultural policy. The agricultural census carried out and directed by Pedro Tomás de Córdoba at the beginning of the nineteenth century failed, in fact, to even mention it. It was the botanist De Grosourdy, in 1863, who focused some limited attention on tannier, and when he did, it was only to pay it a backhanded compliment, as a crop that "it will at least be prudent and useful to have as a secondary crop, for the purpose of supplementing other viandas should their harvest fail or their yield be slight."[29]

Nor was tannier mentioned, either as a tuber that could be eaten by itself or used as the basis for another dish, in the signature mid-nineteenth-century *El cocinero puertorriqueño*. Early twentieth-century cookbooks and cooking manuals continued largely to ignore it. There were no recipes for tannier in the 1909 *Porto Rican Cook Book* and only three in the 1914 public school-adopted manual, *Home Making* (for inclusion in salads, in *tortitas*, and, as an "agent," in soups.)[30] More than likely, the tannier's preference for the fresh yet still wet climates found at higher altitudes, its propensity to be harmed by pests, tuber rot, and the like more than other tubers (for which reason farmers later took to calling it "the disease"[31]), and its long period of maturation (from eight months to a year) all contributed to its decidedly low profile.

However, we should not be misled into thinking that, because it was hardly mentioned in the literature, tannier was not a part of people's diets. It was, both as a tuber boiled in salted water—the primary form in which it is still eaten today—and as the central ingredient in cooked or fried specialties, such as the tortitas included in *Home Making*. To make these, the skin had to be grated off the tannier, to which beaten eggs were added. Spoonfuls of the mixture were then fried in hot fat. As with many other delicacies made with viandas, it required considerable expertise to make tortitas well. The dough had to be kneaded by hand, so that it had the proper smoothness and consistency, a task at which the cooks with African blood excelled, not just with tannier but, as we shall see, also in the preparation of dishes based on the yam.

The general lack of recognition accorded the tannier throughout the nineteenth century and the early twentieth came to an end in 1931 on the initiative of the University of Puerto Rico's School (then department) of Home Economics. The department distributed to nutritionists, cooks, and others associated with the preparation of meals a bulletin devoted exclusively to enlightening them about the tannier plant. It described twenty-six ways of preparing the tuber, including recipes for pies made with tannier and plantains, and empanadas made with tannier and capers. These were recipes that had been known, informally, to street vendors and domestic cooks for a long time, but to this point had not figured in cookbooks because their preparation hinged more on personal ingenuity, happenstance, and the transmission of recipes orally than on codified accounts and the written word.[32]

At the end of the 1930s, troubled by the over-representation of foods high in starch in the diet of many Puerto Ricans, the island's Agricultural Experiment Station began to focus more intently on varieties with greater nutritional value. The station also introduced and promoted the cultivation of new types of tannier, such as the "Kelly" or "yellow," imported from the English territories in the Caribbean. The rebirth of the tannier, in particular the enthusiasm for the yellow varieties (prized for their excellent flavor and smooth texture), as a highly valued vianda in the 1940s owes a great deal to this work by the Agricultural Experiment Station.[33] By the start of the following decade, tannier had leapfrogged all the other root vegetables and was now the preferred type among Puerto Rican consumers.[34]

Sweet Potatoes

In his description of the sweet potato (*Ipomoea batatas*), Oviedo refers to it as a "fruit or delicacy," intending that it be understood in the same way that the European aristocracy thought of fresh fruits and the finest jam: as products that stood out above other food because of their delicate flavor, their soft flesh, and their capacity to be made into preserves.[35] Oviedo, in fact, used "marzipan" as his point of reference to describe the texture of the sweet potato: "A sweet potato [that has been] preserved is no less appealing in taste than the most suave marzipan." He suggested that a sample of one be sent to King Charles V.[36]

In 1636, during his tenure as the bishop of San Juan, Juan Alonso de Solís placed the sweet potato on a par with the few tropical fruits that, for him, were "incomparably better than those of Spain."[37] His successor as bishop, Damián López de Haro, also saw the sweet potato as a fruit, and he linked it to others on the island, such as the citron, which were made into preserves, "because sugar does not hurt them."[38]

In contrast to other indigenous tubers such as tannier and cassava, the sweet potato, which aboveground takes the form of a leafy vine or creeper, has a property that simplifies its planting and stimulates its growth, hence strengthening its role as a secure, accessible food. It can be propagated in two ways: from seeds (*de semilla*), that is, from bulbs or small cuttings coming from the root itself, or from shoots taken off the vine (*de sarmiento*), a method also known as *de bejuco* to those cultivating it in the wilds.[39] By using the latter method, campesinos could assure themselves both of a source of food for years on end and of the spontaneous propagation and growth of new plants, as it was only necessary to rake the soil, cut the tubers, and leave the roots of the vines intact to obtain new shoots.

In line with almost all the viandas—apart from the cassava—the sweet potato was categorized as a "regular subsistence food" in listings and descriptions of edible foodstuffs available on the island during the seventeenth and eighteenth centuries. It was therefore placed in the larger group of "edible roots." While these featured prominently in the islanders' diet, were recognized as important by the colony's administrators, and sometimes warranted mention in the travel accounts written by persons who visited the island, they garnered little attention otherwise. One of the few references to sweet potatoes was made by Bishop López de Haro in the critique that he offered to the Council of the Indies in 1644 on the state of the island and bishopric, after which the tuber was rarely if ever mentioned by those treating the subject of food and daily life in Puerto Rico. In the eighteenth century, even Iñigo Abad y Lasierra, who wrote at length about the characteristics of the cassava plant and the plantain within the island's agriculture and husbandry, had very little to say about this aspect of the sweet potato.

Abad y Lasierra identified it as one of the common crops cultivated in the fields of farmers and campesinos. In his investigations, the sweet potato appears as a substitute for rice (the "heart" of the meal) or is included as just another vianda—one more item in a serving of food. Abad y Lasierra writes: "Their vianda [the term is used to mean a meal or common, daily subsistence fare] comes down to a kettle of rice or sweet potatoes, yams, squash, or all of those together."

Moreover, in Abad y Lasierra's observations on the supper meal, the sweet potato is included—together with the plantain—as an alternative when a more substantive, robust food is lacking: "Supper is very modest: some little bit of rice or some land crabs, and absent this, some plantains or sweet potatoes suffice as a family's supper."[40]

By the start of the nineteenth century, the amount of land devoted to the cultivation of sweet potatoes was substantially higher than the acreage allotted to other tubers (8,367 cuerdas for sweet potatoes versus 4,698 for yams and 767 for cassava.)[41] The number of quintals of sweet potatoes produced likewise sharply exceeded the number for yams, which in this period seem to have been second in importance to sweet potatoes.

The sweet potato was cooked in much the same way as other tubers, that is, by boiling it in salted water or by adding it to stews or casseroles. What distinguished it from other root vegetables was its natural sweetness. While the cassava and yam both had a comparatively high sugar content—1.5 and 0.7 grams per 100 hundred grams of an edible portion, respectively— these paled in comparison to the sweet potato, for which the comparable figure was 5.7 grams.[42] Moreover, baking sweet potatoes over an open fire, a practice widely followed in the twentieth century,[43] elevated their sugar content, as did steam-cooking them. The latter method was widely used in Africa and must have been repeated in a number of Puerto Rican households.[44]

The preference that Puerto Ricans have for the sweet potato over other tubers is not accidental but, rather, stems from how it interacts with other foods by virtue of its sweetness. This quality, which becomes even sharper when the sweet potato is baked, complements the hot, spicy seasoning characteristic of Arawak and African cooking, as well as of the mestizo gastronomy that began to assume a distinct form in the seventeenth century. The effect is seen today in the island's less commercialized lechoneras (stands where pit-roasted pig is sold by the portion or pound, or restaurants specializing in pork and roast suckling pig), such as Lechonera Bruno, in the Tres Puntos district of Humacao's Mariana neighborhood, and in similar establishments in the municipalities of Las Piedras (with its annual celebration of the Festival de Lechón Asado), Yabucoa, and Guavate, where the first accompaniment to well-seasoned pork is roasted sweet potato.

Its inherent sweetness also gave it pride of place among the various desserts made with roots, tubers, and plant stalks. El cocinero puertorriqueño contains sixteen recipes involving the use of sweet potatoes, whether as an ingredient (in soups and stews), side dish (in this case it could be fried, baked, or boiled in salt water), individual sweetmeat, or complement to other sweets and preserves. Of the sixteen recipes, there are six involving the preparation of sweets: buñuelos, malarrabia, dulce de jícama, bocado de batata, cajeta de piña cubana, and a delectable dessert, made with sweet potatoes and grated coconut cooked in sugarcane syrup, known as alfeñique. In mid-twentieth-century Puerto Rico, sweet potatoes were still the core ingredient in what were called pastas—to distinguish them from fruits preserved in syrup—such as nísperos de batata, pasta de batata, and pasta de batata y piña, and also served as the main sweet element in Puerto Rico's most unusual and complicated dessert—cazuela (literally, earthenware).

The sugary taste of the sweet potato made it a favorite among those inclined toward food having a soft, creamy texture and sweet flavor, and the facility with which it blended with other ingredients likewise enhanced its popularity. Today on the island these qualities have a particular cultural resonance: they denote someone who attains a government job without possessing the qualifications for it. The name given to such an appointee is *batata política*.

Yams

Native to other lands, the yam belonging to the *Dioscorea rotundata* species seems to have first appeared in the islands of the Caribbean shortly before 1540.[45] Well before Columbus's voyages across the Atlantic, however, this tuber had acquired ceremonial and gastronomic importance across large areas of West Africa,[46] and the *rotundata* seed appears to have entered the New World along with the Africans themselves as part of the food they surreptitiously carried with them. On this point Oviedo commented: "It came [here] with this unfavored caste of blacks, and has done very well, it is beneficial to the blacks and excellent sustenance for them."

The way in which Oviedo holds the yam at arm's length—"it is beneficial to the blacks and excellent sustenance for them"—suggests that, like some of the foods indigenous to the island, it failed to receive the attention accorded the cassava plant.

Throughout the centuries, this fruitful tuber became a complement to the island's native viandas, eventually overtaking them, particularly cassava. The knowledge that the Africans possessed regarding its cultivation, and the desire to replicate at least part of the diet with which they were familiar, aided in its dissemination. For example, the yam was soon used to make *gachas de ñame* (a yam porridge), and yam tortitas—in sweet or savory versions, kneaded and fried, or cooked over a griddle—as well as *fufu*, a preparation made out of boiled, mashed yams that was found (and is still found) throughout the Caribbean. Fufu, which incorporated a good many other viandas, was kneaded into a stiff dough until it resembled a loaf of bread.[47] A food traced back to the West African Yoruba people, fufu was apparently the origin of what in contemporary Puerto Rico is called *mofongo*, though the latter is made with plantains, not yams.

As time passed, the yam's position as a complement to other foodstuffs strengthened, because it enjoyed an agro-ecological environment not dissimilar to the West African, could be stored and conserved for extended periods—either reburied in the earth itself or piled up, mixed with wood ash and kept well covered in a dry location,[48]—lacked the poisonous hazards associated with cassava, and suited the conditions that helped mold the diet of most Puerto Ricans until the advent of the twentieth century. Yams added volume to the intake of food and were a good source of energy: 93 percent of the calories obtained from each 100 grams in a serving of yams derived from carbohydrates.

That yams, either boiled or steamed and wrapped in banana leaves, are little seen in Puerto Rico is somewhat surprising. This way of eating them, a recurrent sight to travelers visiting different areas of West Africa, must have been common among those West Africans who became cooks after arriving on the island. Once established, cooks used yams instead to make pounded dishes with other tubers and fruits, such as plantains, bananas, and tannier. This practice possibly gave rise to the *pastel navideño*, a dish associated with Christmas-season festivities which brings together the gastronomic heritage, techniques, and resources of all the groups that have peopled the island, Afro–Puerto Ricans in particular.[49]

Vianda in the Form of a Fruit: The Plantain

Plantains, as well as bananas, were apparently introduced into the Greater Antilles in 1516 from the Canary Islands,[50] the outcome of what Ferdinand Braudel called the maritime integration of the world,[51] or, when examined from a different angle, what might also be termed the migration and exchange of food.

While specialists agree that the plantain (*Musa paradisiacal*) and the banana (*Musa sapientum* and *Musa cavendishi*)[52] are of South Asian origin, the trajectories they followed as they moved west, into the Middle East, Europe, Africa, and the islands of the Atlantic Ocean, are extremely difficult to trace and reconstruct.[53]

For my purposes, I will restrict myself to discussing only the plantain. Although it qualifies as a fruit, Puerto Ricans saw the plantain as a vianda, perhaps because it functioned like one—it was a filling food, readily available, a staple of the daily diet. Bananas, on the other hand, were seen to be what they are: a food to snack on between mealtimes or a dessert fruit.[54]

The plantain reached the Antilles first, and its cultivation began as early as 1516.[55] As a treelike perennial herb of tropical origin, accustomed to hot, humid regions, the plantain could adapt easily to the island ecology and environment, and its reproduction did not require an involved process of experimentation, as occurred with other types of fruit, like peaches, pomegranates, and plums.[56] To the great advantage of the colonists, it germinated spontaneously, spreading from its first New World home, Hispaniola, to other islands of the Caribbean, and then outward, to Central and South America.

The common plantain (*Musa paradisiacal*) is an herbaceous, typically seedless plant. It propagates by means of shoots or suckers that sprout at its base, or from the underground portion of its trunk that has rhizomes, or yams, as the most rustic farmers in the nineteenth century called these seedlings produced by the plant's torso.[57] All that is necessary, then, to begin a stand of plantains is to plant several rhizomes. When planted on virgin land, its initial period of germination is extremely short, with new shoots appearing in a matter of four or five weeks. What seems to our eye to be the trunk of the new plant is actually only a tightly bunched clump of leaves wrapped around themselves.

As this "false trunk" grows, the oldest leaves are pushed outward by the younger leaves emerging from within, revealing the growth of a real trunk—shiny, solid, and firm. Depending on the fertility of the soil, the first set of large leaves, intensely green in color, begins to appear some twelve months later. The fruit, growing in bunches, emerges from a bud that in turn sprouts from the heart of the trunk. The first harvest is usually ready after twelve months, depending—again—on the condition of the soil, as well as on the climate and the variety of *musa* that has been planted.

In terms of agricultural productivity, however, the most remarkable thing about the plantain is that as the plant grows, baby plants start developing at the base of the false trunk. This manner and cycle of reproduction proved decisive for the wild propagation of plantains throughout the island starting in the early sixteenth century. The plant spread first through coastal valleys and flatlands, followed by its appearance on the savannas and in the mountainous interior.[58] So rapidly did it disperse across the island and so quickly did new groups of settlers take to it as a staple food that any shortage of it was exploited to argue that the fleets should put into the island's ports more frequently with supplies of food from Spain, especially after hurricanes had struck.

The manner in which the plantain grew and propagated itself captured the attention of the most studious, well-informed naturalists, such as the Jesuit friar José de Acosta, whose ecclesiastical duties took him to different parts of both viceroyalties in the 1570s and 1580s.[59] During the eighteenth century, interest focused on the plantain's productivity and marketability; these became (at least for some) the touchstone of its value. By then, however, for the majority of islanders, its role in the diet had taken on a life of its own, helping outline the contours and content of a distinctive culture of food and cooking. This role, as we shall see, would be vilified, made the object of deeply derogatory interpretations, in the administrative, moral, agronomic, and culinary spheres.

Plantains as Basic Sustenance and Plantains as a Rural, Uncouth Food

During the course of Puerto Rican history, no dietary staple has stirred more comment and reflection than the plantain. As colonial officials, successful settlers, and informed visitors sought to find a phraseology indicative of its uses and characteristics, this fruit came to be defined in two broad ways: as basic sustenance (*plátano mantenimiento*) and as food consumed by the uncultivated rural population (*plátano rural y bárbaro*). Precisely when the two perspectives became firmly embedded is not clear, but at certain times they were held simultaneously.

In the sixteenth century, for example, as the cultivation of the plantain took hold, encompassing more and more land, the more prosperous settlers who came into contact with plantains began to think of them as a basic, everyday food that was essential for the physical well-being and reproduction of social groups whose circumstances, material and otherwise, differed from their own. In being perceived as "the sustenance fare of others," the plantain was put on a par with corn and cassava, to form a trinity of foods that were cooked in great batches and parceled out to those who had little or no prospect of ever choosing themselves what to cook and eat.

The first known reference to plantains dates to 1597. In that year, the island's governor, Antonio de Mosquera, requested reimbursement of the funds that he had invested in a farm devoted to growing corn and plantains "as a source of food and sustenance for the blacks who must work on the island's military fortifications."[60] Ángel López Cantos, in the study he made of the food consumed by slaves during the eighteenth century, notes that plantains and cassava were the core part of meals eaten by prisoners confined in El Morro, as well as by a certain class of soldiers detailed to the fort.[61] His research further showed that by the start of the nineteenth century, plantains had become a "principal part" of the diet of those sectors of the population, such as slaves on the sugar plantations, least capable of meeting their own food needs.

In this same period, as noted earlier, those who governed the colony came under the sway of certain ideas emanating from the late stages of the European enlightenment. As part of this movement, both the state and slave owners altered their thinking about security and work productivity in order better to regulate life on the plantation. To this end, the nature of the relationship between master and slave needed to be spelled out more clearly, especially as concerned the provision by slave owners of adequate nutrition to their slaves. Focused above all on maximizing slaves' productivity in carrying out the work of the plantation, versus the attention slaves might give to cultivating their own small plots, slave masters strictly limited the mobility of their slaves, thereby suppressing what opportunities they had to supply their own food.[62] Chapter 3 of the 1826 Reglamento esclavista pertained to the question of slaves' food and diet, that of children as well as that of adults.[63] On this subject, three matters were addressed: the number of meals, the minimum amount, and the type of food to be provided daily. Within this scheme, the role of plantains was paramount, exceeding even that of rice. As the chapter states: "Masters must provide their slaves with two or three meals per day, as they best see fit, but they must be sufficient, not only to keep the individual going, but to reenergize him after his labors. It is stipulated that as a daily fare, six or eight plantains (or their equivalent in sweet potatoes, yams, and other root products), eight ounces of meat, salted codfish, or mackerel, and four ounces of rice or some other common vegetable, must without exception be provided to each and every slave."[64]

The wording of the regulation leads one to think that the state and slave owners conceived of a slave's diet not in charitable terms but as a matter of the bloodless calculation of basic nutritional requirements. It was left to the slave owners to decide how many meals per day their slaves should get, though the criterion "sufficient" was specified, that is, enough food for what the situation required. In the mind of the slave owner, this quantity could ensure a continued population of slaves, since it helped facilitate the conditions under which new generations could be born. At the same time, however, this "sufficiency" of food had to equal the minimum necessary to recharge a human body thought of as an engine of work, whose efficiency and functionality depended on both the amount of food ingested and the frequency with which it was supplied.[65] Obviously, from a strictly commer-

TABLE 5.1 Daily Rations and Approximate Energy Value of Plantation Food, 1826

Food	Daily Ration	Approximate Daily Energy Value in Calories	Annual Total
Plantain or equivalent root vegetable	6 to 8 units	1,443*	2,190 units
Meat, salted cod, or mackerel	4 ounces	303.9**	91.2 pounds
Rice or other vegetable	4 ounces	392***	91.2 pounds

In calculating approximate energy values, I have used the food composition table compiled in 1935 by the nutritionist Rosa Marina Torres. An extended version of the table appeared in the *Revista de Agricultura de Puerto Rico* 43 (January–June 1952): 279–81.

*Calculated on the basis of six medium-size green plantains, each 6¼ inches long multiplied by 2¼ inches in circumference, according to Torres's table.

**Calculated on the basis of 4 ounces of cooked pork meat, boneless but containing fat. Pork was chosen because it was much less expensive than beef during the nineteenth century. Were the calculation made using 4 ounces of beef, the calorie count would come to 285.

***Calculated in terms of whole rice minus the fat or lard with which under these circumstances it was cooked. On this point see the chapter on rice.

cial standpoint, this body ought to be kept operating at the lowest cost to its owner. Although the regulation did not confront the issue directly, the calculation of a slave's nutritional intake tried to obviate the possibility that slaves would step out of line or act defiantly over perceived insufficiencies of food.

The key role played by plantains in the diet of the slave population is evident in the pages of the *Reglamento esclavista*, where it not only ranks higher than other tubers but is placed ahead of meat, salted codfish, and rice as well.

If one measures its relative value in terms of nutritional content and capacity, acknowledging margins of error caused by irregularities in the quality of products as well as the difficulties inherent in projecting such values back in time, it stands as in table 5.1.

As can be seen, the plantain became not only the principal "sustenance" fare of slaves, the central component of their diet, but also the food that their masters relied on to replenish their lost energy and give sufficient bulk to their meals. For the slaves, the chemical composition of the plantain was the pillar on which their nutritional needs and expectations rested. Such was the situation at the beginning of the nineteenth century; subsequently, and running to the end of the century, cornmeal and imported rice would become secondary, complementary foods.

The plantain was also identified by more educated elements as something consumed not by a refined, urban-dwelling population but, rather, by rural, backwoods, uncultivated types. In one sense, the very bounteousness of the plant, the little discipline required to care for it and to harvest its fruit, and the poor prospects of marketing it in Europe helped mold a negative stereotype about the capacity for work and the way of life of those living in the countryside.

In commenting on his experiences, during 1644, sampling the different foods of the island, fray López de Haro referred to the plantain as "rural y bárbaro": "They do not lack for various biscuits and buns, and a fruit they call plantains, which are found abundantly and in different varieties in the countryside, they are ordinarily what sustains the blacks and even many poor whites, because the riper ones serve them as bread and fruit, the green plantains are roasted over the embers of a fire like sweet potatoes or carrots, the farm workers eat them like chestnuts and make lots of stews out of them. . . . They are a healthful food."[66]

Although he considered it to be "the king of all the food that is eaten" because it predominated in so many parts of the island, and further granted that one could truly speak of a "gastronomy of the plantain," the historian López Cantos, writing about the eighteenth century, essentially cast it in the same light. In documenting references to the plantain, Cantos found it labeled as "the black man's bread," "the common bread of the very poorest," "the only thing that sustains the poor," and "the crude bread of the island." These associations were rooted in and reflective of an educated, urban outlook, an outlook disdainful of the culinary world inhabited by those living in the far hinterlands.

The association persisted. In the nineteenth century, the Frenchman De Grosourdy's assessment of the plantain vied between the agroindustrial orientation, to which he was sympathetic, and the immediate value it had for those living in rural areas of the island: "In the high, cold part of Puerto Rico, we have seen very extensive, magnificent groves of plantains, producing large yields, which on that island is the food almost exclusively of poor people and even those of somewhat limited means: it aids considerably in maintaining slavery."

Looking outward, he championed the idea of commercializing the green plantain, by converting it into flour, so that it could "perhaps find a place in the European diet," and by the same token, he was taken aback by how cavalierly it was wasted (in his opinion) by campesinos who used it as fodder for their pigs: "Green plantains, cut into small pieces and sun-dried, form a quite viable part of the trade on some Antillean islands, such as Jamaica, all the more so when the fruit yields an abundant harvest, for which reason it is very inexpensive in many places in the interior of Puerto Rico, where it goes for a farthing, such that at times it is used even to fatten up the pigs."[67]

In the entrepreneurial spirit of the nineteenth century, the botanist saw a market for plantains. If they were processed on an industrial, or even semi-industrial scale, they could be made into a specialized product that would hold appeal for Europeans hungering for more exotic tastes and aromas: "In this way they could be exploited for exportation or for sale on the island itself, and so be put to more beneficial uses. The green plantain should be cut when it has developed fully and reached its maximum size, the hard outer skin or rind removed at that point, whether by hand or mechanically, and sliced into pieces that will dry in the sun . . . , or better perhaps in a stove used for that purpose . . . : dried thusly they can be pulverized and the powder passed through a sieve, they will then have turned into plantain flour, called 'coquina tay' in Jamaica; in that state, the plantain has acquired a special fragrance, one akin to that of freshly cut hay or tea from China."[68]

Yet for the majority of the population the plantain meant something entirely different. It was food, pure and simple—the chief component of meals and, in extremis, what kept starvation at bay. Hence it was seen more as a vianda than as a fruit. Iñigo Abad y Lasierra pointed out that campesinos applied the term hartón to the plantain in the eighteenth century, a term later clarified by the agronomist López Tuero, who explained that campesinos called the plantain by this name "because a man is stuffed to the gills by its fruit or because it produces more fruit than any other variety [of plantain]." A rich and colorful lexicon sprang up around the plantain. The use of names such as plátano hembra and plátano macho (that is, female and male plantains) to distinguish between people who had "heart" and those who did not (usages resurrected by El cocinero puertorriqueño in the mid-nineteenth century); chamaluco or malango to signify, according to López Tuero, the "less nourishing," "more faithless," "last to bear fruit" banana, and matahambre (hunger-killing), recorded by the botanist Oratio Fuller Cook at the beginning of the twentieth century, bear eloquent testimony to the "saving," protecting nature of the plantain in the mind and imagination of Puerto Rican campesinos.

Moreover, as the Spanish state tried to stimulate and reorient the island's agriculture at the end of the eighteenth century, the plantain began to be seen as an obstacle to the commercial development and profit potential of this sector. Both foreign visitors and the island's own critics interpreted the all but effortless way the plantain reproduced on the steep hillside tracts of the poorest campesinos as a metaphor for their weak appetite for agricultural work and their general way of life. As Iñigo Abad y Lasierra wrote in the diary that he kept during his travels: "The strangest thing is that despite the great fertility of the land and how it lends itself to growing these and other fruits, which can be planted in any season and weather, and be re-sown at least three times per year in the same soil, a great many of this island's inhabitants desire no more than to live at the expense of the plantain groves."[69]

Several years earlier, the Irish-born Spanish officer and military reformer Alejandro O'Reilly had conveyed a similar impression. Although he placed part of the responsibility on the government's inability to foment agriculture and on the disinclination of immigrants who took refuge in the mountainous countryside during the eighteenth century to apply themselves to exploiting the land, O'Reilly, too, cited the abundant fertility of the land as one of the reasons behind the lax development of commercial agriculture on the island. He observed, ironically, that the very prodigality of the harvests worked against the interests of campesinos, by luring them, as it were, into a permanent complacency. Insofar as they lacked ambition to improve their circumstances and remained satisfied with the little they had, the plantain was the chief culprit: "With five days of work a family has enough plantains to last an entire year. With these, [and] cow's milk, some cassava, sweet potatoes and wild fruits, they are more than contented."[70]

This notion of the plantain as a plant whose ease of cultivation and propagation stagnated the colony's development, on the one hand, while it nourished an indolent, undisciplined work ethic toward agriculture, on the other, also informed the thinking of the sharpest agronomic minds in Puerto Rico a hundred years later, at the end of the nineteenth century. Out of such thinking came the expression *aplatanarse*, which found its way into learned discourse and meant: to idle time away unworried, to accept apathetically things as they are, and to do nothing in the face of adverse circumstance.

Subsequently, as realignments and accommodations among social and political sectors spurred the formation of a distinct Puerto Rican national consciousness, an educated elite employed the term to refer to a change in attitude on the part of some foreigners, Spanish immigrants in particular, who—on first arriving in the colony—affected a boastful superiority but later took to ethnic and racial intermarriage and to adopting native ways. That was how the *costumbrista* author Miguel Meléndez Muñoz used it, through the voice of the black woman María, who sells her sweets on the street and lectures Hipólito Velázquez, a recently arrived Spanish pedagogue who seems tempted by her preserves: "And afterwards you *all make your peace*, go native: you marry here, have your family, booze it up a little, lose your light skin color and your old way of talking, it's just the same for everyone and the differences are washed away."[71]

Nevertheless, those who saw the plantain as the cause of backwardness and lax ways would, to their way of thinking, be vindicated by the low production of foodstuffs in coastal areas at the end of the nineteenth century, a development ultimately brought on by the expansion of sugarcane cultivation. Indeed, as Puerto Rican agriculture was redirected over the course of the century toward the production of sugarcane and coffee, critics again took up the idea of systematizing the cultivation and processing of the so-called *frutos menores* (essentially, any agricultural product other than sugarcane and coffee [and tobacco]) for culinary, medicinal, and industrial purposes.[72] This time, in a much more precarious agro-food context—one that was understood as potentially affecting the ability of everyone,[73] at all levels of society, to maintain an adequate diet—the proposal put forward by the agricultural vanguard to modernize the production of domestic foodstuffs clashed with the ways in which campesinos cultivated and used plantains. The engineer-agronomist Fernando López Tuero's 1892 monograph on the plantain and the coconut palm attests to this friction. While concluding that both fruits were vital to the diet, he saw little chance that better techniques of cultivation could be introduced for either one as long as they continued to be planted where they were— on high hillsides. This circumstance hindered progress, preventing both fruits from realizing their potential as "greatly important contributors to the province's overall [agricultural] production." Vicente A. Fano, the president of the agricultural section of the Economic Society of Friends of the Country and the author of the prologue to López Tuero's book, bore in on this point: "When and if they are cultivated in a rational way, [the plantain and the coconut palm] are sooner or later destined to be greatly important contributors . . . compelling [us] to recognize the importance of plants whose fruits men harvest with an unparalleled lack of concern for their needs and chances of success . . . it is to be hoped that our campesinos will once and for all rid themselves of the indifference with which they treat certain plants; afforded better conditions and cultivated in an orderly way, these plants will for certain contribute to bettering lives now held back."[74] In the period between 1850 and 1900, the plantain completed its definitive migration to the upland areas of the island's mountainous interior. Its pilgrimage was not caused purely by its exceptional fertility and spontaneous way of reproducing. Campesinos, displaced from lower-elevation land by the steady expansion of sugar plantations in the coastal plains and valleys, transported its seedlings, or "yams," in their baggage. Around 1891, 187,500,000 quintals of plantains were harvested in Puerto Rico,[75] a figure more than two and a half times greater than that for tubers, rice, corn, cassava, oranges, mangoes, coconuts, legumes, and produce combined (which equaled 70,455,000 quintals). In these years, the mass of people whose lives and diets were so closely bound up with the plantain may have had little grasp of the "rural and uncouth" meaning that members of the intelligentsia attached to it, but they indeed recognized and extolled its bounteous nature and great worth as food.

The Plantain in the Kitchen: Mofongo and Pastel

Plantains lend themselves to being cooked and eaten in a variety of ways: they can be baked, boiled, fried, or used even when they have become *podrido* (overly ripe). In contrast to tubers, they can be eaten without having to ripen first. In their pre-ripened, or "green" state, as it called in Puerto Rico, plantains can be roasted or baked over the coals of a fire, or cut into slices, fried in fat, flattened, and fried again to make *tostones*. Similarly, their flesh can be shredded and fried to make an appetizer or side dish known as *arañitas* in Puerto Rico.

It was in the plantain's green state, too, that over a long stretch of time people encountered its one negative quality—the little moisture that it contains. Of all viandas, in fact, the *musa paradisíaca* contains the least amount of water, only 167.3 grams for each 291-gram portion consumed.[76] On the other hand, people took advantage of this aspect of the plantain to experiment with it. This was how they arrived at the practice of pounding, or crushing, the plantain with a mallet after it had been baked, boiled, or fried; and then either adding some liquid to it, moistening it with fats, or incorporating pork crackling (*chicharrón*) into it. Out of these innovations came the interesting custom of shredding the plantain and, with the palm of one's moistened hand, shaping pieces of it into "little balls" to add to soups or broths.

The array of ways in which the plantain can be eaten increases incrementally as it ripens. It qualifies as *pintón* when its peel, heretofore completely green, begins to change color, turning yellow, as *maduro* when the peel has turned completely yellow and develops its characteristic dark spots, and as podrido, or *pasaíto* as it known in Puerto Rico, when it has become overly ripe. As the plantain gradually ripens, its flesh changes texture, becoming spongier and moister. The softer and sweeter the flesh of the plantain, the more appealing it is to the palate; it then begins to look as though it could be eaten just as is, as if it were a "banana." Through this entire process of ripening, in addition to being fried, or grilled, or boiled in salted water, the plantain can also be dried out in the sun and stored, to be preserved in a sweet syrup or—if left to ripen and ferment—made into vinegar.

With time, the use made of plantains—green, pintón, or maduro—and the accumulation of knowledge about what worked well or badly in how they were cooked and in what state (boiled, fried, baked, or podrido) created a corpus of recipes and preparations, each of which came to have its own name. Those on the island who had the greatest hand in planting, cooking, and consuming plantains, namely, groups of Africans and their mestizo descendants, were instrumental in passing these dishes, with their names, "upward," that is, into the diet of a privileged minority for whom cooking and all that transpired in the kitchen was lower-caste work. The situation was fraught with irony. On the one hand, for reasons of social distinction, this minority prided itself on sitting down to a more cultivated cuisine, one that highlighted how different it was from those who labored in the fields to produce food and in the kitchen to prepare it. On the other, however, the plantain began to show up on the tables of the more privileged, even as they persisted—well into the future—in thinking of it as an uncouth food.

To examine the plantain in the wider culinary context is to discover that, for all that it was disparaged for centuries as "rural y bárbaro," it was central to a set of beliefs and associations that an educated minority, during the nineteenth century, drew on in forming the idea of a distinct Puerto Rican nation. In that new entity, food and cooking stood out as emblematic, a fact to which El *cocinero puertorriqueño* perhaps paid homage by devoting a full chapter exclusively to the plantain.

Moreover, in the shaping of this idea of Puerto Rican nationhood, two dishes—mofongo and pastel, acquired a special significance. Throughout the island's nineteenth-century literary production, both were treated as signs of Puerto Rican identity, the embodiment of authentic local custom and tradition. For example, in the 1843 publication, El Aguinaldo puertorriqueño, pastel de hoja is given as one of the dishes prepared to celebrate the Eve of the Three Wise Men, or Three Kings Day, in opposition to the Christmas season dishes and sweets that come from other regions of Spain and the Caribbean.[77] Three decades later, in La leyenda de los veinte años, Alejandro Tapia y Rivera depicts a scene in which mofongo is part of a lunch prepared by the cook, María Francisca, on the finca of Gurabo, a lunch which "not [simply] because it was called criollo, was no longer European."[78] Still another example of using mofongo and pastel to define the authentically Puerto Rican was provided by Ana Roqué, in her novel Luz y sombra, when Matilde—the wife of a yeoman farmer—serves her husband the two dishes after he returns home from a day in the fields.[79] To cite a last example, pastel is one of the delicacies offered by a suitor to a young woman at a ballroom dance in Bonafoux Quintero's "El carnaval en las Antillas."[80]

The origin of mofongo goes back to the most rudimentary methods that the various Angolan ethnic groups who populated the island employed for preparing food, in particular the technique of using a mallet to mash great quantities of starchy foodstuffs, then softening the mixture by adding liquids and bits of fat. Indeed, the word "mofongo" appears to stem from the Angolan Kikongo term mfwenge-mfwenge, which means "a great amount of anything at all."[81] Similarly, the noun mfwongo, meaning "plate" or "flat surface," is also found in another variant of the Kikongo spoken in Angola. Álvarez Nazario suggests that this latter word, "mfwongo," is closely related to the act of crushing or mashing, which of course is what is done to the plantain to make mofongo. The contemporary custom of using little mortars and pestles to prepare "snack" style "homemade mofongos" has the effect of obliterating the image of the colossal mofongos that were prepared with enormous mortars in the slave quarters to feed a great many people at the same time.

As Puerto Rican national identity, and within it a distinctive culture of food and cooking, assumed firmer shape, mofongo continued its ascendancy, with all the African overtones its preparation and consumption carried, in a context in which what people cooked and ate helped set boundaries of social class and standing. The 1859 publication of El cocinero puertorriqueño marked the debut of mofongo as a formal, written recipe.

In that period, it entailed a preparation similar to that of the Dominican mangú, in which the plantain was boiled—not fried, as in Puerto Rico—in a broth containing veal, chicken, bacon or fatback, and ham, after which the mixture was mashed in a pilón and then formed into "large balls, on which a little bit of broth was flicked so they would not stiffen."[82] The cookbook also included the recipe for a similar dish, funche de malanga y plátano.[83]

After being excluded from the 1914 manual Home Making, mofongo reappeared in the 1948 publication The Puerto Rican Cookbook.[84] Here the recipe called for using butter and milk to soften and moisten the plantain, an example of a new gastronomic sensibility in which old fears about pork being an unhealthy meat again came to the fore. From this point on, mofongo unfailingly turned up in all the cookbooks, just as it undoubtedly had in home-cooked meals for a very long period of time. The recipe for the version of mofongo followed today in most Puerto Rican kitchens dates to 1950, when the first edition of Berta Cabanillas's cookbook, Cocine a gusto, came out. In this new, post–Second World War context, in which cooking had again come to be seen as a mark of Puerto Rican identity, mofongo still fulfilled its role as a simple dish, but one that now existed in an urbanized, industrialized environment. Whether fried or baked, its plantains were mashed in a mortar, with half a pound of pork crackling worked into the mixture. The mofongo could be eaten as a separate dish or—once formed into balls—used to thicken soups.[85]

The history of pastel de plátano and guineo, or pastel navideño, is not so easily traced. It does not appear in any of the cooking manuals or recipe books published prior to 1930, an omission that seems odd given that, like mofongo, it features prominently in Puerto Rican fiction and other writing of the nineteenth century. As distinct from mofongo, however, it may have been ignored because of its deep-seated African roots, telescoped in how the dough was wrapped up inside "banana leaves."[86] Yet its long absence from cookbooks seems in fact to be tied primarily to another factor—the many involved steps needed to make it. Whoever has made pastel, in one form or another, is well aware that the task is complicated and requires considerable focus, organization, and judgment, along with something that cannot be planned—an intuitive sense of how the dish will best come together. There is no single accepted way of making pastel. For example, the first step in the process—softening the banana leaves prior to enfolding the dough in them (or, amortiguarlas)—has always been the subject of differing interpretation. The preference in some kitchens is to accomplish the operation by suffusing the banana leaves in the smoky heat given off by a wood fire. In other kitchens there has been a preference for boiling the leaves slightly, and in yet others for exposing them to steam.

The same lack of uniformity characterizes the preparation of the dough and the filling. In preparing the dough, some cooks prefer to mix the plantain, in equal parts, with the variety of short banana known as *mafafo*, others with particular viandas, such as the yellow tannier (nowadays rarely encountered), or "the mother" of the white tannier, the part that is used as a seedling. Some prefer to mix it with squash and "green banana," but only the variety of green banana called *malango*. Still others do not use plantain at all, preferring to limit themselves to bananas and other viandas.

The filling, too, varies from kitchen to kitchen, its content often determined by what food happens to be on hand at the appointed time, as well as by the likes and dislikes of household members. Some prefer to use garbanzo beans, while others do not. Some like to include raisins but draw the line at hot chili peppers. Others will avoid using the *empella de cerdo* (meat from the topmost part of the pig's foot) but happily include carne *magra* (a lean cut, such as pork loin) or a part of the pig called *carne flaca*, which comes from the animal's hindquarters. The question of whether the dough should be colored or not also enters the picture. Some like to put achiote in the lard, and others do not. That opinion about the proper way to make pastel varied so widely, indeed that no official, proper way ever really existed, meant that the art of making it was generally learned firsthand, in the kitchen, by watching and imitating others, or was transmitted orally, or—in some cases perhaps—was acquired by reading the casual jottings on a slip of paper. These, however, were a far cry from an organized set of uniform written recipes, set down for posterity, which the most educated cooks may have wanted to see in print but realistically had no chance of doing so in the face of such powerful countercurrents.

In trying to account for the absence of published pastel recipes much before the mid-twentieth century, yet another factor should be considered— that pastel was typically made only on special occasions, or to celebrate particular holidays. Moreover, the complicated, multistep process needed to make pastel no doubt discouraged people from expending the effort unless the occasion seemed sufficiently important, for social, religious, or other reasons. Thus pastel was associated most closely with the meals eaten during Christmas celebrations, the festivities of the Three Kings in particular, and not with the meals traditionally consumed on other annual holidays. The custom also exists of making pastel to present it as a gift, much like the traditional acceptance and presentation of *tamal de maíz* in different parts of Mexico and Colombia and of *hallaca* in Venezuela.[87]

Pastel resembles sofrito in two respects: the way in which it evolved and its bricolage-like character. A more or less standardized version of the dish emerged only after a long period of experimentation and improvisation, in which inherited preferences for certain foods and diets, as well as ways of cooking and preparing meals, were tried, rejected, accepted, blended, and modified. Hence pastel ultimately became a dish whose ingredients genuinely mirrored and combined the gastronomic traditions of the island's major population groups, incorporating Arawakan chili peppers, tannier, and achiote; Iberian garbanzos, raisins, olives, and pork; and plantains and bananas from the Canary Islands and parts of Africa. If one focuses, however, on what truly makes pastel unique—the mashing of the dough to give it a certain texture and its being wrapped in leaves and cooked by boiling, three features that were constant—then the African element seems especially prominent.

When a recipe for making pastel finally debuted in written form, it was not—like mofongo—in a cookbook but in a 1931 home economics cooking manual devoted to the tannier, underlining the frequency with which this tuber was used in its preparation. The belated appearance of pastel in a culinary publication may have been inspired by the spirit of *puertorriqueñidad* (the belief in and assertion of a distinct Puerto Rican cultural identity) associated with the island's generation of 1930. Nearly two decades later, in Dooley's 1948 *The Puerto Rican Cookbook*, pastel was included as a Christmas-season dish, along with majarete, hallacas, pastel de arroz, arroz con dulce, and cazuela.[88] The recipe that Dooley used was credited to one América Gaztambide, yet another indication that the dish could be made in a variety of ways. When it came to pastel, each cook had her own protocol.[89]

With respect to the plantain as a basic item of food, an interesting historical parallel emerged beginning in the late 1920s. At that time, coincident with efforts (as we shall see) to introduce more elaborate ways of preparing and cooking tubers, the perception and classification of the plantain as a foodstuff started to change. It began once again to be thought of as a fruit, as it had been—according to the impression left by some early visitors to the island—in the sixteenth and seventeenth centuries. Little by little, cooking manuals and cookbooks began to treat the plantain differently, separating it from viandas and grouping it with banana and other tropical fruit recipes.

As a more urban and sophisticated gastronomic sensibility took hold in Puerto Rico, new ways of preparing and cooking plantains began to appear, expanding the options beyond the traditional practice of either baking or boiling them. For example, one recipe in the 1914 manual *Home Making* called for adding cheese to ripe fried plantains; and another called for preparing green plantains in the form of tostones or arañitas.[90] In *The Porto Rican Cookbook* of 1948, the plantain is relegated in some recipes to playing a secondary role as an ingredient in dishes centered around meat, such as *pastelón de plátano horneado*, in which layers of plantain, first ripened and fried, are topped with chopped meat, then covered with beaten egg whites; or soups that as their centerpiece contain little meat-filled plantain "bolitas," or the iconic *piononos*.[91] The cookbook also has a recipe that calls for using baking powder to make fried plantain *arepitas*, and it describes how servings of plantain might be dressed up by adding olives and chopped, hard-boiled eggs.[92] The widening of gastronomic horizons in Puerto Rico from the early 1900s on, the spreading influence of a more inventive home economics curriculum, and the publication of cooking manuals and recipe books between the mid-nineteenth century and the early twentieth afforded greater opportunity to the island's wealthier inhabitants to adapt, enrich, and disseminate plantain-based recipes that had earlier attained their fullest expression in the kitchens of Afro–Puerto Ricans and among mestizo cooks who followed their own intuition and imagination.

Breaking with the Past: A New Gastronomy for Viandas

Within the food culture of urban Puerto Rico, the appeal and value of dishes made with other viandas was not well appreciated during the early years of the twentieth century. However, the scientific study of family and home life, now more attuned to the realities of the island in the agricultural and food-related spheres, endeavored to bring their potentialities to light, in part by seeing that students in home economics classes learned about them. Within the University of Puerto Rico, by the end of the 1920s, considerable strides had been made in this direction. By then, viandas were not only seen as central to a well-rounded diet but as products that could also be prepared in more targeted, sophisticated, and attractive ways. With this outcome in mind, two studies were issued, under the supervision of home economist Elsie Mae Wilsey, in a series entitled *Tropical Foods*. The first volume appeared in 1926 and focused on the malanga, *lerenes* (guinea arrowroot or sweet corn root), *apio* (arracacha), *pana* (breadfruit)—all four had been ignored in earlier cookbooks—and cassava.[93] The second volume, published in 1931, was devoted exclusively to the tannier.[94]

The publications encouraged the preparation of dishes that until then had occupied a distinctly minor place in the daily fare offered in the majority of households: salads, croquettes, viandas cut into strips and embellished with a cream sauce, purees, with various seasonings also proposed to serve as dressings for them. It was even recommended, notably in the text devoted to the tannier, that there be servings of vianda—a series of different vianda dishes—corresponding to each of the courses that constituted a complete meal: viandas as the appetizer, side dish, and main dish. At this stage, both home economics and nutritional science recognized the versatility of viandas as a foodstuff and their importance as a core part of the diet, in contrast to how persons concerned with such matters had viewed them at the end of the nineteenth century, when they were associated with poverty and squalor.

While the majority of the population continued to prepare viandas in the simplest way possible, the proposals put forward by the University of Puerto Rico team and by others unquestionably marked an important transition in terms of how viandas were used in the long run. Many of the new recipes, involving purees, seasoned dressings, cream sauces, and more, were not merely taught to the students enrolled in public school home economics classes; they also served as the basis for dishes that the students themselves cooked and enjoyed. Subsequently, they found their way into such cookbooks as the 1948 *Puerto Rican Cookbook*, and not many years later were given their due, along with other recipes for vianda dishes, in the first two major books on Puerto Rican cooking to be published since *El cocinero puertorriqueño* in the nineteenth century: *Cocine a gusto* (1950) and *Cocina Criolla* (1954).[95] In turn, the vianda recipes in both these publications have been altered and modified in more recent cookbooks. In broad terms, however, the recipes inspired by the reevaluation of viandas on the part of home economics specialists in the 1920s set the pattern for how they are prepared and served today.

Viandas: The Comforting Food of Motherhood

In similar fashion to other venerable foods, such as cornmeal and rice, whose position in the daily diet has eroded, there has been a gradual but persistent shift away from the consumption of starches. While the downward trend has not been as sharp as that affecting either salted codfish or beans, it is nonetheless unmistakable. First, the bromatology of viandas has itself impeded their integration into a more cosmopolitan, elegant way of preparing them. In addition, like rice before them, they are fully at the mercy of an indifferent global market. None of the viandas, excepting perhaps sweet potatoes because of their pleasing flavor, have managed to pass any of the culinary tests thrown at them, at least not in the environment of the home kitchen. All in all, and despite worthy attempts at converting viandas into flans or using them as a filling—it has become very fashionable to stuff turkeys and roast chickens with varieties of mofongo—they are still often fried or, even more commonly, boiled in salted water.[96] This latter method of preparing them has likely remained dominant because, for most people, it is the simplest and most economical.

Yet in accounting for such loyalty to tradition, other elements seem to be at play, some of which appear to be grounded in the close relationship that the population has historically maintained with viandas, extending back to times when dietary options were much more restricted.[97]

Moreover, for many years viandas enjoyed popularity as a food to give to infants after they came off breastfeeding. This attraction derived in part from their high water and starch content, which allowed them to be converted into soft, digestible food during a period in the infant's life when he or she lacked any hard, permanent teeth. During this stage, as the French sociologist and philosopher Pierre Bourdieu contended, one's sense of the taste of food registers an indelible impression. According to Bourdieu, it is during this early time of development that the things one first learns "withstand the distancing or collapse of the native world and most durably maintain nostalgia for it."[98]

If one considers that the development of a sense of the taste of food comes through a mother's offerings of it—a mother confined until the 1950s, in Puerto Rico, within a narrow gastronomic world—as well as through the "learning derived from observation," the "influence of fellow youngsters," and the "internalization of certain rules and norms," then the daily presence of viandas in the diet must have been decisive in the formation of what has come to be called the "palate's memory." At this stage in the child's development, the senses begin to test and try, to reject or accept, various tastes, smells, colors and textures.

Furthermore, during this early phase in the formation of a sense of taste, children tend to be drawn to sweet flavors, as opposed to those which are bitter, salty, or sour. The pronounced sweetness of viandas could thus have drawn the infant back to them, creating a clear preference in his budding sense of taste. The same power of attraction could have been exerted by the color of viandas, similar as they are to the color of a mother's milk, and by their soft texture as well.[99] Thus, when viandas were given as a baby food or puree to infants, they must have played this deeper, normative role, both attenuating, if not negating, what pediatric science might have recommended and forestalling the inroads of industrial baby formulas.

In addition, more directly than any other food, viandas—before being fed to the infant—were checked by hand, fingers, and mouth to make sure the temperature, consistency, and texture were right. The constant repetition of these actions doubtless strengthened the conviction, lasting until the middle decades of the twentieth century, that these were the proper types of food for infants. In this way, by these means, viandas were long instrumental in helping mold standards of taste in food among many Puerto Ricans.

Furthermore, as infants progress through successive culinary phases, they become part of a relationship, grounded in feelings of affection, which also seems to contribute to the development of their sense of taste in food. Claude Fischler points out that taste is "a sense strongly marked by affectivity, colored by emotion."[100] Thus the diminutive form that is still used to name various preparations made with viandas—*bolitas, tortitas, buñuelitos, tortillitas, bocadito de batata*—signifies not only their physical form or size but also the realization, via the diminutives themselves, of feelings of tenderness and affection. This mutual exchange of feelings and sensations nurtures a reciprocal relationship, a bond, between mother and infant.

Finally, viandas are also considered by many as an appropriate food for certain cycles in life or certain conditions of poor health, such as gastrointestinal illnesses. In earlier times, when medical care was often inaccessible, viandas were taken as "dietetic and therapeutic cuisine." It is still common to recommend them in the case of delicate stomachs and intestinal problems.

In sum, viandas were part and parcel of the food that a Puerto Rican mother fed to her child (*la cocina de las madres*), and that act, according to Fischler, constitutes one of the key means by which a sense of taste is developed. Clearly, beginning some five decades ago, the influences that might shape a child's food tastes widened dramatically on the island. Likes and dislikes, as we know, can be affected by social context, by the range of choices available—far more extensive today than in earlier decades—and by the level of cultural or educational attainment that exists in the family or school environment in which the child grows up and comes of age. Theorists such as Fischler suggest, in contrast to Bourdieu, that the origin of the most deep-rooted or lasting tastes do not necessarily lie in the foods that were tried, by way of a mother's cooking, during infancy.[101] He further notes that a certain element of nostalgia can lurk in the very idea of "everlastingness" propounded by Bourdieu. Or perhaps, interwoven in the whole analysis, one encounters both elements: the central position that viandas have occupied in the infant diet, and, for the oldest segment of the population, the image of certain food that is evoked by the longing for earlier times when, though the choice of what to eat was much more limited, there was an abundant supply of fresh products to be harvested from the country garden.

Viandas within the Global Supermarket

Figures for the per capita consumption of the most popular tubers show a significant decline in the last quarter of the twentieth century against comparable figures for the late 1930s. It can be hypothesized that the gradual loss of a market for viandas resulted from a change in favor of potatoes, a change caused by the power of the foreign import market, which increased the availability of potatoes in relation to tuberous viandas. In 2000, the amount of imported potatoes came to 127,471,005 pounds (64 million from Canada and 62 million from the United States).[102]

The figures for 2003 were even more compelling. By July of that year, 357.6 million pounds of imported "treated" potatoes had entered the local market. The consumption of these alone, exclusive of "fresh" potatoes, equaled an annual per capita consumption of 91.9 pounds.[103]

The plantain, in contrast, maintained its popularity and market share. As mentioned before, it is a much more versatile food than the viandas. In addition to being prepared in the form of tostones, amarillos fritos, mofongo, and arañitas, a side dish of plantains has always been an accompani-

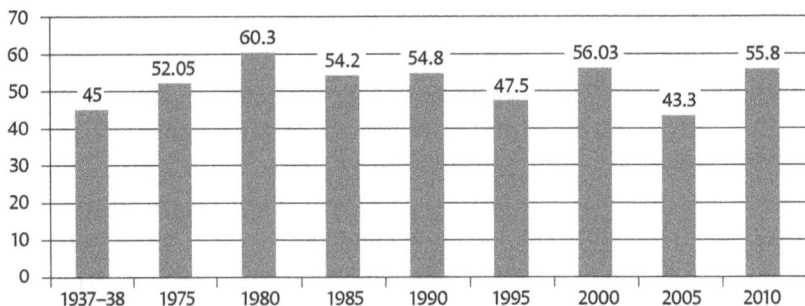

FIGURE 5.1 Annual per capita consumption, in pounds, of plantains

Sources: Descartes et al., *Food Consumption Studies*; and Departamento de Agricultura de Puerto Rico, Oficina de Estadísticas Agrícolas, *Consumo de plátano, 1975–2010*, Ffolder 1657b24.

ment to a full meal. This convention has enabled the plantain to hold its own against the incursion of fried potatoes, which have come to be central to meals in Puerto Rico.

Although consumed today in much smaller quantities than before, there is an expectation about tubers similar to the one that attends rice: namely, that if they are not a part of daily meals in the home, they will at least be an everyday item on the menus of restaurants specializing in local fare as well as in Cuban and Dominican dishes.

In contrast to rice, however, viandas have not moved with the times, such that one finds them prepared in cosmopolitan or "exotic" ways. There have been attempts, recently, to use them differently, in particular with respect to the cuisine known as "nuevo latino," "nuevo caribe," or "fusion." For example, an attempt was made to use sweet potatoes in a novel way, by whipping them up and putting the emulsion as a topping on roast meat, but this recipe and form of presentation proved to be no more than a passing fad. Then, at the end of the 1980s, it became fashionable to stuff sweet chili peppers with pureed tannier and serve them as appetizers, a recipe launched by the chef of the newly opened Café Central in San Juan. Its life, however, was as short-lived as that of the restaurant.

It is becoming increasingly evident that viandas have been relegated to the status of an accompaniment or side dish, left to compete in this role with plantains, when fifty years ago they were the centerpiece of a meal that had peripheral food, such as salted codfish or dry, cured beef as accompaniments.

In the present dual context of the "global supermarket," in which products from anywhere in the world are at the reach of consumers through-

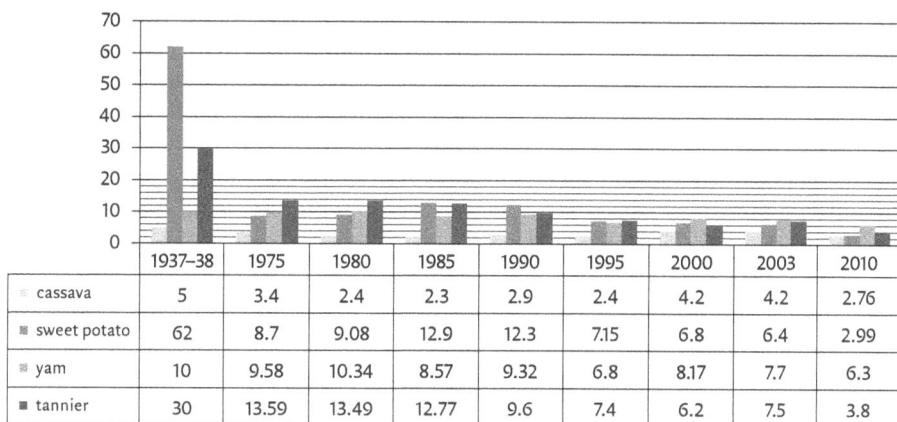

	1937–38	1975	1980	1985	1990	1995	2000	2003	2010
cassava	5	3.4	2.4	2.3	2.9	2.4	4.2	4.2	2.76
sweet potato	62	8.7	9.08	12.9	12.3	7.15	6.8	6.4	2.99
yam	10	9.58	10.34	8.57	9.32	6.8	8.17	7.7	6.3
tannier	30	13.59	13.49	12.77	9.6	7.4	6.2	7.5	3.8

FIGURE 5.2 Annual per capita consumption, in pounds, of viandas

Sources: Descartes et al., *Food Consumption Studies*, and Estado Libre Asociado, Departamento de Agricultura, Oficina de Estadísticas Agrícolas, *Consumo de Alimentos Farináceos*, 1975–2010, folders, 16-57b16 (cassava), 16-57b21(sweet potato), 16-57b22 (yam), y 16-57b23(tannier).

out the island, and local production of these same products has declined precipitously, viandas have come to represent the "delocalization" of food-stuffs and what results from it: the weakening of ties (economic and cultural) between food and the land we know.[104]

The viandas that Puerto Ricans consume, including those not yet treated or processed, come not only from the island but from Central American and South American countries as well. The case of cassava illustrates this trend. Around 2000, for example, Puerto Rico received 161,911, 4,462,097, and 16,187 pounds of frozen cassava from Colombia, Costa Rica, and Ecuador, respectively; Puerto Rico itself produced only 16,531 quintals of fresh cassava. On the other hand, in 2001, the island imported 7,053,853 pounds of fresh cassava (primarily from Costa Rica, which accounted for 6,967,556 of the total), while producing only 1,653,100 pounds locally. In 2000, Puerto Rico produced 6,026,800 pounds of sweet potatoes, but imported more than double this number, 12,986,278 pounds, the following year, 94 percent of which came from the Dominican Republic. The same imbalance applies to yams; 16,547,462 pounds of this tuber were imported (almost entirely from Costa Rica) in 2001, while in the year before, less than half this number, 8,076,800 pounds, were harvested on the island. In 2000, 289,349 quintals of tannier were imported into Puerto Rico and only 29,706 produced locally.[105]

The phenomenon of delocalization, together with the ever-shrinking production of viandas on Puerto Rican soil, have created an image in people's minds of a kind of past golden age of food production on the island, during which the majority of the population planted and harvested what they consumed. In turn, this attachment to the land and the self-sufficiency it provided became the cornerstone of the highest human values, with the capacity for work standing out among all others. In this idealized image, nothing better represents the campesino and the agrarian life as supposedly lived in Puerto Rico prior to 1950 than the viandas arrayed on a plate of food.

What is more, the image has produced a counter effect, causing Puerto Rican consumers to make prejudicial, sweeping judgments about the quality of viandas based simply on where they come from—if they are from Santo Domingo, they do not taste the way they should; if they originate in Costa Rica, they are *jojotas* (bruised and on the verge of spoiling) and *amarran* (having a very unpleasant, astringent flavor); if yams, unlike rice, are not produced locally, they are deemed inferior (ignoring that the island's rice comes from India), a criterion that—curiously—is not applied to any other basic foods. Negative opinions are also expressed about those who have turned their backs on local agriculture. Indeed, viandas have become the vehicle for expressing a new sense of identity about the island as homeland, a development taken to absurd lengths when the viandas that enter Puerto Rico from neighboring islands or other countries are rejected out of hand or judged to be inferior on that basis alone.

This dynamic suggests that the cultural, physiological, and culinary moorings rooted in viandas, as part of the complex of Puerto Ricans' contemporary expectations about food and diet, have loosened only fractionally. It likewise illustrates that they are operative—though not to the degree they were in the past—when people ponder what to order in a *fonda* (modest eatery or pension) or what to cook and eat at home. The decline in their consumption notwithstanding, viandas will assuredly be part of the diet of Puerto Ricans well into the future, boosted by the expectations that people from other Caribbean islands—who are settling in growing numbers in Puerto Rico—bring with them. Dominicans, who have maintained a similar relationship with tubers, are a case in point. One of these tubers, the yam—harvested between November and January—has been a favorite food to eat during the Christmas holiday, preferably accompanied by roasted meat from one of the animals examined in the next chapter—the pig.

6 | Meat

Rice, please! . . . There's a load of meat.
—Contemporary Puerto Rican saying

During an interview that took place more than a hundred years ago, Vicente Muñoz—a planter and former mayor of the municipality of Caguas—was asked by Henry King Carroll, a U.S. Treasury Department official, whether the order issued by General Guy V. Henry, the island's American military governor, prohibiting the leveling of taxes on consumer products had helped reduce the price of bread and meat after the U.S. invasion. Muñoz replied: "The order preventing the collection of the consumption tax appeared at first a very beneficent one, but it was really quite the other thing. We are buying bread and meat at the same prices we were before, and instead of the people of the city, who consume the bread and meat, paying the tax the extra taxation has been put on us."[1]

Then, the two proceeded to have the following exchange:

Dr. Carroll: What do you pay for bread?
Mr. Muñoz: Six cents in town, I pay seven cents in the country.
Dr. Carroll: How much was it before?
Mr. Muñoz: It was eight cents for a pound, light; now they sell a full pound for 6 cents.
Dr. Carroll: It was eight cents in San Juan, and now it is four cents.
Mr. Muñoz: But the agricultural laborers do not eat either bread or meat.[2]

Beyond the question of whether certain prices were rising or falling, Muñoz made two points about the food situation in Puerto Rico that should be emphasized; first, that a clear divide existed between cities and towns and rural areas—meat and bread had become part of the urban diet—and second, that agricultural day laborers had little chance of eating either meat or bread.

In 1899, when Carroll interviewed Muñoz, the saying quoted at the beginning of this chapter would not have carried the suggestive meaning it does today. "Rice please! There's a load of meat" ("*Arroz, que carne hay*") is charged with sexual innuendo and, as with many other double entendres related to food—for example, "*tanta carne y yo comiendo bacalao*" (so much meat, and I'm just eating salted codfish)—the act of eating becomes a metaphor for the sexual act. As a rule, one hears them exclaimed when a man is captivated by the physical charms and attractiveness of a woman. In a society in which the rules governing male-female relations are defined very differently for men and women, it is the man, as the aggressive, dominant party, who is the recipient of the meal and the woman—as the object of pursuit—who constitutes it.

Since popular sayings, however, represent a response or reaction to particular lived experiences, their meanings are transmuted as the wider social and cultural context surrounding them changes. The saying "arroz, que carne hay," as well as "tanta carne y yo comiendo bacalao," could be the surviving elements of expressions coined in an environment characterized by limited dietary options, rather than by the appeal to sexual, and sexist, intimations and word play, as is the case today. In the past, meat was scarce, but when it was there, it was accompanied by rice; thus the saying could originally have referred to that brief moment of plenty, which—as conveyed in the imperative tone of its words—needed to be seized without reservation.

Whether or not earlier generations of one's family managed, at one time or another, to have meat in their diet does not concern us today, nor despite all the warnings issued about it, does the health danger posed by the fats contained in meat seem to be of great nutritional concern to many in the population, even those who otherwise live in fear of fat. The consumption of meat by Puerto Ricans is such that neither outbreaks of hoof and mouth or of mad cow disease have given them much pause to worry.[3] The sole exception to this aloof reaction may have come from the Agriculture Department, which rose to the defense of Puerto Rican meat products. No one, however, evinced the same kind of fear that was witnessed in other countries, the European nations especially.[4] Put another way, meat is a food that today people take for granted.

This situation, however, in which meat can be consumed frequently and abundantly, indeed in which the consumption of certain types of meat is equated with power and prosperity, is the end point of a long historical process marked by three stages: one that began in the sixteenth century and lasted until the mid-1700s, during which meat was easily obtained as a result of the spread of the pig and cattle populations across the open, wild territory of the island; a second period characterized by sharp shortages and inequalities, brought on by economic and demographic changes occurring between the end of the eighteenth and the middle of the twentieth century; and a third era, of post-1950 recuperation, sparked by advances in the U.S. cattle industry and the canned and processed meat industry, as well as changes in the nutrition politics of the modern welfare state.

The disparity noted by Caguas's former mayor first appeared around 1780 and gradually became institutionalized over the next century. To understand how the possibilities of consuming meat first shrank and then closed for a large number of islanders it is necessary to describe the relationship that existed, prior to 1780, among animals killed for their flesh, the forest system, the island's inhabitants, and the state.

The Early Emphasis on Pork and Beef

The need to keep cattle as draught animals and as a source of hides, as well as the strong impulse to preserve a cuisine heavily dependent on pork, led *encomenderos* and high level colonial officials to promote, at the very outset of conquest and colonization, the introduction and breeding of pigs and cattle. For example, in September, 1512, Juan Ponce de León unloaded 50 cows and 4 young bulls in San Juan.[5] A year later, he delivered 17 cows, 6 of whom were calving.[6] Acting on behalf of Bartolomé Colón, Diego de Bergara also brought 58 pigs to San Juan in September, 1512,[7] and in that same month and year, Ortuño de Archuri added 60 pigs to the domestic livestock population.[8] In May, 1513, 200 male pigs, 73 female pigs, 24 cows and 4 bulls arrived in the port of San Juan on the ship La Magdalena.[9] In all, between 1512 and 1516, 1,191 pigs, 127 cows, 28 bulls, 14 oxen, and 9 rams were brought onto the island.[10] As part of the larger enterprise of establishing a colony and its food supply, the Spanish bore with them a long-held, specific practice vis-à-vis livestock: that of raising pigs for the sole purpose of satisfying the ingrained habit of eating meat. Indeed, the first group of pigs to set foot in the Antilles arrived in 1493, as part of the cargo carried by Columbus on his second voyage.[11] In that year, the relatively small world of animals known to the indigenous inhabitants of the Caribbean was, to their surprise and wonderment, enlarged by the addition of pigs, cows, sheep, and horses.

In 1513, a set of laws was promulgated (the *Ordenanzas para el Tratamiento de los Indios de San Juan*), establishing a regimen of obligations and penalties, aimed at ensuring that encomenderos provided an adequate amount of food to the Indians who made up the labor pools that mined for gold along the rivers. And while these and other such regulations were hardly followed to the letter, the colonizers—if for no other reason than their own self-interest—found it necessary, during the early, more violent phase of the conquest, to build up a supply of livestock in order to sustain the indigenous work force. It is possible that the first animals to be fenced in for this purpose were pigs, or "*puerco de carne*" (pigs raised and slaughtered for their meat), as mentioned in the account books of the office of the Royal Treasury in San Juan, rather than cattle.[12] As Spanish colonization took root and expanded, the raising of pigs proceeded apace, because, unlike other animals, pigs quickly adapted to this new environment. In this connection, archaeozoologist Elizabeth Rietz has posited that rams experienced difficulty in procreating because they became sterile for a full year after being transported to a tropical climate.[13] She further noted that, even post-twelve months, their breeding was not optimum. Conditions for cattle were likewise difficult, as they had first to acclimate on the Canary Islands before later being shipped to the Caribbean.

Pigs, on the other hand, had always reproduced copiously in both humid and forested regions. As omnivores, they tended to adapt easily to a new ecosystem and to being raised "in a corralled" area, rooting around in their muddy pigpens, devouring the native tubers, the corncobs stripped of their kernels, and the skins and rinds of fruits that the Arawaks and Spaniards ate from one day to the next.

It was this domesticated pig that the Spanish carried with them to San Juan during the early years of the conquest. Noting how it adapted to Hispaniola's tropical climate and conditions and could be successfully bred in the settlements that provisioned the mining camps, they continued importing it as a source both of fresh meat for themselves and of salted beef and bacon to feed those working in the mining grounds.

It was a simple matter to breed, raise, and prepare these pigs, because the settlers already possessed an ample understanding of how to salt and preserve pork meat. Indeed, a "*tocinero*," (a master butcher and provisioner of salt pork) or person selling salt pork, was included among the party attached to Diego Colón as it made its way into San Juan in 1513.[14] The abundant deposits of sea salt which the Spanish found along the southwestern coast of Puerto Rico also aided in the preparation of fatback and dried cured pork.[15]

The Pig and the Taínos

The island's indigenous inhabitants first experienced pork in the mining camps, where they encountered pigs not as creatures to be hunted, as was the case with the fauna known to them, but as a breeding animal and a source of food, initially trying salted portions of its meat and meat by-products as part of the communal meals the conquerors furnished them. Moreover, the Taínos' first contact with pork took place under conditions of extreme physical duress and exploitation in a context of restricted food choices. Their initial reaction to this new food was adverse, not because meat was unfamiliar to them—for they indeed ate birds and rodents—but out of genetic and cultural predispositions. In his book *El Dorado borincano: La economía de la conquista, 1510–1550*, Jalil Sued Badillo reasons that encomenderos needed to supplement the insufficient, squalid meals fed to the Indians with both salted fish from Spain and cured pork produced on the island, because of the simple economics of the situation; it was more profitable to impress the native inhabitants into washing the "golden sands" than to allow them to hunt animals for food.[16] If this is true, then—given a known pattern of human behavior, whereby people initially resist eating new or unfamiliar food[17]—the Taínos' first exposure to heavily-salted protein-rich meat and fish had very likely to be unfavorable. That reaction would explain the colonists complaints that some Indians preferred to hunt their own familiar game in the mountains than to eat the food supplied by encomenderos. In nutritional terms, Badillo suggests that because of the meager rations they were fed as well as their difficulties in ingesting them, the Indians' diet in this early period did in fact lack sufficient protein. Yet in the context of the food insecurity that pervaded the mining camps, a mutual exchange of food took place between the Indians and their Spanish overlords. That is, whether out of convenience or necessity, both parties—despite strong innate aversions—accepted some foods that were alien to their diets.[18] The alternative was starvation.

Of course, this accommodation occurred gradually and brought with it both cultural and genetic clashes. Moreover, we can adduce two things from Badillo's line of argument: first, that because of the division of labor introduced in the mining camps, Indians had to become familiar with breeding pigs; and second, that whether its proportion to the total was large or small, pork constituted the major protein component in the rations given to the indigenous laborers.

Evidence of these developments can be found, for example, in the 2,500 hogs that the encomendero and treasurer Andrés de Haro was raising on his properties at the time of his death in 1519. De Haro's large population of hogs may have been attended by some of the 300 Indians who served him as a labor force. The 342 pigs that were slaughtered and consumed between 1517 and 1518 in the camp of the encomendero Lope Conchillos are a second example, since it stands to reason that not all of them were eaten by the Spanish alone.

Indeed, the confusion that overcame Oviedo, in trying to comprehend the relationship that a Taíno maintained with his pigs—on the one hand treating them as pets and on the other using them as wild beasts to hunt other pigs in order to have food to feed himself and his own pigs—is one instance of the chronicler's inability to recalibrate his views to accommodate the cultural realities and contradictions emergent from the conquest. This anecdote that so puzzled and troubled Oviedo, however, does not conceal the relationship that the Indians early on worked out with the new animal in their midst. In a setting of physical exploitation, power offsets, and food insecurity, in which the fine line between living and dying depended on eating unfamiliar foods, the Indians learned how to "relate" to hogs, albeit in ways that struck the conquistadores and colonists as aberrant and bestial.

In time, what Alfred Crosby observed in his study of the biological and cultural exchanges that accompanied the colonization of the New World— that its indigenous inhabitants, who otherwise ate little in the way of animal flesh, found it easier to adapt to meat, and especially to pork, than to other types of food introduced by the Spanish—came to pass on the island.[19]

The Unbranded Hog

For all this, however, what proved most decisive—in terms of setting a dietary pattern and enabling people to obtain animal flesh quickly—was the appearance of another type of pig. From the earliest days of the conquest, stemming from the voluntary efforts of conquistadores to endow occupied areas with animals whose flesh could be eaten, a "feral pig" began to reproduce within the island's hills and mountains. In Puerto Rican history, the leading example of such efforts was that of Vicente Yáñez Pinzón, who in 1505—before committing himself to colonizing the island—opted to let free various animals, among them pigs, along its coasts.[20] Thus in time, aided by a number of factors—the fruit that fell from the guava and corozo palm trees, the remains of cattle shot by hunters, the low population density of much of the countryside, and its own insatiable predatory practices—a pig characterized by its lean meat, and similar in appearance to a wild boar, began to proliferate in the mountainous regions, becoming a ready source of animal meat for backwoods settlers, runaway slaves, and others who lived on the margins of society. As the consumption of meat became more central to the diet of the urban population, this pig began to be called "*orejano*," or unbranded, to distinguish it from domesticated pigs. For example, Oviedo states that in 1540, the mountainous parts of Hispaniola were populated by "wild, untamed pigs, which are found in great numbers on this island, and which spring from the pigs, brought from Spain, that clambered off into the mountains."[21]

The effects of this early practice reverberated in San Juan. By the beginning of the seventeenth century, the orejanos had become such a fixture in the mountains that they became an object of trade and exchange in the capital's butcher shops, where they were brought by "*monteros*"—the men who hunted these unsociable animals. San Juan's municipal councilors considered their meat to be distinctly inferior in quality, so much so that they passed an ordinance in 1601 penalizing any montero who, by cutting off their ears, tried to sell them in the city as if they were pigs that had been "raised," or "fattened up." City officials then went further, declaring "that nobody who hunts or kills a pig in the mountains [should] cut off its ears, but instead [should] leave them intact, so it will be clear if it is feral or tame."[22]

Yet, because its habitat stayed essentially unchanged and unspoiled, while the population of the island continued to expand, the orejano still counted as both an important source of meat and of commercial trade and exchange in the last quarter of the eighteenth century: "Great packs of pigs live and reproduce in the forests," wrote Fray Abad y Lasierra in 1770, "but they are small, with long, bristly hair like small wild boar, whose tusks stick out two or three finger lengths from the jaws, fierce in nature; some people trap them and tie them up in the palm groves where they go to gorge on fruit from the trees. If they are kept for a long time, they get fleshier and more pleasing to the palate. This line of animal has degenerated notably from its counterpart in Spain; for which reason people try to exchange them for the ones carried on passing ships, offering three or four from the island in return for one of the others, in order to improve the line; without such recourse, they reign completely wild, inferior in quality."[23]

Wild Cattle

A similar pattern occurred in the case of cattle, the difference being that it was tied to the growth of agriculture, the widening arc of settlement over the land, and the market for hides that developed after the initial phase of conquest in the Caribbean had subsided.

The expansion into sugarcane production in the post-1530 period, with its requirement for teams of cattle to pull loads, as well as the incorporation of African slaves as a plantation labor force that not only needed to be fed but that in many cases had long experience in pasturing and caring for cattle,[24] favored maintaining a system of "fenced in" cattle. Moreover, when Puerto Rico ceased to be a profitable source of gold, and expansionist energies got directed out toward the South American and Mesomerican land masses, the island's role in Spain's New World empire became that of a military post and port used for re-provisioning vessels and personal supplies. While their ships were anchored (there were fewer such calls into port in later decades) passengers supplied themselves with cattle, hides, and edibles, before moving on to other destinations. As a rule, travelers brought their own supply of food on board ship before sailing out of Seville.[25] Since it was frequently exhausted during the long crossing, they took advantage of their stay on the island to acquire the two foodstuffs known to preserve best—corn and cassava, along with cured pork and beef. This demand acted as a stimulus to the business of raising cattle in pens near the ports of Aguada and San Juan, for the purpose of selling them to sailors and passengers.

Concurrent with these developments, a type of wild cattle—deficient as a source of meat but valued for its skin and hide—began to flourish amid the dense vegetation of the mountains. Its reproduction in the wild resulted from the method by which vast tracts of land were divided and parceled out for grazing herds of cattle and from the lax regulations for maintaining such herds within enclosed areas.[26] In 1542, when the island's fields, mountains, and waters were declared open resources, available for common use, the areas devoted to pasturing cattle became the lightening rod for opposition to the new policy on the part of ranchers who owned large herds. In the arguments advanced by San Juan's municipal council and the cathedral's ecclesiastical chapter, the degree to which domestic cattle had wandered into and spread across unoccupied wilderness came to light: "The freedom, now, of each person to set himself down wherever he wants can only cause hurt. The land is rugged, very mountainous; the cattle tough and difficult to bring out of the mountains and hills, which, with lots of dogs around, many inhabitants would not be able to do, denying them that advantage."[27]

According to historians who have studied the matter, it was the market in hides—highly prosperous after 1530—that mainly benefited from the presence of wild livestock. But this conclusion assesses matters from the commercial perspective. From the perspective of food and diet, the principal beneficiaries were the aforementioned "monteros" as well as people living in more remote rural areas. During the first years of colonization, when people struggled to find enough food to survive, meat complemented both the native foodstuffs and those, like plantains, yams, and rice, which were originally foreign to the island. In this scheme, meat played a supplementary role in the diet of the majority of islanders, a role which it continued to play throughout the seventeenth and eighteenth centuries.

If, in speaking of the formation of a food culture, or cultures, what Sidney Mintz called the "intensification" and "extensification" of the consumption of certain foods, that is, the force or forces which provoke the adoption of a new food that gets added to a basic complex of foods and over the long term becomes integral to who we are and how we define ourselves, has to be taken into consideration, then in the case of pork and beef two factors must be considered: the eventual social and economic primacy of a traditionally carnivorous human group and the circumstances that arose affecting agriculture and livestock in the years following the conquest.[28] Both factors served as the foundation upon which the practice of and meanings ascribed to consuming meat soon spread across the colony.

Carnivorous Island

The Spaniards who deliberately introduced pigs and cattle to the island hailed from a culture in which the consumption of meat was a sign and symbol of distinction and a confirmation of one's religious faith and heritage; it reinforced and consolidated an individual's power and his social and religious associations.[29] Equally important was the principle that the quality of meat, and its type, should correspond to the social standing of the person consuming it.[30]

At a basic level, however, the consumption of meat in the colony was not solely a privilege of the few from the sixteenth through most of the eighteenth century. The majority of Spanish settlers who commanded power during that era indeed sought to reproduce all the forms, rituals, and practices—including that of eating meat—which had confirmed their high social position within the metropolis. Yet in broad terms, the powerful did not monopolize either access to or the consumption of meat. The ecology of the island permitted rural inhabitants, runaway slaves, and persons eking out a living from the land to obtain animal flesh without undue strain. The move away from these free conditions toward a far more restrictive environment, in which access to meat was largely confined to the powerful, resulted from two major developments occurring between the mid-eighteenth and the first half of the nineteenth century, first: the inversion of the balance between the human population on the island, which steadily grew from the mid-1700s on, and the population of animals whose flesh could be eaten; and second, the restraints placed on hunting animals within forested zones in order to provide both Crown officials and soldiers garrisoned in the capital city with a constant supply of meat. The reception banquet staged by San Juan's municipal council in 1766 to honor the arrival of the colony's new governor, Marcos Vergara de Lupo, marked the point at which the colony passed definitively into this new era.[31] To comprehend the magnitude of the modification that was soon made to secure meat that was fresh—something which (as will be explained below) the majority of the population would find beyond its capacity until the middle of the twentieth century—it is first essential to delineate the several ways in which animal flesh was obtained.

During the sixteenth century, to find it possible to eat meat was not simply a day dream, as it would become by the middle of the nineteenth century. All the same, it is notable that during the 1530s, within a society of pronounced social inequalities, meat—like cassava and corn—was seen, and treated, as basic sustenance for the African slaves who were deployed to search for gold in the island's rivers.[32]

Hence meat, which prior to the conquest had been exclusive to a select segment of European society, became a food consumed by all social ranks in the colony of Puerto Rico.[33]

On this point, the communications sent at the beginning of the 1530s by the San Juan municipal council to the ecclesiastical authorities requesting that people be allowed to consume meat on days set aside for fasting reflect not only the strictness with which the liturgical calendar was observed and the concomitant fear of violating Church rules and doctrine,[34] but demonstrate as well how abundant meat was during the first decades of colonization. Even for those persons whose religious practices were a decisive influence in cementing their social position, and underscored their fidelity to the Catholic Church, the options for consuming meat were dietary realities that had to be negotiated. On this matter, the San Juan municipal council made the following appeal to the Crown in 1534: ". . . we beg of your majesty, in that in this city and island meat is inexpensive and fish dear, and the inhabitants are in need, and when they ask license of the island's bishop so they can eat the salted meat with which they give alms; and likewise black folk during Easter [and Christmas] and other fasting days have no fish to eat, and being out in the campo; and because they are badly nourished start to go missing, become shiftless and troublesome . . . may your majesty's will be done . . . that while fish are lacking or cost dearly in the campo we are able to consume meat without giving offence."[35]

The conditions addressed by the council illustrated two parallel things: that incoming supplies of salted fish—especially mackerel and herring— which had been common enough during the initial years of colonization, were now only intermittent; and that the number of cattle grazing both nearby fields and mountainous areas had multiplied rapidly, thus enabling people to obtain meat relatively easily.

Entries made in his diary by Francisco López Mendoza, chaplain on the expedition led by Pedro Menéndez Valdés, also afford a glimpse into these circumstances.[36] The fleet captained by Menéndez Valdés put into port in 1556 to refresh its stores of food and load some horses before sailing on to Florida. López Mendoza, who was offered the chaplaincy during the brief layover in San Juan, devoted considerable space in his diary to recording impressions of life on the island based on his interactions with its inhabitants. "And here the men who are rich," he wrote, "are so because of the cattle, there are men with twenty thousand and thirty thousand cows and a good many mares."

Although the cleric expressed the opinion "that if it were not for their hide the cattle would have no use nor be worth anything in any other way" (that is, could neither be harnessed for work nor sold live in the cattle market), both he and the crew proceeded to do the same thing that many of the local population did when they wanted to consume meat: they went out to hunt cattle, and afterward made "some special items, very good dried beef, to have at sea. . . . We did a dozen cow's tongues and cured some tender parts and we did so because when we got there I understood the needs that go unmet at sea."[37]

López Mendoza's observation about the massive herds of cattle owned by colonists was seconded some years later by another cleric, the chaplain John Layfield, who served as a member of the English squadron led by Sir George Clifford, Count of Cumberland, that attempted to capture San Juan in 1598. In his diary, Layfield referred to the rumor that a leading resident of Aguada, in the western part of the island, had 12,000 head of cattle, adding that the number of cattle on the island grew with "unlimited license." He also noted that at one time, so belief held, "because of the great abundance of cattle, it was permitted, in keeping with the law, that a man could kill as many as he required for his use if he was honorable enough to bring the hides to his master(s) . . ." On these points, Layfield may have been exaggerating, but he was not spinning tall tales.[38]

Comments made by Bishop Damián López de Haro in 1644 also allude, indirectly, to the ability of most islanders to have meat as part of their diet. Although complaining about how infrequently he was able to consume meat, the prelate's account included a revealing marginal note, in which he disclosed that one of the reasons he was motivated to accept the bishopric was the rumor, which had circulated among his friends in Spain, that San Juan often had supplies of meat "*de balde*," that is, meat whose handling was not subject to the municipal council's regulations, because it came from cows in the campo that were killed by slaves as well as by breeders who wanted "purely to realize profits from the hide and [enjoy] the delicious sweetbreads."[39] The picture left by López de Haro does not entirely square with the incessant complaints made by colonial administrators during the seventeenth century about the lack of meat in the colony, complaints which historians have appropriated to undergird the idea of an island that was poor in resources and abandoned to its own fate by the metropolis. Viewed from another perspective, these complaints were more the expression of the central place that meat had in the diet of each new contingent of administrators than evidence of the absence of meat beyond the seawalls of San

Juan. Colonial officials were accustomed to adorning their tables in a way that accorded with their high social standing, and the simple fact that meat was lacking on one day or another, for one reason or another, clearly does not mean that it was available only on rare occasions or that the population beyond the walls of the city scarcely ever encountered it. If anything, conditions—as reported by López de Haro and via the testimonies of others—suggest that meat, even during periods of fasting, such as Lent, was as available as fish in the city market.[40]

Likewise, the frequent prohibitions instituted against using beef and pork as goods to exchange on the contraband market reflect the concern of San Juan's administrators that the supply of meat inside the city might run short, rather than any difficulty that the rest of the population had in securing meat.[41] Pointing up its importance and availability, meat was one of only three foods, apart from cassava and plantains, that San Juan's residents could secure, over a period of several days, in order to feed a group of families from the Canary Islands that the governor, Juan Fernández Franco de Medina, had brought with him in 1700.[42]

From the sixteenth until the last quarter of the eighteenth century, however, the availability of meat did track divisions of caste and class within colonial society. If the consumption of meat was to serve as a clear measure of superior social standing, then a disequilibrium had to obtain between the island's population on the one hand and the supply of meat on the other, and the relations of production and ownership would need to evolve such that the mass of society could not freely exploit animals found on wild lands. Until these changes happened, though, those who lived far outside the city's walls, beyond the pale of urban life, developed a close connection with the island's forests, hills, and mountains.

Forest Lands and the Monteros

From the middle of the sixteenth to the end of the seventeenth century, as sugarcane production became less profitable, the estates on which the cane had been grown were converted into farms, or ranches, with a more stable agricultural base. These enterprises, which flourished on land either close to the two ports, San Juan and Aguada, where the fleets anchored or at other points along the coasts, supplied food to both registered ships legally in transit and to vessels, carrying contraband, that sailed from and between other Caribbean islands.

The ranches, whose possibilities of marketing tropical products (such as ginger and cacao) to Europe were in part circumscribed by restrictions placed on the use of ports other than San Juan and by Spain's commercial tilt toward other products, benefited in the long run from the demand generated by Caribbean markets for foodstuffs, cow hides, and livestock. They managed, via this channel, to insert themselves into a market that favored and stimulated not only a furtive agricultural production but also the raising of cattle and hogs and the spread of feral livestock into mountainous areas.[43]

Until well into the eighteenth century, pig and cattle raising on ranch land occupied a middle ground, between domestic rearing of livestock for consumption and draft animal power at one end, and hunting them in the mountains at the other. By 1716, the monteros who hunted cattle in Puerto Rico had already made a name for themselves among the English colonies of the Caribbean, where they were described as a kind of "banditti," or outlaw population, living in the island's mountain wilderness.[44] The circumstance of an agricultural system still in the making (in part developed but also still characterized by simple gathering), complemented by low population density, exerted little pressure—for the time being—on the island's cattle resources, nor did it create pressure either to open up virgin territory in wilderness forest areas or to enact regulations aimed at reserving the use of land for agricultural purposes. Ultimately, however, these changes would come about, upsetting the equilibrium of a system which since the sixteenth century had promoted the reproduction of wild cattle and pigs and, as a consequence, given many islanders an easy, or easier, path toward filling out their diet.

The extensive areas of pasture land and the abundant variety of fruit, legumes, and roots, nourished the wild cattle and enabled them to reproduce throughout the eighteenth century. The thinking that opposed the destruction of these herds beginning in the middle of the eighteenth century invariably refers to how simple it was for cattle living along the island's mountain ranges to get enough to eat.[45] During years when hurricanes struck, the food chain could be broken, adversely affecting the reproductive cycle of animals, that of pigs especially. At one point in the eighteenth century, addressing this problem, San Juan's cabildo declared that "in sterile years, which generally occur when there are hurricanes, the arrival of new litters is set back a great deal, because the fruit on which [the pigs] depend is lost . . ."[46]

Hurricanes, however, could also produce an opposite effect, their gale force winds scattering banana and plantain leaves and fruit of various kinds across the landscape, providing a windfall of easily obtained food for many a wild pig.[47]

Such circumstances led the rural population to forge a close relationship with different livestock and to develop a keen appreciation for the most effective ways of raising, feeding, and fattening them. The observations made by Field Marshal Alejandro O'Reilly in 1765 reflect the experience that generations of herders, ranchers, monteros, and runaway slaves had by then built up with respect to animals that were raised for their flesh: "The cattle are large and beautiful and when very fat, which is how they are when slaughtered, their meat is thick and very tasty: the pasture land that the island produces could not be better: in fattening up the cattle and caring for them on their ranch lands, these native folk prove themselves more intelligent than they do at anything else."[48]

In parallel fashion, the experience they had accumulated in pursuing wild livestock enabled the monteros to pinpoint their hunting grounds in the mountain ranges. In 1772, while en route toward the southeastern part of the island, a delegation representing Bishop Manuel Jiménez Pérez spent the night in "a miserable hut that serves as a hideout for the blacks when they go out to hunt the cattle in these forests."[49]

Accompanied by their hunting dogs, the element of the rural population that lived most removed from any semblance of city life was also accustomed to pursuing wild pigs, as occurred, for example, in the forests around Arecibo.[50] A similar pig, whose flesh was very tasty because it fed on branches of wild oregano,[51] is the type that Abad y Lasierra identified, in his account of the island's inhabitants, as being eaten by those settlers who were most rustic in their ways: "Those who live in the wild are accustomed to going off at certain times in the year to kill pigs, from among the pigs that live and forage in the forests, they greedily consume this meat, only half cooked, until it is gone."[52]

It should also be stressed that the island's ranches, together with the great herds of cattle, provided a continuing source of meat for portions of the population.

O'Reilly's figures, recorded on the basis of information coming from the owners of domestic livestock, round out to some 101,000 head, split among a population of pigs, oxen, cows, heifers, goats, and rams. The true distribution of domestic livestock among all of the island's inhabitants

TABLE 6.1 Types of Domestic Livestock and Their Distribution in 1765

Livestock	Quantity	Number of Head per Person
Oxen, cows, and young bulls	44,633	0.99
Rams	5,735	0.12
Goats	2,683	0.05
Pigs	47,906	1.06
Total head count:	100,956	2.20

Source: Alejandro O'Reilly, "Relación circunstanciada del actual estado de la población, frutos y proporciones para fomento que tiene la Isla de San Juan de Puerto Rico, con algunas ocurrencias sobre los medios conducentes a ello," 1765.

and their specific use cannot, of course, be corroborated, but on the basis of O'Reilly's data, there would have been 2.2 head of livestock per person on the island. Without counting the numbers that lived in mountainous regions, the figure ought to have been, on average, at least 4 head of livestock for each of the island's inhabitants. In O'Reilly's listing of the type of domestic animal, the figures for pigs and cattle are significant within a food context very different from our own.

Owing to various occurrences, the panorama sketched out by O'Reilly, Abad y Lasierra, and others would change, slowly but perceptibly, in succeeding decades. One of the most influential developments was the growth and consolidation of San Juan as a dependent city, a "ciudad garganta" that had to be supplied with food.

Meat for the City, Meat for the Militia

It might be thought that the formidable "*carnivorismo*," or strong predilection for consuming meat, that Puerto Ricans display today has its origins in the availability of meat in the past, and there is doubtless some truth in this. Yet in the formation, and constant change and reforming, of food cultures, absences count as much as presences. The insufficiencies experienced at a certain juncture influence and contribute to the physiological urge to eat particular foods, above all food that has a high fat content and is thus pleasing to the palate. When such food is not there, it becomes something longed for, an object of desire. Other forces, too, have contributed to the "carnivorismo" that continues to pervade the Puerto Rican table. In the current social-cultural context, when the craving for meat can be relieved simply by making a trip to the supermarket, or by having a meal in one of the *Ponderosa* or *Bonanza* steakhouses located across the island, it challenges the imagination to realize that there was once a time when the consumption of meat had become an activity monopolized by the privileged few. At the end of the eighteenth century, the possibility of obtaining meat became increasingly difficult for the general population, and by the close of the nineteenth century, it was all but impossible.

From the vantage point of enjoying meat as part of one's diet, the last quarter of the eighteenth century marks a break from the pattern which had prevailed up to that point. For the island's most rural inhabitants, and for its thousands of immigrants—whether illegal, voluntary, or involuntary, whether military deserters or exiles—all of whom contributed appreciably to the rise in the colony's population at this stage of Puerto Rican history—the possibilities of obtaining meat would become more and more difficult as livestock began to be guarded so that the burgeoning population of the capital could continue to be fed. Between 1775 and 1800, San Juan reaffirmed its role as a "ciudad garganta," ever more dependent—as the population of slaves, soldiers, and free individuals living within its walls continued to grow—on foodstuffs brought in from the mountains ranges without.

The opening wedge of the break first appeared in 1757, when the colony's military governor, Felipe Ramírez de Estenós, presented a plan to San Juan's municipal council and to the island's other administrative entities, for converting the colony's cattle ranches into ranches devoted to agricultural production.[53] In his proposal, Estenós argued that the cattle ranches closest to San Juan should be converted into ranches having combined production, that is, the production of crops as well as the raising of fattened cattle. He claimed that the meat from the cattle in the wild or open range herds was not of optimal quality "since the greater part of the land and the richest and finest parts are occupied by the herds and breeding operations which belong only to special individuals and, as is notorious, serve no purpose beyond what the weak and exhausted cattle contribute."[54] Estenós's argument contained an additional plank: that the military garrison in San Juan needed to be assured of a supply of both meat and products farmed from the land.[55] Over the coming years, however, his proposal would encounter opposition and a mountain of bureaucratic obstacles.[56] Only some three decades later, around 1786, did the boundaries of these enormous holdings begin to get demarcated and the land redistributed.[57]

According to Aida Caro Costa, it was during this period that San Juan's municipal council decided to adopt the system of "*reparto*" (a distributive system) in place of that known as "*exclusivas*" (a monopoly-based system), which had been used until then to furnish meat to the capital.[58] Traditionally, the latter gave a monopoly to a single *vecino*, or group of vecinos (typically, the vecinos of a municipality had more privileges—often serving on its council—than did simple residents, or *moradores*), to supply the city's butcher shops for a year, exempting this person or group from having to turn to any other proprietors, ranchers, or owners of large herds to guarantee such supplies. This system had its advocates, but the council went against them and adopted the system of reparto. Caro Costa explained the essentials of how it worked: "The system operated in the following manner. Once a year the cabildo, taking into consideration the number of vecinos living inside and around the city, including its detachment of soldiers, prepared an estimate of how many cattle and pigs it would be necessary to sacrifice in order to assure a daily supply of meat. Armed with this estimate, the cabildo proceeded to calculate, on a pro rata basis, the total number of livestock required from the administrative areas falling under its jurisdiction, taking into account the number of cattle herds, ranches and their sizes, as well as the breeding operations for cattle and for sheep, pigs, and goats, within each administrative area."[59]

She further noted that the reparto system acquired an obligatory character. Livestock owners, whether operating on a large or more modest scale, were required to participate in the system and supply their assigned quota. Quite apart from whether they were able to do so, the transition to this system more than likely meant that, whatever the size of their herd or ranch, they would need to maintain greater vigilance over the pigs or cattle they kept on their land, in order both to prevent the monteros from hunting and killing them and to meet their obligation. By comparing the number of cattle that particular municipalities contained with the corresponding number that the cabildo required them to supply each year, one can get a sense of just how carefully the livestock must have been watched over once this reform was implemented.[60]

In the reparto of 1764, for example, the number of cattle needed to keep the city supplied with enough meat for a year was estimated at 2,400 head. In the years just following, the jurisdiction of Aguada had to send three hundred head of cattle to help feed the residents of San Juan, a number that represented approximately 6.8 percent of its cattle population. The municipality of Toa Alta, located along the northern coast of the island, slightly to the west of San Juan, found itself in the same situation, as the reparto called for it to supply the capital with 6.1 percent of its total head of cattle.

Moreover, the demands made upon Aguada and Toa Alta were less severe than some others. For example, Toa Baja, which according to the 1765 census had 1,996 head of cattle, was obliged to send 240 head, or 8 percent of its total cattle population, to San Juan. The administrative jurisdiction of la Tuna, which the same census recorded as having barely 469 head of cattle, was required to part with 25, or 18 percent of its total number. The reparto system, which left cattle owners no option but to send a significant portion of their herds to San Juan, thus denying them the opportunity to sell those cattle to the highest bidder, led to regular, careful inspections. In this respect, the inclusion, in the ordinances issued for the capital in 1768, of proposals to organize and rationalize cattle-related matters outside of San Juan are most revealing.

Until the members of San Juan's municipal council issued this new set of ordinances, the regulations that governed the supply of food coming into the city had been in force, unrevised, since 1626. With respect to the provision of meat, the old statutes illustrated that the cabildo's concerns were more about where the meat was to be slaughtered and sold, and its prices, weighing, and quality, all calibrated within the context of an urban market. The only concern expressed regarding the supply, per se, of meat coming from the campo to the city was that "those who handle the livestock to be weighed in the butcher shops . . . bring it at the time that has been indicated."[61] Scarcely any mention was made, in the original statutes, about the breeding or hunting of animals beyond the city's walls, or—more particularly—about who could hunt them and where.

An important change was made in the statutes that the council issued in 1768. A lengthy chapter was added, entitled "*Del Gobierno para el Recinto y Fuera de la Ciudad*," that broke new ground.[62] The chapter included four subsections aimed at hedging in and regulating the breeding and hunting of animals in rural regions. The two most relevant to the city's concerns over its supply of meat are worth quoting at length:

> . . . In that many with the pretext of being owners of hunting operations, without possessing livestock nor a breeding operation, enter these areas to hunt, causing grave damages to the owners of the said property, and that the former are totally in possession of the benefits

of killing the livestock in them by constant hunting in times that are prohibited . . . no owners . . . even if they are in possession of them can enter the said hunting grounds to hunt without license from the owners of the said pastures, and under these conditions they cannot kill by hunting an animal that has been incorporated with the tame stock until such time as it separates from them and does not form a part of the herd with unleashed dogs under the penalty of a fine of fifty reales . . . in that the division of hunting operations into many and small groups has caused their complete ruin and eradication it has resulted in the former, who are the least interested in their worth, being those who generally take advantage of them, the hunting operation has no owner . . . he that would not be interested in it the quantity of twenty-five pesos . . . and that they cannot kill a female animal at times of bearing or nursing under the penalty of a fine of twenty-five reales . . .[63]

The conflict, although it certainly involved the interest of owners of livestock and breeding operations in protecting their herds and the physical integrity of their property, was more complex than it appeared on the surface.[64] At bottom, it had to do with the relationship that had evolved between campesinos and the colony's wild, open lands as well as with the ways in which they dealt with and hunted the animals that lived on these lands: there were thousands of rural settlers who would pass themselves off as owners of territory for the purposes of raising and hunting animals, although they never actually owned any livestock or breeding operations. Ultimately, however, the most far-reaching part of the 1768 statutory reform was that henceforth greater vigilance was exercised over who could hunt, where hunting could take place, how domestic livestock were to be raised and when they were to be killed, which wild animals might be killed, and more. The council's action marked a sea change, since for the first time in the island's history access to animals eaten for their flesh came under official regulation.[65] Meat began to be a foodstuff of the city, and within it, a luxury of the privileged few.

Paralleling this development was an effort made by the colony's capital to guarantee, at least "on paper," the provision of meat to the military garrison.

The island experienced a considerable increase in its military population during the last decades of the eighteenth century, when the threat of an

TABLE 6.2 Types of Food and Quantity of Same for the Military
Population*

Type of Food	Days during the Month	Quantity	Annually, in Pounds
Fresh meat	16	1 pound	192
Salted meat	9	10 ounces	67.5
Salted cod	5	5 ounces	18.7
Rice	30	3 ounces	65.6

*The soldiers also had to be furnished the following: oil (1 ounce when fish was served),
wine (approximately three-eighths of a liter per day), salt (1 fanega for each 1,000 men),
rum (approximately one quarter liter for each 6 men), firewood (3 pounds), and one
ounce of tobacco. The calculation is based on a 350-day year. See Ángel López Cantos,
"La vida cotidiana del negro en Puerto Rico en el siglo XVIII: Alimentación," 149.

English invasion was always close at hand. Bibiano Torres points out that,
starting in 1765, San Juan's standing battalion was reinforced on various
occasions by other regiments, including those from León, Toledo, Vito-
ria, Corona, Brussels, and Naples. As Torres notes, however, none of these
remained permanently on the island but were reassigned, at one stage or
another, to Spain or to other Spanish colonies in the Caribbean. In addition, although Torres does not specify the number of soldiers who made
up these regiments, he cites a figure of 12,000 militia during the times of
greatest military activity.[66] While their total doubtless fluctuated, 2,000
plus would be a decidedly conservative estimate of the number of soldiers
who were stationed in San Juan during periods when the prospect of invasion was greatest.

Table 6.2 shows the types of food and the respective quantities that were
furnished, on a monthly basis, to the garrison's soldiers during these years.
As can be seen, the garrison's leaders arrived at the figure of 260.5 pounds
of meat, salted and fresh, for its soldiers annually, with fresh meat much
preferred over salted. It is possible that this total, and its breakdown, were
intended to cover the standing battalion, and not the volunteer forces and
trained militia that the different administrative jurisdictions deployed, beginning in 1765.

Since Spain's colonies in the Caribbean were the scene of serious armed
conflict in the coming years, one can reasonably posit that the number of
soldiers stationed in Puerto Rico stayed at 2,000 or more. Thus, in the wan-
ing years of the eighteenth century, San Juan's authorities would have tried

to see that the garrison received close to 521,000 pounds of meat annually. This quantity was the equivalent of some 1,302 head of cattle directed, over a twelve-month period, to the military force alone.[67]

In 1770, San Juan's cabildo estimated that 10,000 head of cattle would be needed to supply the city with meat, "in the event it came under siege." That figure represented 73 percent of the large domestic animal population (cattle, horses, mules) on the island. It also meant that San Juan's population required annually, per person, 1.3 head of cattle within a total estimated population for the capital, in 1776, of 7,429. This provision of meat, albeit proposed to cover an emergency situation, lays bare San Juan's by then entrenched position as a "ciudad garganta." The expectations of the city's administrators, relative to the supply of meat that the capital needed, likely led the island's cattle ranchers to guard the cattle on their properties even more closely. That the colonial administration considered this matter to be of the utmost importance is evident in an order issued by the island's governor, Miguel de Muesas, categorically threatening anyone who sold cattle to foreigners with the death penalty.[68] Through such measures, the possibilities were sharply curtailed that those who lived in distant rural areas might obtain meat from time to time.

In their totality, these new policies entailed a profound shift in the social and economic history of Puerto Rico. Until this point, they were unforeseen and uncalled for in the thinking of the state and its administrative jurisdictions, since a balance had always existed between the island's human population and the animals that were killed for their flesh, and because—given the circumstances—the rural population had from a practical standpoint never found it necessary to use agricultural resources to their full capacity. The new policies, however, had an even wider effect, for they presaged a decisive turn in the history of nutrition and dietary practice on the island.

As the state began to reorient its thinking, viewing the campo as a source of food organized around the dual enterprise of "agriculture and livestock breeding and raising," with a handful of cities designated as the recipients of these fruits, the colony's general dietary pattern was reordered, socially and qualitatively. From this point on, the island's rural inhabitants began to rely on agriculture and what they themselves could farm, while meat products were increasingly redirected into urban areas, San Juan in particular. The rural diet revolved more and more around crops that produced good yields and had nutritional worth. Meat consumption in the campo became more sporadic, an event connected to rituals of social solidarity and the celebration of unexpected good fortune or of festival days. The practice followed by rural families of keeping some pigs fenced in, to assure themselves of the occasional meal of pork, must have started in this period as well, giving rise to the traditional image of the pig roasted on a spit as a ritual and centerpiece of festive celebrations. Along with these trends, the opportunity of rural folk to consume fresh beef shrank more and more, until it was seen to be out of reach, a privilege denied them.

Within urban populations, the provision of food from the campo—and of beef in particular—came to be seen, in time, as a nutritional prerogative; a natural expectation that assumed the aura of the inevitable. Nevertheless, for those living in cities, the distribution of meat was characterized by clear inequalities, inequalities that were destined to become more sharply defined during the first decades of the nineteenth century.

Meat: The Fulfillment of a Food Fantasy

In 1826, more than a hundred day laborers from the area surrounding the neighborhood district of Algarrobo, located in the western coastal municipality of Mayagüez, decided to divide up the meat from a cow that had fallen ill and just died from "*llaguita*" (subcutaneous infection caused by flies laying eggs on the animals's hide) The workers decided to share the meat among themselves, despite knowing full well that the local cattle were suffering from this strange illness. A description of their action forms part of the report that Andrés López Medrano, a physician and the health officer for the jurisdiction of Mayagüez, sent to the island's governor, Miguel de la Torre, who had tasked the physician with investigating the epidemic.[69]

> At the beginning of the month of March . . . , in the district of Algarrobo, not very far from this pueblo, in an area near the estate of the deceased D. José Salinas . . . , a cow that some people were milking suddenly fell down dead, having just suffered, for a minute or two, a tremendous shuddering. The milkers, taking in its healthy size and good build, and wanting to believe that it had not perished from a disease, requested permission from its owner, Gaspar González, to make use of the meat; and he replied that after they gave him the hide and tallow, they could do what they wished, averring that he would not like any food such as that. Hearing this, some became suspicious about satisfying their appetite at the cost of being in the dark; but the

less fastidious, or the most eager to have the free food offered by this turn of events, had made up their minds, and with others from the vicinity coming around to carry off their own portion, the cow was distributed among more than one hundred individuals.

In another part of the report, Medrano stated that the day laborer Alejo Matos, who helped to "skin" the cow, took some pieces of meat that had been torn off the animal so that eight members of his family could enjoy a meal. All those living in the area, as well as Matos's family, were sickened and poisoned by the flesh. The physician ended his report by alluding to another incident of food poisoning, caused by the ingestion of the remains of a cow infected by the same illness, that occurred in the area surrounding Mayagüez's beachfront. According to Medrano: "[O]ne of the seven oxen that died on the estate of don José Vigo was thrown into the sea; during the night, the waves having washed it up onto the shore, or its having run aground in the sand, four blacks, their master not having warned them, sliced off a piece of the flesh and ate it, and soon thereafter they began to entertain the unfortunate consequences of their little repast."[70]

The question looms—why lose control, suspend judgment, give way to the irrational impulses of the moment, in order to share and eat the remains of some meat known to be contaminated? The events described by Medrano suggest an almost frenzied desire on the part of day laborers and slaves to satisfy their unfulfilled cravings for meat, brought on by having endured prolonged periods without the presence of any meat or fat in their diet. They further suggest that such satisfaction lay in the meat from cattle. The behavior vis-à-vis food reported by Medrano marks two beginnings: the unequal and sporadic access to meat, especially beef, among the Puerto Rican population, and the adoption of the pig as the vehicle through which to fulfill a gastronomic fantasy.

The vicissitudes surrounding the availability and consumption of meat in Puerto Rico during the nineteenth and early part of the twentieth century are closely bound up with a series of broad-scale developments: population growth; the development of export-based monoculture along the island's coasts, which in turn altered and redirected the use of land heretofore given over to ranches and breeding operations for livestock; the transformation of the historic habitat of wild pigs owing to the development of coffee cultivation in the mountainous interior of the island; the failure, by and large, to renew cattle herds by introducing new species, which caused the degen-

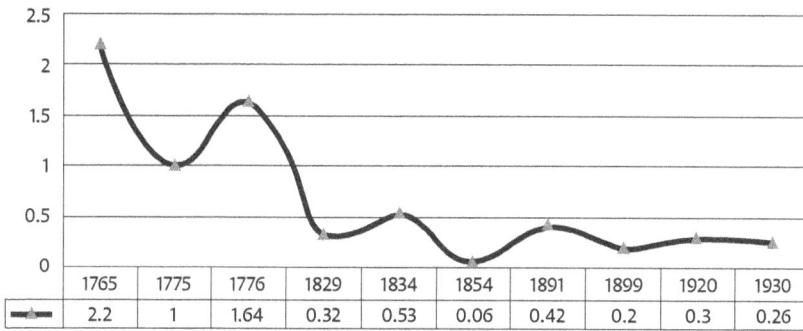

	1765	1775	1776	1829	1834	1854	1891	1899	1920	1930
▬▬	2.2	1	1.64	0.32	0.53	0.06	0.42	0.2	0.3	0.26

FIGURE 6.1 Per capita availability of heads of livestock for consumption, in rough numbers, 1765–1930

Sources: O'Reilly, Miyares, Iñigo Abad, Pedro Tomás de Córdoba, Acosta, López Tuero, Henry K. Carroll, and United States Bureau of the Census, 15th Census, 1930. Note: To calculate Miyares's figures, I have used the number of inhabitants reported by Iñigo Abad because the former excludes both slaves and soldiers.

eration of the breeds and resulted in cattle that were weak and unhealthy; the lack of emphasis on treating the raising of cattle used in agriculture as a business; and the practice of breeding cattle not for their use as a source of meat but for their employment as draught animals in agriculture.[71] Between the end of the eighteenth and beginning of the twentieth century, the number of cattle potentially available to be slaughtered for consumption was significantly reduced.

Consequently, throughout the nineteenth and into the first part of the twentieth century, beef as a source of meat in the diet became a distant prospect for the rural population. It is not that it ceased entirely to be consumed in rural areas, but that families in the countryside turned instead to breeding and raising pigs as the way of having meat to consume throughout the year, if only sporadically.

Under these circumstances, pigs became virtually the sole source of meat for both campesinos and urban day laborers. From this point forward, moreover, pigs ceased to be game that were hunted in the mountains and brought back, admiringly, as the fruit of a collective effort; rather, they were understood in strictly functional terms, as domestic livestock that got raised for a certain period of time and then killed, always in the satisfaction of some purpose deemed to be more important than their own lives: to provide sustenance and nourishment, or help bolster the family budget, or make some community celebration, and the meal that accompanied it, a more pleasurable occasion for all. In the hands of campesinos, the killing of a pig, the seasoning of hefty pieces of pork, and the preparation of blood sausages, white pudding, and spicy sausages, always had a communal aspect and were done, by friends and neighbors, with the intention of preserving the meat and sharing what was left. The pig might also be used in trade, sold to the company store of a plantation or in the city market. Toward the end of the nineteenth century, around 1890 and after, it became the custom among the affluent young to breakfast on—among other fine foods—roast pork, crackling and blood sausages, which were brought to San Juan's market square by "*madamas cangrejeras.*"[72]

At other times, undaunted by possible future shortages of food, people slaughtered a pig, in order to express their sense of communal spirit and because they simply felt like celebrating the joy of being alive. Everyone reveled in this moment of plenty, filling themselves until their stomachs ached: "The plates were licked all clean / stuffed to the gills we were / no more than the pig bones left behind / also those from the ham / . . . What a bellyful a Christian had! / who said no more can I / Oh what a gullet full! / to touch the food I can / that with the fingers of my hands!."[73]

So strong was the impulse to indulge that the pig was consumed even though it was known to be ill or carrying a disease. Perillo, the rustic from the heartland in the comic theatrical piece "La triquina," falls sick for having gorged himself at his uncle's wedding: "They had killed a plump one / spicy sausage, crackling pigskin / and plantains and tostones / meat pies of the finest / and for each blood sausage chunks / . . . with half an almud of lard / and of broth a cask-sized portion / that so Christ can tempted be / to have a gluttonous feast.[74]" By the close of the nineteenth century, however much they may have dreamed of eating beef, the island's rural inhabitants had settled contentedly on pork.

When organized by the wealthier farmers, the slaughtering of a pig was a way to make good on unfulfilled promises; it was a paternalistic gesture, symbolizing power and conveying kind-heartedness, the ensuing feast always taking place under the realization, known to all, that the campesinos' options for consuming meat had become little more than a dream. Indeed, it was this reality that underlay the traditional festival of "*acabe*" held annually by the large coffee plantation owners, in the highlands of the central mountain range, to celebrate the end of the harvest.

On the sugar plantations along the coast, beef—in contrast to pork—was offered as a way of soothing and tamping down the grievances of slaves who were never given more than skimpy amounts of meat. In 1843, the hacendado José Martínez, accused by the slave Blas Candelario of not providing those who served him an adequate diet, rose to his own defense, arguing that on Thursdays and Sundays, his slaves received "*mondongo de res*" (the cow's tripe), and that "during the Christmas holidays he had a cow killed just for them, on top of their usual portion of food."[75] When—as was the case in Puerto Rico—access to meat products was sharply differentiated along class and geographic lines, the pig's entrails—kidneys, heart, liver, lungs, tripe—the so-called offal—the innards—or the extremities—feet, tail, ears, head—almost always ended up on the tables of the most disadvantaged.

The fantasy continued unabated. In addition, as the population of the cities kept expanding, the image of the pig as an unclean animal whose meat was insalubrious[76] gained wider currency. In line with this development, the pig not only came to be viewed as repugnant within urban settings, but it was also associated with diseases such as trichinosis and cholera. If the only prohibition in 1821 was that un-penned pigs could not freely root about through the streets of villages and towns, by the middle of the nineteenth century more stringent regulations were in place, and pigs were not allowed to be bred and raised inside city boundaries. In 1859, three years after an outbreak of morbid cholera spread across the island, taking 10,000 lives, pigsties were declared to be unhealthy and, as a consequence, could legally be located only on the outskirts of pueblos, at a distance of no less than 160 meters from any residence.[77]

A school of thought which viewed the consumption of beef as a measure of the civil, moral, and physical advancement of campesinos cast a further shadow over the image of the pig: "Mastery over the world belongs to those who eat beef and draw in oxygen for the satisfaction of their lungs, Pelletan has stated . . . , and beef is a luxury item for Puerto Rican campesinos."[78]

The negative view held by some about eating the meat of animals already compromised by their appearance and condition also came into play, and in this regard, pigs—given their potential to transmit trichinosis—were exhibit A. In his booklet, *Cartilla de higiene para las escuelas públicas*, the physician Francisco del Valle Atiles recommended that: "Meat that comes from sick animals should not be eaten; nor is it suitable to make use of the meat of animals that are scrawny or exhausted from overwork, nor of meat that has not been bled, and even less so meat that has gone bad or begun to decompose. The veterinarians are in charge . . . of seeing that cattle invaded by illnesses are not slaughtered . . . In addition to this practice, which has been adopted by all civilized countries . . . where there is any doubt it serves to subject the meat to being cooked under a high temperature, in order to kill any germs, such as those associated with tapeworm, trichinosis, etc. [sic] dangerous as they are to our health."[79]

Among those who weighed in on the matter, the agronomist López Tuero was the only one who viewed pigs differently, but he qualified his more positive outlook by declaring that pigs should be fed with corn, which produced a healthier meat, in the form of "hams and well prepared sausages, like those of Extremadura and Murcia." Only if consumed in this form would "pork make a contribution to the public diet, even though there are many people who have an aversion to this meat."[80]

The unlikelihood that meat would be part of meals became progressively greater during the last decades of the nineteenth century, until the wave washed over *jornaleros* within even more distant, rugged areas of the cordillera. A study made of wills registered in the central-western mountain municipality of Lares during the period 1849–1899 reveals a decline, as of 1870, in the number of livestock passed down to family members or others. The downward trend, which persisted until the end of the century, affected the inheritance of pigs especially.[81] Around 1898, for example, the small mountain town of Adjuntas, to the east of Lares, counted relatively few head of cattle—only 980—but the number of pigs found in the community was dramatically lower, a mere 21, in a population that exceeded 18,700 inhabitants.[82] As Fernando Picó has underlined, the opportunities that jornaleros had to consume meat were essentially reduced to days, and only those days, on which a domestic pig was slaughtered.

Now, however, the meat from the slaughtered pig was less likely to be shared among the community, but instead was increasingly secured by some profit-minded cynic, the *"mata puercos"* (pig killer) who in turn sold it either to middlemen or directly to jornaleros anxious to fulfill their craving for the taste of meat. The infrequency with which meat, above all pigs, figured in the diet at times distorted the consumption of roast pork into a grotesque Rabelaisian affair in which every part of the animal was wolfed down in a communal feast. The images of indulgence and festiveness which suffuse roast pig and its consumption in contemporary Puerto Rico trace back to the fervent desire of campesinos to take every advantage of the rare, splendid occasion on which the animal was there to be eaten, a momentary abundance associated with the powerful in society, those who enjoyed the luxury of eating fresh meat regularly. It was these extremes and antecedents which drew the following observation by an anonymous critic: "What people really love in Puerto Rico is to eat roast suckling pig; no one imagines a country outing, a picnic, or a meal among friends without a roast pig being the main attraction or sometimes even the only dish; but it is not the six or seven-day old suckling pig, weighing a kilo and a half, that gets eaten on the peninsula [Spain], but a pig that is a good many months old and weighs more than one *arroba* [24 to 36 pounds], and, by the way, those Puerto Rican women who are close to the soil do it up and season it with real flair."[83]

Other Options for Consuming Meat

During the nineteenth century, those who either had no hope of obtaining fresh meat (excepting pork) or found it beyond their capacity to preserve very effectively what little they had,[84] turned to salted meat of one sort or another. For example, "tasajo" (dried cured beef) or the extremities of the pig were exported from countries with more developed agricultural and food processing industries to countries, colonies, and territories like Puerto Rico.

Both Brazil and Argentina seem to have been sources of dried beef for the island.[85] The amount of it imported increased as the size of the population subject to regulated, homogeneous diets increased on Caribbean islands under Spanish control,[86] as the possibility of raising domestic livestock decreased for most of the rural population,[87] and as the food importation market penetrated and drew in other commercial networks, those encompassing Uruguayan and Argentinian dried beef in particular.[88] Selected nineteenth-century import figures are shown in figures 6.2 and 6.3.

Near the end of the nineteenth century, a pound of dried beef could cost between 6.4 cents, as it did in the municipality of Aguadilla in 1896, or 8 cents, as in the municipality of Ceiba, or up to 9.8 cents—the amount it cost in the municipality of Cabo Rojo in 1895.[89] At the same time, 4 ounces of dried beef—the amount that ordinarily would be found on the plates of the poorest Puerto Ricans—cost approximately 2.4 cents. For many families on the island, dried beef came to function much as salted cod had; it was added to other food purely as a way to increase both taste and fat content.

Throughout the nineteenth century, the extremities of the pig, or smoked pork, or pork conserved in brine, took their place alongside dried beef as a way to consume meat when fresh meat was too costly for the fam-

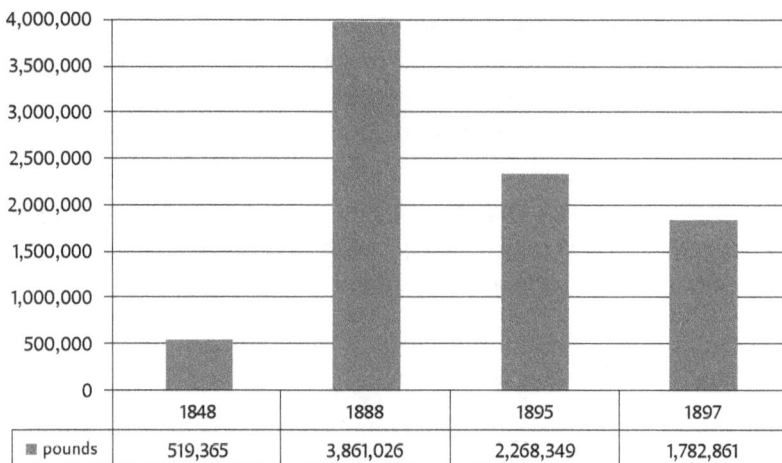

■ pounds	1848	1888	1895	1897
	519,365	3,861,026	2,268,349	1,782,861

FIGURE 6.2 Dried (jerked) beef imports in millions of pounds
Source: Centro de Investigaciones Históricas de la Universidad de Puerto Rico, *Balanzas mercantiles*, Selected Years, 1848–1897.

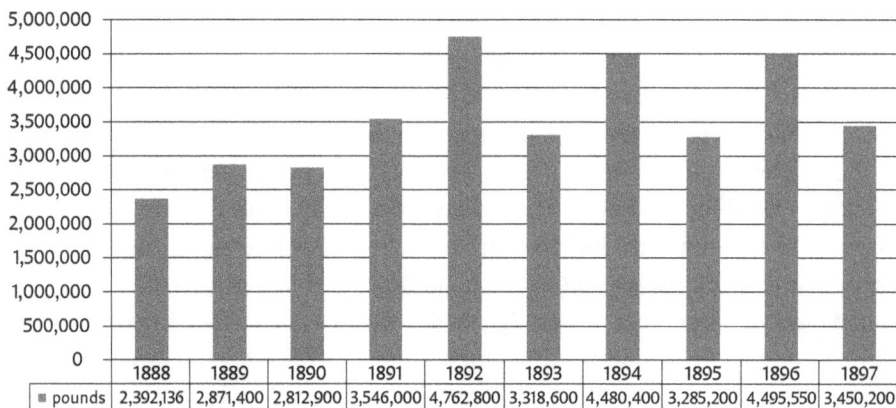

■ pounds	1888	1889	1890	1891	1892	1893	1894	1895	1896	1897
	2,392,136	2,871,400	2,812,900	3,546,000	4,762,800	3,318,600	4,480,400	3,285,200	4,495,550	3,450,200

FIGURE 6.3 Pork by-product imports in millions of pounds
Source: Frank H. Hitchcock, *Trade of Puerto Rico*, Washington, D.C.: Government Printing Office, 1898, 33.

ily budget. The main supplier of these products was the United States. Although figures for their cost no longer exist, import data indicate that the extremities of the pig found a solid market in the last years of the century, overtaking—in numerical terms—the use of dried beef among the population.

Meat: A Ticket to Progress

In one of the last measures that it took before Spanish rule came to an end on the island five years later, San Juan's municipal council allowed the price of meat from pigs, goats, and sheep slaughtered in the city to float free of the price set on the basis of auctions of beef, whose cost was always the highest.[90] As much as anything, this generous move on the part of the cabildo underscored the inequalities in the patterns of meat consumption among the population, a dietary problem which only a few years hence would have to be confronted by the colonial administration installed by the United States.

The General Order of 18 July 1899, issued by the island's U.S. military governor, George W. Davis, permitting the unfettered killing and sale of livestock, was evidently designed to calm the clamorings of the public with respect to the difficulty of purchasing meat at reasonable prices. The first part of the Order prohibited the sale of fresh meat through auctions, and the third allowed refrigerated meat to be brought into any municipality without the levying and collection of duties.[91]

The idea first elaborated by enlightened elements in nineteenth-century Puerto Rico, that the consumption of meat by a society formed part of its march toward progress, continued not only to find adherents during the first decades of the twentieth century but to get argued even more emphatically as classes in cooking began to be introduced into the public school curriculum. While it was thought that Puerto Rico's hot climate probably made it best to eat meat in moderation, the capacity of meat, as opposed to vegetables, to produce a sturdy musculature was an article of faith: "It [meat] builds firmer muscle in the human body than a diet of vegetables, but is more heating" stated the cooking manual, Home Making.[92] Coupled with this belief that the right food helped pave the way to social and material progress[93] was an interest, anchored more in practical than theoretical and moral considerations, in experimenting scientifically with the basic Puerto Rican diet.[94] Similarly, the first recipes compiled for cooking classes in the public schools were gathered from upper class homes, where meat was a regular part of the diet.[95] As a result, meat continued to be thought of as essential to the formation of a sound constitution, even though most Puerto Ricans consumed it only occasionally if at all.

This view of meat as utterly necessary to a successful diet moderated some during the years of the First World War, when the public school home economics curriculum deemphasized it to a certain degree, while elevating the importance of other foodstuffs produced on the island, such as milk, eggs, and beans, which could be used as substitutes for meat.[96] Viandas, too, were endorsed for their nutritional value in home economics classes.

However, the old idea that no meal was complete without a prominent serving of meat returned to the fore at the end of the 1920s, when the island's school dining hall program was launched. A guide prepared for the public schools, the *Manual del comedor escolar*, set out a menu of thirty meals, with meat as the central food in six and an important component (replaced in certain dishes by some extremity of the pig) in a number of others.[97]

The Naked Reality

Despite this renewed focus on meat and a visible increase in the importation of salted, refrigerated, and even canned meats,[98] the true picture of meat consumption on the island was quite different. Department of Agriculture studies carried out between 1937 and 1940 estimated the annual per capita consumption of fresh beef and fresh pork at 15 and 6 pounds, respectively. When broken down by geographic area and region, the per capita consumption of fresh beef was much greater in San Juan—56 pounds annually, or approximately 4.66 pounds per month. In twenty-two urban areas outside of San Juan, the comparable annual figure was estimated at 35 pounds, or 2.91 pounds per month. In the island's rural zones, the estimated annual per capita consumption of beef declined sharply, dropping to 2 pounds, or only 0.16 pounds per month.[99] The tale can also be told in terms of the island's hog population, which at the beginning of the 1930s was estimated at 69,266,[100] versus a figure of 47,906 at the end of the eighteenth century, when the number of people living in the colony was much smaller.

Domestic animals continued to dot the landscape, but—for the majority of Puerto Ricans—raising and making use of livestock was increasingly associated not with personal consumption but with some other modality, for example, using the few pieces of meat from a slaughtered pig to obtain other food that spoiled less easily and went further in terms of volume. In a study she carried out several years after the Second World War ended, the nutritionist Lydia Roberts discovered that in a sample group of 601 families in the rural zone, 33 percent bred and raised pigs.[101] Yet only half of this smaller group, or 16.8 percent of all the families, killed pigs as a source of food for themselves, and only 11.1 percent, or some 67 families, kept three-quarters or more of the pig meat for their own consumption.

The figures for poultry were roughly the same. While 70 percent of rural families raised hens, only 24 percent used ten or more of their hens as sustenance for their table.[102] Less than a quarter of rural families, or 23.1 percent, raised cows, the majority of which were kept as milk cows, but they produced remarkably little: Roberts found that only 4.2 percent of the families in her sample group obtained, per cow, at least three quarts of milk per day—a comparatively meager amount.[103]

The situation in the cities contrasted sharply with that in the campo. Out of a sample group of 443 families (2,107 individuals), only 7.9 percent raised pigs. Roberts concluded that "in the urban zone, most of the few pigs kept are sold rather than killed, except in the top income bracket where about half of the families kill some for food."[104]

With regard to the purchase of meat in urban zones, 37 percent could afford the luxury of buying meat at least once per week. On the other hand, nearly a fifth of urban families, or 19.5 percent, found it impossible to buy fresh meat and were categorized, in the sample, as those who purchased it "seldom or never."[105]

For a great many Puerto Ricans, then, the consumption of meat was increasingly tied to another dietary question: what food provided the greatest volume at the lowest cost. This and related considerations operated in the context of low wages and salaries, seasonal unemployment, internal migration and population shifts, and an agricultural system organized around latifundia. From the start of the twentieth century until well into the 1940s, obtaining and eating fresh meat, even if only on Sundays, became a veritable luxury: "Pigs are usually regarded as an almost certain asset of farm families, and even urban families on the edge of town with space to keep them frequently do so. Pigs can be fed largely from food waste; they grow rapidly; and when killed, they supply fresh meat for the family table and lard to be used for cooking." Thus did Roberts introduce the section on pigs in her study of food and daily life in late 1940s Puerto Rico. She was careful, however, to add the following qualifier: "In Puerto Rico, however, only a small proportion of families, even rural ones, have this home source of food."[106]

The image of the roast pig as the center and high spot of fiestas and celebrations continued to be reinforced, and to eat it in the glow of such events demonstrated that conditions of plenty were still possible, if only for a passing moment.[107] One year after Roberts completed her study, Eric Wolf—while in the midst of his own investigation of a Puerto Rican coffee community—recognized the symbolism of festive communal celebration associated with the sacrifice and consumption of a pig. Yet he also saw that the campesino population, in order to have pieces of pork to eat at a celebration, had come to depend on the "mata puercos," the small-time rural businessman who, in the context of a general absence of meat, intervened (as we saw earlier)—by cynically using his power and money—to make the dream of tasting and eating meat a reality for poor peasants and townsfolk. Among these people, the mata puercos was a despised figure:

> In addition to the small rural shopkeeper and to the itinerant trader, a third type of person concerned with marketing in the rural area is the pig-killer (*mata-cerdos*). He buys pigs from the peasants, slaughters them, and sells their meat in pieces for festive occasions. Usually the pig-killer produces only on order, rather than for an open market. His occupation carries a slight stigma. The term *mata-cerdos* is usually pronounced with contempt, perhaps because the pig-killer is an agricultural laborer who ekes out an income by tapping the resources of peasants who are in bad financial straits and who must sell their pigs. A pig is not only an animal. It represents about twenty dollars of accumulated savings. The pig-killer benefits by the financial misery of his neighbors.[108]

The increased availability of salted meat, or of less desirable parts of animals, expanded the options for eating meat, with much of this alternative selection imported from the United States. Toward the end of the 1890s, 3,450,000 pounds of salted pig, or pig preserved in brine, were imported from the U.S., a figure which less than four decades later had jumped to 11,752,000 pounds.[109] The availability of such processed meat, however, was tied to the priorities of the import trade and to price oscillations in the food commodities market.[110] Canned meat proved to be the best option, and by 1935 7,799,000 pounds of it were imported into Puerto Rico.[111] Under the war-time food rationing policies of the 1940s, as the uncertain supply of other types of meat took its toll on public school dining halls, canned meat was able to fill the gaps. The importance of public school dining halls was underscored in studies carried out by Luz Loriana Aponte, who compiled figures showing that during the 1945–46 scholastic year, the school lunch program in Puerto Rico served 29,603,203 lunches annually to a student population numbering 179,812.[112]

From the point of view of the consumption of meat by Puerto Ricans, however, the most surprising part of her study was her finding that the lunch program enabled a majority of students to eat certain types of meat for the first time, among them such canned meats as "beef stew," "chopped ham," "corned beef," "corned beef hash," "pork and luncheon meat," and "Vienna sausages." By the end of the 1940s, many students between the ages of twelve and eighteen managed to try small offerings of meat which, quite possibly, they had never had the opportunity of eating before. In the research leading to his essay "Cañamelar," Sidney Mintz also came to this realization, when he detected the clear difference between what the children of sugar estate workers ate at home and what they ate in their school dining hall:

> The school lunch program provides hundreds of Cañamelar children with their lunches everyday. The menus are worked out centrally, put together with emphasis on what is dietetically regarded as a "balanced" diet. It is a common experience to find children refusing some items of these lunches which are unfamiliar to them. But the rule has it that a pupil must eat all his lunch in order to get the lunch at all. Granted that this may occasionally cause discomfort to a child, it is usually possible to develop in children a liking for the new diet. Families in Barrio Poyal are extremely enthusiastic about the school lunch program. Children continue to eat the "culturally standardized" diet at home and the school lunches at school.[113]

Toward the Shaping of a New Meat-Consuming Society

When the focus is shifted to more recent times, we are confronted with a central question: how and why have Puerto Ricans, on average, come to consume some 45.7 pounds of beef annually, as occurred in 2010?[114] Similarly, why has the annual per capita consumption of pork risen, as it has, to 52.4 pounds?[115] Obviously, the answer does not lie in a sudden reprise of the favorable conditions which prevailed between the sixteenth and eighteenth century, yet the ability of Puerto Ricans to consume meat on an almost daily basis seems to have occurred virtually overnight. Broadly

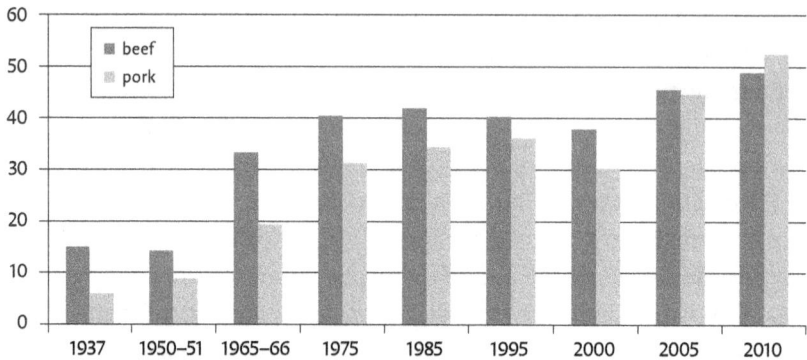

FIGURE 6.4 Annual per capita consumption, in pounds, of beef and pork

Sources: Descartes et al., *Food Consumption Studies*; Departamento de Agricultura, Oficina de Estadísticas Agrícolas, *Consumo de alimentos en Puerto Rico, 1950/51–1973/74*, vol. 2, *Productos pecuarios*; ibíd., *Consumo de carnes en Puerto Rico, 1975–2010*, folder 1158c9 (beef and mutton, fresh and frozen), folder 1159c10 (pork, fresh and frozen).

speaking, in the mid-1930s, the per capita consumption of fresh beef and fresh pork was 15 and 6 pounds, respectively;[116] by 1957–58, the comparable figure for beef and veal combined was 18.5 pounds, and 12.1 for pork. In subsequent decades, the figures continued to climb.

In terms of how Puerto Ricans relate to the food they eat, on both material and symbolic levels, as food pure and simple and as an image representing something else, it is undoubtedly meat—out of all the categories of food treated thus far—which has experienced the greatest modification. These changes run the gamut from a more frequent appearance in the daily meals of a majority of Puerto Ricans, to an improvement in the quality and variety of cuts of meat, to the adoption of new ways of eating, preparing, and representing meat socially and nutritionally. A series of factors analyzed in earlier chapters underlay some of these changes.

Yet, when meat is examined from the dual perspective of being a "desired food" as well as a nutritionally complete food, the origin of its high rates of consumption and its new symbolic meanings lies in the democratization of the diet which began to take shape at the end of the 1950s. With this development, the majority of Puerto Ricans could begin to experience the satisfaction of sating their appetite for particular foods. The social leveling of the diet was crystallized in the nutritional policies adopted as part of a campaign to reform and modernize the island's economy. These policies were also tied to an image of meat as a symbol of progress—an image, as we have seen, first popularized in the late nineteenth century—and to its association with the virtues of productivity and efficiency. The urbaniza-tion of society also aided in democratizing patterns of food consumption. As having meat and other once-scarce products became a reality for the majority of Puerto Ricans, a new etiquette toward food emerged, born out of the desire to eat what for so long had been the privilege of the few. This complex of factors was buttressed by other critical developments: the agro-industrial advances of the 1950s, which made it possible to acquire different grades of meat, free of the loop that had historically enclosed its consumption (hunting, killing, slaughtering, preserving, distributing); the "specialization" of the economy of food in Puerto Rico, linked to the devel-opment of supermarkets, with their shelves of fresh and frozen meat, be-tween 1955 and 1965; a rise in the general standard of living, which created better opportunities to eat well outside the home; and the implementation of nutritional assistance programs by the state.

Together, all of these factors were a necessary but not sufficient answer to the question: why did the diet of most Puerto Ricans include so much more meat so quickly? Claude Fischler contends that the longer the human organism goes without eating, the more it is inclined to prefer both some type of meat and food that is high in fat, in contrast to how it manifests its preferences when it receives food every day. Fischler asserts that "whether we feel full and satisfied or deprived and dissatisfied has a palpable effect on the formation or evolution of our tastes in food."[117] Could the marked preference for food, such as meat, that is high in fat and calories be the human organism's immediate response to a perennial state of uncertainty over the availability of meat, thus leading to our present elevated state of "carnivorismo," or pronounced urge to consume meat? There is a certain logic and coherence to this idea, since the ingestion of lipids does impart a sense of satisfaction in the person consuming them. In broad terms, how-ever, when was the desire to satisfy the hunger for a particular food ever laid to rest? Is not the hungering for such tastes and flavors always renewed?

We will find a cogent answer in the cultural sphere. In centuries past, the nineteenth in particular, the consumption of meat—above all beef—was associated with health, dietetics, and a certain idea of what it meant to be "civilized." Indeed, meat—like wine—was one of the foods that was recommended for treating people who were ill or who felt lethargic. Eating meat was prescribed as the way to gain "weight," or "fatten up." It was a sign of success, of economic solvency, and of family stability; linked—in a lasting way—with those who enjoyed social and economic advantage. For this same sector of the population, the rules of good practice, of dietary common sense, also dictated that meat should be consumed in moderation.[118] Advice to this effect, however, was evidence more of its excessive consumption by the wealthy than their observance of a disciplined restraint.

The democratization of the diet likewise created the possibility of making meat one of its central components. For the majority of the population, eating meat not only entailed satisfying the hunger to taste a particular food; it also represented something higher, more intangible—that one was in tune with the spirit of the times, had advanced socially, had partaken of the progress brought by urbanization and enjoyed the fruits of improved nutrition. All of these changes, material and otherwise, took place within the span of some thirty years.

The vertiginous growth in the intake of meat has engendered and helped shape new thinking and practices with respect to its consumption. One of these is its shift from playing a peripheral role in meals to becoming a principal component. Moreover, as eating meat ceased, starting in the late 1950s, to be a sign and symbol of privilege,[119] a new food ethic has emerged and gained a footing on the island. Its proponents, drawn from different sectors of Puerto Rican society, believe it wrong to eat meat on the grounds that doing so harms the ecological balance, violates the natural rights of animals, is nutritionally unsound, and furthers world-wide inequalities in the distribution of food. The proposals they have made to remedy this situation[120] have received a cool greeting on the part of most Puerto Ricans, who find the premises and justifications too inflexible and too insistent on a radical separation of nature and culture.[121] Those who are receptive to part of the message, but either cannot make the switch to full vegetarianism or find the claims about the dietetic wonders that accompany a complete renunciation of meat to be exaggerated or utopian, have sometimes taken a middle course, limiting themselves to eating poultry, fish, dairy products, and nuts.[122] Ultimately, all of these standpoints, and the tensions between them, reflect a shared desire to improve and rationalize diet and nutrition generally.

Yet so long as the effort persists to spell out and concretize a new relationship between humanity and meat—the food so prominently missing in the diets of the majority of islanders from the early nineteenth century on—the saying quoted at the top of this chapter, "Rice, please! . . . There's a load of meat," will still receive its due in Puerto Rico.

7 | Are We Still What We Ate?

In the four decades from 1960 to the start of the new millennium, Puerto Rico experienced a groundswell of socioeconomic development that helped transform the gastronomic landscape, radically changing the types and variety of foodstuffs available, as well as the ways in which they were acquired and then prepared, cooked, and brought to the table. Since the mid-1950s, Puerto Ricans have come to know firsthand the blessings (or otherwise) of consumer capitalism, their lives ever more intertwined with automobiles, private residences, television sets, and—not least—new kitchen appliances. Indicative of this trend were the figures for refrigerators and freezers imported onto the island for domestic use. During 1956–57, the total reached 35,327; by 1961–62, it had climbed to 58,271. A similar rise occurred with respect to electric stoves imported from the United States. The figures for 1956–57 and 1964–65 were 9,182 and 17,250, respectively. The inclination on the part of Puerto Ricans to replace and upgrade cooking and kitchen appliances, stoves and refrigerators in particular, has continued into the new century. In 1999, 21,654 stoves were imported from the United States, and in 2001, the island received 77,332 refrigerators from that country.[1]

Similarly, whereas in 1956 only thirteen markets in Puerto Rico were classified as *supermercados*, by 1998 there were 441 such establishments, 221 of which fell into the category of *hipermercado*.[2] In addition, food assistance programs were augmented significantly during this period. In 1960, 120,000 Puerto Rican families benefited directly from nutritional aid provided by the government; by 2007, this figure had more than tripled, to 509,339 families, or about 1,078,822 recipients.[3]

In contrast to past eras, when changes in the basic diet came about slowly and seemed all of a piece, or were constituted by only one discreet thing (the appearance of a new food, or a single structural transformation), the decades between 1950 and 2010 have been the scene of multiple, complex, and overlapping changes, including: the mass production and supply chain distribution of foodstuffs produced in Puerto Rico and on the mainland; higher personal and family income levels—especially between 1950 and 1980, though the pattern has reversed in recent years, with a rise in the number of families living under the poverty line;[4] the increased availability of foodstuffs, in comparison to earlier times when hunger and the possibility of famine confronted large segments of the population, which in turn has boosted the number of overweight and obese adults and children to 66 and 32 percent of the population, respectively;[5] the development of a distinctly urban food culture, which has borrowed from, adapted, and absorbed the cuisines of other countries and regions; the "specialization" of cooking; the emergence and embedding of a new and almost uncontrolled fast food restaurant culture; and the expansion and homogenization of food production. Furthermore, these and other challenging and sometimes contradictory transformations have taken place against the backdrop of a stagnating local agricultural output and a lopsided dependence on food imports. In 1950, 1,904,000 *cuerdas* of land were dedicated to agriculture; in 2007 this figure had been reduced by more than two-thirds, to 557,530.[6] Unsurprisingly, then, in 2008 Puerto Rico imported 740.2 million pounds of food, while producing only 147 million pounds on the island.[7] The transformative effect of these changes is everywhere visible; yet if one enlarges the field of vision and examines them in light of other factors, such as notions about food in the popular imagination, the use and consumption of traditional foodstuffs, and a wider ambit of rules governing gastronomy and the culture of food, certain fissures and inconsistencies can be discerned.

In this last part of the book I have two main objectives in mind: first, to assess and interpret key dimensions of food habits and practices in present-day Puerto Rico in light of certain contemporary theoretical perspectives on diet and food consumption generally, perspectives that are rooted in history, philosophy, and different social studies fields; and second, to employ Alan Warde's model of "culinary antinomies" to describe the most visible aspects of the relationships that obtained between the Puerto Rican population and food, cooking, and diet at the end of the last century and during the early 2000s. Warde's thesis provides the clearest lens through which to view and understand contemporary attitudes and habits toward food and the tendency they display toward smoothing out differences and divergences.

Finally, I plan to offer preliminary answers to two questions: whether what we are eating today is what we used to eat, and whether certain features that defined and characterized our cookery and diet in the past will retain their prominence in future years. By drawing some tentative conclusions to these questions, we can better judge what has been modified or transformed, or has simply remained unchanged, with respect to our past food habits and practices.

Food Consumption Today: Some Theoretical Perspectives

Studies focusing on food and diet in the contemporary context agree not only that diet and approaches to eating in the most developed countries have gone beyond the simple need of satisfying the body's basic requirements for survival but also that the changes affecting food cultures have been profound, have occurred at an accelerated rate, and have originated on different levels. While scholars studying such changes have approached them from different theoretical and methodological angles, and thus classified and categorized them differently, their analyses have clustered around the same factors and processes, in particular the restructuring of the production and distribution of food; the development of new ways of acquiring it and of cooking, preparing, and presenting meals; and of relating to and representing food symbolically. The following is a brief review of the principal ideas expounded by the authors whose studies I have found essential.

In Stephen Mennell's view, as a result of the major advances in agroindustry that began in the mid-twentieth century, it becomes difficult to discern—during the last quarter of the century—any clear, unitary set of tendencies either in culinary activity as a whole or in the consumption of food per se. For Mennell, what is most evident is that as the number of foodstuffs got ratcheted up and—in contrast to past eras—got distributed more widely, two phenomena emerged and ran parallel to each other: "diversity" (in the variety and availability of food products) and a "narrowing" of the socioeconomic "differences" that had historically prevailed in the distribution of food and in the ability that people had to consume it. He describes these dual phenomena as "diminishing contrasts, increasing varieties."[8]

Although Mennell's model places considerations of production before those of consumption, it nonetheless opens up the possibility of changes in our food tastes and in future culinary practices to the extent that agroindustrial advances erode historic contrasts or differences via the genetic altera-tion of food, the increase in the "value added" element of food products, the standardization and expansion of food production, and the distribution of its fruits on a worldwide scale.

For his part, Claude Fischler believes that we currently live in a state of "gastro-anomie," a clever trope representing the anxiety we feel that stems from the greater possibility we enjoy of exercising what he calls food freedom (autonomy). According to Fischler, such autonomy makes us prey to uncertainty because, as we step up to make choices about what to eat, "there are no clear-cut and coherent criteria," as there were within the rural society of earlier times.[9] Insofar as they are omnivores, human beings can consume all manner of food, but under present conditions they no longer know just what, how, when, or where to eat, since hand in hand with the increase in diversity have come genetic changes in food, ambiguous and contradictory medical and nutritional advice, changes in the way in which food is cooked and meals are prepared in the domestic sphere, and the progressive disappearance of the traditional meanings placed on different types of food. As Fischler sees it, the old rules regarding food, the rules that were passed down from one generation to the next, have been loosened or upended, leaving the modern diner to ask himself which among them can offer effective guidance about what to eat and related culinary matters—a situation he calls the "paradox of the (h)ominvore."

A still different perspective is taken by Massimo Montanari, who claims that the price of having gotten beyond the "fear of famine" is that a "friendly and intelligent" relationship no longer exists between ourselves and the food we consume. He underscores that in Western societies, the European in particular, "the abundance of food . . . creates new and diffi-cult problems—once it becomes a permanent and socially widespread phe-nomenon—for a culture we know to be marked by the fear of famine."[10] Montanari believes that contemporary attitudes and comportment toward food are conditioned by this cultural inheritance. Sounding a decidedly pessimistic note—similar on that score to Fischler—he speculates that the current abundance of food is nurturing nutritional contradictions. In Montanari's words: "The irresistible allure of excess, impressed upon our bodies and minds by millennia of famine, has begun to shock us now that abundance has become a daily reality. In wealthy countries, the diseases of nutritional excess have come to replace those of nutritional deficiency."[11]

These maladies, Montanari asserts, have spawned dissonant attitudes and thinking, which he believes are reflected in the very language and terminology we use to describe food and dietary practices. For example, the word "diet" has gone from meaning "daily nutritional regime" within a broader regime "of life" to mean "the limitation or denial of food."[12] While it is true that Montanari thinks that the success of current dietary regimens can signify the adherence to new aesthetic, health, and utilitarian values, he also believes that they hide "certain reticent penitential values, a desire for denial and, we might say, self-punishment, linked to the abundance (or rather excess) of food available."[13] He concludes that, in general terms, we are impelled at present by a "fear of obesity."

A fourth critic, John Urry, argues that a visible transfer is occurring within contemporary capitalist societies, one that is taking us from an organized to a disorganized form of capitalism. Although Urry is concerned not with food cultures themselves but, rather, with the tourist industry and tourism as an object of consumption,[14] his ideas about a society "in movement," crossing over from "massification to specialization," is a useful tool for evaluating changes occurring in the realm of food and culinary practice, above all when they have become more than just a matter of "physiological" concern.

If one applies Urry's model, diet and its modes would not simply be a logical activity undertaken in furtherance of "biological nutrition," but, instead, an activity intersected by values derived from what he calls "post-Fordist" consumption" or "specialization." Such consumption takes the following form:

> Consumption rather than production dominant as consumer
> expenditure further increases as a proportion of national income;
> new forms of credit permitting consumer expenditure to rise, so
> producing high levels of indebtedness; almost all aspects of social life
> become commodified . . . much greater differentiation of purchasing
> patterns by different market segments; greater volatility of consumer
> preferences; the growth of a consumers movement and the "politiciz-
> ing" of consumption; reaction of consumers against being a part of
> a "mass" and the need for producers to be much more consumer-
> driven, especially in the case of service industries and those publicly
> owned; the development of many more products each of which has
> a shorter life; the emergence of new kinds of commodity which are
> more specialized and based on raw materials that imply non-mass
> forms of production ("natural" products for example).[15]

In this way, food habits and practices, and the activities that develop around them, can trigger the quest for and structuring of new identities in the midst of changes in consumer markets.

In Urry's view, although there are elements on the contemporary scene of what he terms "mass consumption," consumption is nonetheless increasingly intersected by "the wish for individuality," the hope of distancing oneself from "massified" consumption, which is also a characteristic of the present moment.

Hence one notes the specialization of production by "market segments," and a constant "volatility" in the preferences shown by consumers as strategies of more individualized action are asserted and pursued. In lockstep with the volatility, production is forced to develop many more products whose shelf life is highly abbreviated.

If the thesis of specialization is applied to food and dietary practices, three hypotheses can be offered: first, that expenditures on food today consume a greater percentage of family budgets—one notes in this connection the widespread tendency to eat "outside of the house" or to enjoy more elaborate and exotic food; second, that certain segments of the population act as "specialized food consumers," that is, they gravitate toward "high-end" or up-market types of food; and third, that contemporary gastronomy and food habits are increasingly marked by food "fashions" and by stylized and individualized practices.

Although Urry sees post-Fordist consumption as biased toward specialization and individualization, his thesis nevertheless recognizes that mass production is a reality and that the consumer of mass-produced products shares an important space with the consumer of specialized products. The modern diner's attitudes and practices toward food are therefore crisscrossed by competing tendencies; on the one hand, the impulse toward cultivating the "high-end," and on the other, the "homogenization" and "standardization" of food, a tension which has drawn the attention of the sociologist George Ritzer.

For Ritzer, such homogenization and standardization are the outgrowth of "McDonaldization," his metaphor for the operational principles—efficiency, calculability, control, and predictability—that drive the fast food business and that are "coming to dominate more and more sectors of American society as well as of the rest of the world."[16]

In Ritzer's view, McDonaldization is synonymous with the application of knowledge and technologies that encircle and command a system of production all of whose elements—of scale, quantity, and quality—are predictable and worked out in advance.[17] Under this system, products can be manipulated to create what he calls "a world in which there are no surprises" for a customer who is likewise entirely predictable,[18] a world such as the McDonald's chain holds out, with its Big Macs readily available in every corner of the planet.

The association between technological control and a "world without surprises," which lies at the heart of Ritzer's thesis, implies that food production today does not necessarily entail a true increase in the variety of products—as Mennell suggests—but, instead, that a highly controlled, routinized technology churns out the same products, adding "value" to them by advertising and offering different sizing, personalized packaging, additional flavorings, reduced amounts of sodium or sugar, and other such enticements. The element of added value camouflages a type of culinary homogenization aimed at creating predictable mass consumers, rather than high-quality food products and services tailored to specialized, individualized consumers. In this sense, the phenomenon of McDonaldization stands in opposition to the core argument of Urry's thesis.

Ritzer's thesis also maintains that the diffusion and adoption of "Mc-Donaldized" methods and techniques, as applied to other types and areas of food services, are causing profound though scarcely perceptible changes in contemporary food habits and practices. For example, the criterion of efficiency, which in the lexicon of fast food does not necessarily mean that meals will be served quickly, has enabled outlets to trim the use of cutlery and table coverings, shrink the menu down to one central type of food, and turn the customer into a combined "waiter-diner," since, in certain establishments, it is the diner who serves himself at the salad bar and cleans up the table when he has finished eating. As Ritzer puts it, the diner functions as an employee who spends rather than collects.[19]

These changes not only dislodge and destabilize food and dietary practices inherited from the past but also create a uniform mass of like-minded diners whose wishes and habits are predictable.[20]

Similarly, the criterion of calculability and the use of chronometric technologies to control the weight, measurement, and size of food portions, and the amount of time used in preparing them, can cause the cooks in McDonaldized restaurants to lose their skills and capacity for inventiveness. They become nothing more than intermediaries between technology at one end and the dispensation of precooked food at the other. In some cases, technology has replaced them altogether.

Moreover, the principle of calculability has led customers to confuse "size" and "quantity" with "quality," although the two frequently share little if anything in common. While many people focus on eating "core" food products, which may or may not be the most healthful, the phenomenon of McDonaldization promotes an undervaluing of more nutritional choices in food and causes people's capacity to distinguish tastes and flavors to atrophy.[21]

Where both specialization and homogenization intersect food habits and practices, an accelerated flow, or displacement, of food and gastronomic knowledge from and between national and regional cuisines can also be discerned. For the geographers Ian Cook and Philip Crang, foodstuffs are "cultural artefacts" that, from one lived moment to the next, inhabit not just the place or region where they are produced but a range of other times and spaces as well. Food takes on and exhibits new meanings in relation to the social and spatial contexts in which it reappears and is used anew.

In this way, Cook and Crang think that in "local" contexts, that is, contexts in which a particular food is, as it were, a "foreigner," different foods, and the culinary culture to which they contribute, are reappropriated to propel what Cook and Crang term "double commodity fetishism."

This expression refers both to the development of understandings about particular places of food production and to the appropriation of heretofore unknown geographical and cultural "knowledges," which at times leads to the appropriation of erroneous knowledge regarding the ways in which different foods are produced.

In general, however, the globalization of food and the movement of food cultures across the world has the effect—within certain social groups—of turning once exotic and unknown types of food into artifacts of consumption in service of "cultural constructions of difference."[22] In today's environment, then, one can experience "the world on a plate," which may inspire reflection about other cultures but can also lead to appropriating and reinterpreting some of their features. It may even cause some types of food to pass over from being strange, odd, and exotic to being familiar parts of the daily diet.

Along these lines, but from a perspective that is centered more on the multiculturalism of the largest Latin American capitals, the sociologist Néstor García Canclini has propounded the thesis that present-day advances in production and in the global flow of capital inspire the formation of "hybrid" cultural practices. According to Canclini, this process signifies that cultures are becoming a "multinational assemblage, a flexible articulation of parts, a montage of features that any citizen of any country, religion, or ideology can read and use."[23] Much like Gretel and Pertti Pelto,[24] Canclini recognizes that products are now freely moved about from one location to another; hence "objects lose their intimate relationship with the place in which they originated." Under these circumstances, he notes, "what gets produced around the world is [found] right here, making it difficult to know whether [a product] is locally produced or comes from afar."

Although Canclini does not address the theme directly, both diet and cooking are focal points of change within urban societies worldwide, and while they entail hybrid practices, they can also induce a sense of strangeness with respect to certain types of food and their preparation and presentation.

Canclini's thesis tends to celebrate the virtues of a globalized world, but a fellow sociologist like Warde takes the view that such a world also leads to the spread of massification and homogeneity, which in turn produce adverse effects on our food habits and practices. As such, many governments and state agencies are paying renewed attention to the health consequences of food and dietary choices, establishing, as a by-product of this effort, new guidelines to promote the consumption of healthy food.[25]

Yet well-intentioned as they might be, government-authored nutritional policies and the suggested diets accompanying them tend to be ambiguous and, for many, embody the intrusiveness of the nanny state. In large measure, such "directives" are at odds with the notions of personal and individualized choice so strongly advocated in many contemporary societies, since, in their own wording, these diets are also "a package of items," a preselected listing of food that erases individual choice.

In partial agreement with Fischler, Warde further warns that homogeneity can precipitate not only nutritional disorders but also "informalization," that is, the deflating of certain rules and conventions that governed food and dietary practices and imparted a sense of order and a spirit of shared community. He also notes, as a response to the spread of homogeneity, a tendency to both "re-valorize" and invent food and culinary practices that promote and intertwine with the idea of a "national community" and give life to a sense of belonging to a common historical past.[26]

The anthropologist Arjun Appadurai follows a somewhat parallel course when explaining the increase—observable in "post-colonial" contexts—in the publication of cookbooks that refer to practices termed "traditional" or "authentic" and that associate them with the idea of "cultural homogeneity."[27]

According to Appadurai, this development takes place within a distinctive context, what he terms a "gallery of specialized ethnic and regional cuisine." In the case of India—which is Appadurai's focus of study—the last decades of the twentieth century have witnessed the publication of cookbooks that attempt to merge and link traditional repertoires with new styles of international cuisine, or to forge an adjustment to what he calls the "the social world of new Indian cuisine."[28]

Such creativity notwithstanding, Appadurai notes that a countervailing trend is also apparent in the publication of cookbooks that create a culinary literature based on the experience of exile, feelings of nostalgia, and a sense of loss. In his view, some of these texts construct a national cuisine by highlighting a specific historical tradition that is represented as constituting a unified whole. Others, he states, assemble a potpourri of recipes in which, by focusing on some product unique to a local repertoire of dishes, we are meant, or persuaded, to find a common thread or unity.[29]

Appadurai's thesis seems to lend credence to the idea that in a context characterized by variety, homogeneity, individualization, the globalization of food, and the fragmentation and renewal of culinary norms, traditions are indeed "invented," in the sense in which Eric Hobsbawm explained the practice at the beginning of the 1980s in his influential essay ". . . Inventing Traditions."[30]

For Hobsbawm, the expression "invented tradition" refers to a set of practices, of a symbolic or ritual nature, typically governed by rules which over an extended period of time were overtly or implicitly accepted, which attempt to instill values and rules of comportment by means of repetition. This process, according to Hobsbawm, implies a continuity between the present and the past, given that these inventions attempt, so far as it is possible, to establish connections to a more or less shared history.[31]

Although matters related to food and diet were not within the scope of Hobsbawm's 1983 work, his model is nonetheless pertinent to the study of some food habits and practices in contemporary Puerto Rico, since—as we shall see—festivals and fairs, dishes, cookbooks, and various happenings grounded in a gastronomy "of the poor," or a gastronomy born "of necessity," have now been popularized on the island, when in the past this food and style of cooking were dictated purely by brute routine and the absence of choice.

Interestingly, in both the scholarly studies on gastronomy and the theoretical debates spun off from them, there are few works that view present-day dietary and food practices as something marked by cultural and material differences that play out in the consumption of food. Mennell talks about "diminishing contrasts," but it is not clear if this expression refers to a "narrowing of inequalities" in the access to mass-produced food (since there are now more options from which to choose) or, on the contrary, if it refers to the "lessening of differences" that have long obtained in the use of certain types of food and in the social meaning that they carry as marking off one class of society from another.

On this point, the ideas of the late Pierre Bourdieu are richly suggestive. In his work, *Distinction: A Social Critique of the Judgment of Taste*, Bourdieu approaches the topic of food and its social ramifications from the perspective of class-based cultural practices.[32]

For Bourdieu, our practices toward food mark "distinctions" between social classes as well as between segments within each class. Such practices get shaped not only by economic factors, which play an important role, but also by the habits of class—certain dispositions that form a kind of "system of practice-generating schemes which express systematically the necessity and freedom inherent in its class condition and the difference constituting that position."[33] Bourdieu's practice-generating schemes take the form, in the field of consumption, of "practices [or goods] designated by their rarity as distinguished, those of the fractions richest in both economic and cultural capital, . . . the practices [or goods] socially identified as vulgar because they are both easy and common . . . and the practices which are perceived as pretentious, because of the manifest discrepancy between ambition and possibilities."[34]

According to Bourdieu, our food practices and habits involve something that goes beyond the simple intake of food for survival. They also convey and correspond to social meanings that aspire to be something higher, something like "social marks" or even "social messages," which get molded by taste—inherent in class-based culture—that our habits and practices build up and express. With reference to the symbolic attributes of food consumption among segments of the French middle class in the 1970s, he writes:

> The taste of the professionals or senior executives defines the popular taste, by negation, as the taste for the heavy, the fat and the coarse, by tending towards the light, the refined and the delicate. The disappearance of economic constraints is accompanied by a strengthening of the social censorships which forbid coarseness and fatness, in favor of slimness and distinction. The taste for rare, aristocratic foods points to a traditional cuisine, rich in expensive or rare products (fresh vegetables, meat). Finally, the teachers, richer in cultural than in economic capital, and therefore inclined to ascetic consumption in all areas, pursue originality at the lowest economic cost and go in for exoticism (Italian, Chinese cooking etc.) and culinary populism (peasant dishes). They are thus almost consciously opposed to the (new) rich with their rich food.[35]

Although the changes or states of permanence that can occur over time are not Bourdieu's principal concerns, he believes that the element of distinction will always be present insofar as it serves to reproduce structures of class.[36]

Moreover, while sociologists, like Mennell, who focus on the study of food and diet find Bourdieu's thesis too constraining, too apt to blur the analysis of social transactions and vertical mobility,[37] Bourdieu's argument still resonates, because it forces us to consider that, despite a series of developments—the cornucopia of options offered by the modern supermarket resulting from advances in agroindustry, the marked tendency toward individualization, the spread of other cuisines and "food fads," and the visible rise in personal and family incomes—the differences mediated by food practices will continue to exist, due to differences in cultural capital and in the habits inherent in class divisions, if not to the inequalities in amounts of economic capital.

On the other hand, a sociologist like Warde, who has studied food-consumption practices in Great Britain at the end of the 1990s and has also critically assessed discussions on the nature of contemporary food consumption more widely, believes that among the various tendencies he has observed, no single one predominates, since in modern consumer societies, those of the large metropolises above all, they constantly interact and interweave among themselves.[38] Nevertheless, he does speculate that four of these tendencies are more prominent and conspicuous than the others:

1. Gastro-anomie
2. Specialization by segments
3. Homogeneity-standardization
4. Distinction-differentiation

These are trailed in importance, but still much in evidence and open to corroboration, by informalization (the outcome, in a certain sense, of homogeneity); stylization (or the aesthetic appreciation of food as the result of specialization); and what he calls "communification" (something akin to the invention of traditions and the validation of the shared experiences and intermingling that food and its consumption provide).

In the case of Puerto Rico, one can add the combining or conjoining of culinary rules and types of food that had earlier seemed to clash both tangibly, in the concrete fulfillment of different food and dietary practices, and intangibly, in the various meanings they carried. Put another way, new procedures were elaborated to deal with "old materials" and to transform them into "new exemplars"; or the reverse process took place, with "old procedures" followed in preparing "new materials," again with the objective of creating a new offering. These efforts carve out a space for airing novel ideas, produce understandings (or in some cases "misunderstandings," as Appadurai sagely notes) about food and culinary practice that are unprecedented and, ultimately, result in the appearance of new repertoires and new rules that converge and blend together.

The first-tier tendencies identified by Warde, however, do not operate in a vacuum. Rather, they are supported and maintained by means of a network of forces that help nurture and promote them such as food advertisements; new culinary experiences; the diffusion of nutritional information and up-market gastronomic literature; the personal testimony of chefs, food critics, and others; the professionalization of cooking; and the adhesion to la cocina de las madres—the distinct flavors and tastes associated with the dishes one ate as a child and grew up with.

The expanding reach of the more prominent tendencies may be observed in what Warde and Martens call "contemporary modes of food provision," which encompass the "commercial mode" (i.e., restaurants, hotels, diners, pizzerias, food courts, in-store restaurants, cafeterias, fondas [inexpensive restaurants], unpretentious small restaurants serving local cuisine [restaurancitos ciollos],[39] snack bars, catering services, establishments specializing in take-away food or in food to be eaten standing up, either on the street or indoors); the "institutional mode" (i.e., school dining halls, and the restaurants and cafeterias found in businesses, universities, colleges, and hospitals); and, of course, the "domestic mode."[40] The convergences and blending referred to above have become a recognizable feature of these three modes.

Warde believes it very plausible that all of the tendencies and concomitant blendings coexist, because food and dietary practices are "contingent" and "complex," as is seen above all in the matter of choice, where the market offers each of us a wide range of options.[41]

All the same, Warde is party to some more sweeping conclusions: that there has been an increase in variety, that contemporary food habits and practices do not answer exclusively to physiological needs, that the tight connection many have to a defined "regional" food has been liberalized to include other foodstuffs as well as cuisines from around the globe, that excessive and indulgent consumption of food is manifestly evident, and that distinctions and differences in consumption—at least with the individualization that specialization provides, if not in access to variety—still persist. In the case of Puerto Rico, the last factor is decisive, above all because of the high number of people who receive food assistance from the state, which is regulated so that a large part of the funds are directed only to obtaining food used in the preparation of basic meals.

The Preparation and Consumption of Food in Contemporary Puerto Rico

Based on the writings about gastronomy which he reviewed for his book *Consumption, Food, and Taste: Culinary Antinomies and Commodity Culture*, Warde concludes that during the final decades of the twentieth century—or during "late modernity," as he prefers to call this period—a "series of evaluative categories," or "principles of recommendation," rose to the fore in the discourses surrounding food and its consumption. He further concludes that the importance accorded these principles is relative, not uniform, since it is capable of changing over time. And while not specifically addressing the factors underlying such change, he does think that—when examined as a totality—the "principles" or "evaluative categories" reflect four constellations of oppositions or of fundamental or persistent "antinomies" in the selection and consumption of food. These consist of "novelty/tradition," "health/indulgence," "economy/extravagance," and "convenience/care."[42] Each of these contains within it contradictory or opposed ways of carrying out some instance of food and dietary practice. Warde's model of antinomies captures the debate that Puerto Ricans carry on today with themselves, when—in selecting a meal or some product to eat—they struggle to balance or resolve one or more of these oppositions. Exactly how are these sets of antinomies expressed and represented in Puerto Rican food habits and practices?

NOVELTY AND TRADITION

The possibility to experience previously unknown food or foreign, exotic, and sophisticated styles of cooking is not new, though it was much more likely to have been enjoyed by those in the upper strata of society. During the nineteenth century, the opportunity of upper-class creole youth to pursue their education away from home, and the desire among more advantaged immigrants to reproduce or approximate the gastronomy they left behind, opened avenues to try new recipes and food.

Still, such experiences were only sporadic, subject as they were to the vagaries of the import market for basic foodstuffs, which to a certain degree negated the possibility of creating a more refined gastronomic sensibility. Even the capital and municipalities like Ponce and Mayagüez were hedged in by these limitations, although—to use Bourdieu's terms—they possessed the requisite economic and cultural capital, with specialized businesses and food outlets,[43] and also restaurants, like El Universal, which had promoted such taste and sensibilities starting in the nineteenth century. When advertising his business in the newspapers, in fact, El Universal's owner appealed directly to the sybaritic tastes of the socially privileged, while acknowledging the uncertain conditions bedeviling the island's high-end, gourmet food market: "I give license to any person, whether Spanish, French, English, German, Portuguese, or from the United States or any other nation to request here the most elaborate and delicate dish from Europe, for if the necessary ingredients are to be had in the market, he will be nothing less than pleased."[44]

The products that were needed to fulfill this promise would eventually be reliably in stock, above all in the decade 1950–60, when Puerto Rico was transformed into one of the principal centers of Caribbean tourism. This was a period in which an internationally flavored "haute cuisine" enjoyed great popularity, its "practitioners," according to Jean-François Revel, "produced or specialized in certain dishes that became identifiers for the cuisine of a nation or a region."[45] In Puerto Rico, this development occurred primarily either in luxury hotels in and around the capital or in other spots on the island that attracted a heavy tourist presence between 1950 and 1960. Representative of this trend in metropolitan San Juan were the Swiss Chalet, in the El Condado district; the Chinese restaurant Cathay, located originally in Miramar and still operating on Avenida Ponce de León; and the Top of the First, in the banking district of Santurce. Still others were Trader Vic's and Le Pavilion, in the Caribe Hilton hotel and the Hotel San Juan, respectively; and the restaurant Zipperle's—all of these restaurants received the support of the island's Tourist Promotion program.[46]

In recent years, however, another type of haute cuisine, very different from the 1950s version, has come on the scene. Revel characterizes it as having managed "to integrate, refashion, rethink, and rewrite dishes from every country and every region, and whose cooks know how to exploit them to create something totally novel."[47] Moreover, the rather dreary, cheerless light in which the work of the cook had always been cast gave way to a new image that represented it as admirable and professional. A revolutionary part of this change was that women were able to join men as full-fledged "chefs," something that before had been well-nigh impossible. The home setting also participated in this transformation, since a domestic cook's labors had earlier been valued by young ladies and housewives only as a way of gauging whether she remained constant in her dedication and devotion, albeit that splendid meals were brought to the table as a matter of course.

Other factors have aided these changes as well, among them the contributions of food chemistry, nutritional science, and a heightened aesthetic sense toward the practice of the culinary arts. The corporate character that haute cuisine has acquired has also been well served by the application of business and management expertise to restaurant and culinary operations. The enrollment of cooks from other countries in Puerto Rico's Escuela Hotelera (school for the hotel and hospitality industry), and their service on the staffs of the island's most prestigious hotels and restaurants have also played a part in shaping Puerto Rico's contemporary food culture, as have both local television stations, which now devote more time to programs on professional cooking, and cable television. One of the tangible results of this process of change is the renewal of the competitive spirit and upward ambition displayed by cooks and chefs.[48]

The greater interest taken in gastronomy today has likewise been spurred by a new class of food critics who have not only popularized the appreciation for gourmet cooking but have themselves become celebrity figures, as Fischler explicates in the case of France.[49] In Puerto Rico, a competition, started in 1982 to recognize and reward the island's most accomplished chefs and known as El *Certamen del Buen Comer* (Fine Dining Contest), has become the occasion par excellence for debuting novel dishes and recipes and for validating the new style of haute cuisine.[50] An equally prominent event is the *Gran Cocinamiento*, or Great Cookoff, which has been celebrated annually in the exclusive Bankers Club since 1989.[51]

The celebration of the new and uncommon in gastronomy has led, on the one hand, to a greater appreciation for the aesthetic aspects of food and diet and to the appropriation of culinary styles and techniques from foreign lands, on the other. With this move, as Fischler has stated, "the play on words used in naming dishes is perhaps the most characteristic thing about the new cookery," that is, the element of "the poetic," as well as "the intentional reworking and manipulation of earlier culinary terminology and usage." This manifestation of the culinary arts, both their practice per se and the food that gets consumed, entails an exceptionally high level of specialization. As such, it becomes quite difficult to reproduce them inside the home kitchen. Similarly, a high level of gastronomic education and a very refined cultivation of the senses are prerequisites to establishing a "poetics" of the culinary arts. To spread this understanding and level of appreciation so that they lie within the grasp of everyone may not be impossible, but it does imply that everyone be in the know, be—as it were—part of a culinary elite.

In reality, it is only those with sufficient economic resources who are likely to attain this plateau, since doing so is measured out in the preparation of extremely elaborate dishes and the use of expensive, specialized ingredients from other areas of the globe, along with elegant cutlery, tableware, serving vessels, table decorations, service, and more.[52]

As part of the staging and celebration of the novel, it is also useful to underscore what Fischler called the "high-end effect," which involves a decrease in the amount expended on basic foodstuffs by particular urban, professional, and socially privileged sectors, with a corresponding increase in the amount expended on fancy food products. To be sure, this phenomenon is not new; during the 1930s, for example, many wealthy San Juaneros—in contrast to lower-income families—relegated rice and salted codfish to secondary status in favor of wheat and meat. The same occurred with the potato, in opposition to yams, cassava, and green bananas. Today, however, the practice is more pronounced, because "specialty" food once produced and consumed only on a local (or regional and national) level is now—with the advent of global marketing and distribution—available internationally.

Those in Puerto Rico who are attracted to Fischler's high-end ethos are the equivalent of those in England who have earned the label of "foodies." Not only do these people dine out, in conspicuous fashion, on artfully prepared dishes featuring exotic products or products of unique provenance but they are also conversant with a full repertoire of recipes from other parts of the world and possess a superior knowledge of the techniques of the new haute cuisine. Their tastes are catered to in the gourmet food sections of the large hipermercados, located in neighborhoods and districts populated by the wealthiest Puerto Ricans (or by those who put on the airs of the gastronomically enlightened), such as El Condado, Garden Hills, Torrimar, and Isla Verde. Small shops, like Domeniko's, La Hacienda, and Bottles, which specialize in high-end groceries, have also sprung up in response to the growth of this food subculture. The trend is likewise evident in restaurants, like La Ceiba and Kasalta, offering Spanish cuisine; Compostela and Laurel Kitchen/Art Bar (the latter is located in the Puerto Rican Museum of Art), which specialize in high-end fusion dishes; as well as in restaurants devoted to Thai, Indian, and Middle Eastern fare.

In practice, for some groups—especially those with the greatest wealth, who are able to indulge in high-end "gastro-therapeutic" tourism,[53] the pursuit of the novel opens up (or appears to open up) possibilities for realizing oneself and for experiencing a certain quality of excitement that is seen to be the very embodiment of late modernity. The element of the novel also spotlights the various options that exist today to shape food and dietary practices, a richness of choice that was very difficult to realize before 1950, even for those in the upper crust of society.

In its high degree of specialization, elevated cost, social exclusivity, openness to foreign cuisines still unknown to and unappreciated by many, and, above all, in the great distance separating it from the more familiar gastronomy of the island, this food culture of the novel implies a sharp break with past food habits and practices. The reformulation of the various meanings placed on food and culinary practice which late modernity offers has, of course, not stamped out the traditional meanings and associations;

rather, the two now coexist side by side, with the possibility of each influencing the other.

For example, there is an important element to the embrace of a tonier, more sophisticated gastronomy that in part derives from the invention of tradition and the creation of imagined culinary pasts. It consists in the claim made by specialized businesses and outlets that they are providing consumers with higher quality in certain historically popular products because they add some traditional element to them. This occurs even as the social sectors having the closest relationship, historically, to old-line dishes and types of food break away from them. Generally, the added element is a "technique" (for example, in preparing plantain pastel, the plantain leaves will be softened by exposing them to the smoke from a wood fire), or an "ingredient" (in the case of rice pudding, fresh coconut milk will be used), or a "condition" under which or "particular place" where the product is made (for example, that it qualifies as homemade or as produced inside the country). Through such devices, then, late modernity effectively converts tradition into a fashionable, high-end commodity. Of course, we can also conceive of disparate food practices, each with their own meaning(s), taking place at the same time.

It is possible that these ambivalent tendencies have a decentering effect on certain segments of society, whose members—for whatever reasons—find themselves incapable of participating in this novel, sophisticated food culture in any meaningful, day-to-day way; and that the effect, the sense of disconnectedness, is especially strong when a long-familiar culinary referent is also present. Indeed, the very diversity and variety so characteristic of the contemporary food market can nurture indecisiveness in some people about what meal or type of food they should choose to eat and what they should really be accomplishing in the kitchen. This perplexity promotes a tendency to follow what is familiar and repeated on a daily basis in the realm of food and diet (rice, beans, boiled viandas, mixed rice dishes, the flavor of sofrito, eating at home, serving everything together, and so on).

Consequently, in the interweaving of the novel and the traditional in contemporary Puerto Rico, one regularly observes the "invention of traditions," many of them centered on matters of gastronomy, as Ángel Quintero Rivera—picking up the thread of Hobsbawm's ideas—discovered and recorded.[54]

In general, Hobsbawm thinks that invented traditions are responses to new situations. Moreover, he has the idea that in a distant past an ensemble of "practices" could exist that were sanctioned by convention and routine yet remained bereft of important meanings, since their functions were always technical and pragmatic, more than ideological. Nonetheless, he adds that at some future point they could acquire a critical symbolic value, specifically, at that juncture when they lose their original technical, pragmatic functions. For example, following Hobsbawm's line of thought, roasting a pig on a pole that someone from the hinterland turns by hand over the embers of a wood fire (as opposed to its being broiled in a modern gas oven that rotates it automatically) would not bear the stamp of authenticity that it does today if the forests had remained as filled with trees as they once were and the Puerto Rican population had not become so urbanized.

By the same token, mixed rice dishes (especially rice with pigeon peas and pork), which, as they are cooked, get covered with plantain leaves (*apastela'o*) instead of with the lid of a pot, would not be considered so authentically traditional if it were not so awkward to use them in the pots we have in our kitchens today, when lids of all sizes are standard.

In short, the invented traditions pertaining to gastronomy can be understood as new representations, in new contexts, of old culinary rituals, symbols, rules, and practices that held sway during times of hunger and near famine.

Within this landscape of change, traditional foods and familiar gastronomic practices, defined as preeminently Puerto Rican, have been invested with new, or renewed, meaning. While for some, individualism and stylization have led homemade or traditional food to be considered food that dates to some long-ago past, for others, the McDonaldization and informality of new food consumption practices, the advances in genetic engineering achieved by the agro-food industry, and the dialectic of "global" versus "local" produced by the opening of food markets and market systems are re-creating a new quest for roots that are seen to be genuine, natural, and tied to a sense of belonging. Familiar food habits and practices play an important role in this process, coexisting as they do with the novel, the exotic, and the extravagant; and food and culinary routines and techniques from past eras have acquired the status of national symbols.

This dynamic interplay is evident in the numerous festivals dreamed up in recent years that, as Quintero Rivera notes, have historic dishes as well as "poor men's fare" as their theme.[55] He identified a total of thirty-two festivals, held annually between 1975 and 1988, whose purpose was either to celebrate gastronomy in general or to commemorate some particular foodstuff or historic dish. The more notable festivals and their sites in-clude those featuring cassava (Coamo), breadfruit (Humacao), the plantain (Dorado), the land Crab (Maunabo), roast pig (Las Piedras), "traditional dishes" (Guayanilla), stewed pork's feet" (Guaynabo), "Puerto Rican dishes" (San Juan), spicy pork tripe, (Orocovis), and the pigeon pea (mu-nicipality of Villalba).

The Festival de Comida Típica de Loíza, begun in 1995 and celebrated in the high-end Caribe Hilton Hotel, or the Competencia de Comida Criolla sponsored by the Puerto Rican Hotel and Tourism Association, are excel-lent examples of the invention of tradition. In the former, the most creative professional chefs use the knowledge and experience accumulated by the women most versed in cooking over outdoor griddles and open-hearth wood fires to prepare food and dishes unique to the culinary traditions of the island's black coastal populations. The purpose of the latter festival is "to make people aware of the best criollo restaurants in Puerto Rico."[56] These two events (as well as the more recent Comidas Puertorriqueñas fes-tival held in San Juan, under the sponsorship of the state-run public corpo-ration the Compañía de Fomento Turístico) illustrate Warde's point that "to have a distinctive national cuisine has become an important stratagem for the tourist industry and, often with the support of governments, traditional national dishes and even cuisines are either exhumed or invented for the purpose."[57]

Clearly, modernity itself, the social-temporal context in which they are pursued, has drained these activities of a sense of authenticity, if—in fact—a culinary past can ever truly be reconstituted or reproduced. In place of the genuinely authentic, we are made to reinvent it or to accept the standard-ized. The original versions of these activities have been turned into a series of extravagant museum pieces, in which different foods and ways of prepar-ing them are transformed into objects of curiosity, just one more consumer product occupying its allotted space in a world of such products.[58]

This phenomenon can be better understood if one considers such over-blown gastronomic creations as the *supermofongo*, the *super asopao de gandules* (super pigeon pea stew), and the *superpastel*, all of which are also inven-tions.[59] The supermofongo, for example, was produced in the "food court" of Ponce's Plaza del Caribe mall, where—on 23 July 2001—20,000 people gathered and stood in line to sample it. An assistant (presumably speaking for many if not most in the throng) termed the gigantic heap of mofongo "wonderful, a thing of beauty."[60]

The tension between the "fast food" orientation operative in the school dining hall program in 1988, when pizza and hamburger concessions were installed in public school cafeterias, and the orientation, toward nutritional food, of the students' mothers, who insisted that rice and beans should be the foundation of lunches served by schools, helps illustrate another cornerstone of the game of invention: the notion that food consumed in the past was much more beneficial to one's health. The publication of the book *Elogio de la fonda*, by the Puerto Rican writer Edgardo Rodríguez Juliá, is yet another link in this chain of invention.[61] Finally, in her manner of expression, Giovanna Huyke—among the most renowned of contemporary Puerto Rican chefs—unwittingly puts her finger on the phenomenon of invention in the introduction to one of her well-known cookbooks: "Before forgetting those recipes and dishes so representative of us by invoking the excuse of the little time left by modern life . . . our wish has been to rescue and adapt them to the realities we face today. In similar fashion, native ingredients, and variations on old recipes, have been incorporated into new recipes, which are now part of the authentic native cuisine . . . but without forgetting our history for one moment. . . . And in memory of our past and of our ways of cooking, this book shall be there for future generations."[62]

What is perhaps most peculiar and paradoxical in all these instances of inventing tradition is the tendency to search for (and find) authenticity in products, in the ingredients of dishes, and in the dishes themselves that oscillates between nostalgia, a chauvinism toward one's native soil, and—quite often—outright culinary mediocrity and the loss of a dedication to taking genuine care in the preparation of food. The tendency even reaches the extreme of giving certain types of food and dishes names that would create the illusion they were native to Puerto Rico, when in fact one of the central features of our diet and cookery is that much of it did not originate on the island. As a further indication of this hybridization, some products that historically lay at the heart of criollo cooking are now obtained via the import market, rather than from local farms and home plots, but the various dishes that are made with them are still labeled authentic or traditional. This practice is what some theorists refer to as eating "glocal," that is, mediating or effecting a balance between the universal (the availability of standard food products known to and recognizable in Puerto Rican cooking) and the particular (culinary practices and cuisine considered distinctly Puerto Rican).[63] Such imagined authenticity is but a series of historical constructions, the result of one bricolage built on or folded into another, although some might want to see it as emerging pure and whole cloth out of the national cultural discourse.[64]

On the other hand, within the circumstances of the global supermarket and in the midst of the phenomenon of McDonaldization, it would be ingenuous to think that traditional food habits and cuisine are going to be completely leveled down by the "delocalization" of culinary practices and the "massification-homogenization" of the diet. Casual observation will confirm that food preferences and a standard repertoire of dishes, as well as culinary rules and principles taken as traditional, change very slowly. Indeed, restaurant chains themselves grasp this fact, as is seen, for example, in the strategy followed by diners and fast food chains to include some familiar offerings on their menus. In 1997, the McDonald's that opened in the student union of the University of Puerto Rico opted to offer rice and beans in addition to its Big Mac,[65] and the Bonanza chain recently launched an advertising campaign with the theme "Here you eat criollo."[66] The same approach has been taken by Burger King, which recently introduced a sandwich called the *bisteking*. On this point, Fischler observes "that the giants of the agro-food industry need to take into account certain particularities when they seek to impose their universal products."[67]

Still, if these globalized forces have not swept away certain foods and special preparations, such as sofrito, pork, and rice, and have in fact grafted new combinations onto the repertoire of domestic dishes, the absence of fresh ingredients—along with the erosion of a feeling of culinary pride that can accompany their use—is increasingly evident. Today, the persuasiveness of food and agroindustrial advertising has led many people to believe that cooking is simple and that everyone can accomplish it just as easily as he or she can sit down to a meal. Regrettably, this simplistic thinking carries three dire risks that have already begun to bear fruit: the loss of basic ideas and principles of cooking, the absence of an appreciation of culinary practices on an emotional level, and the shaping, or reshaping, of local cuisine and cookery into something mediocre and superficial.

HEALTH AND INDULGENCE

Nobody can reasonably deny that Puerto Rico, at least as concerns its food supplies, is a society characterized by abundance.[68] At the same time (and perhaps because of such abundance), discussions about food are often characterized by a seemingly paradoxical or contradictory double obsession: on the one hand, incessant talk of cuisine—high, vegetarian, nouvelle, fusion, criolla, and home fare—and on the other, an excessive concern for following a constricting nutritional diet. In contemporary Puerto Rico, in contrast to how things were before, one experiences what Fischler refers to as the divorce between cooking and dietetics.[69] What was once a whole has now been separated or divided: in the past, cooking was undertaken and meals consumed simply to live; they were part of the regimen, the connective tissue of one's life, on a basic level, and the pleasurable, sensory aspects of cookery and food scarcely figured, if they figured at all, in recipe books. Such, at least, was true for the cooking manuals born out of the Puerto Rican home economics initiative in the first decades of the twentieth century. Today, by contrast, cooking, the kitchen, and food belong to the world of pleasure and indulgence. The "regimen," its meaning now inverted, belongs to the field of health, of ensuring one's physical well-being. The word "diet," as Montanari explains, has come to mean the limitation or denial of food, self-punishment, and the fear of gaining weight and becoming obese.

The separation in question is reflected, in Puerto Rico, in the element of "gastro-anomie," which runs through discussions about and references to matters of food and diet. On one side, advertisements for food inveigle people with its aesthetic and pleasurable aspects; and on the other, warnings are issued against the dangers of obesity. In 2002, Puerto Rico's health secretary, Johnny Rullán, reported that five of every ten Puerto Ricans were clinically obese and, more shocking still, that six of every ten Puerto Rican children suffered from obesity, with rising levels of Type II diabetes, which normally afflicts obese adults. The secretary found these statistics to be alarming, to say the least.[70] As a sign of the times, however, an article about a restaurant in Chicago serving a six-course meal to celebrate its anniversary ran in the same source as Rullán's report, and both stories were flanked, on the same date, by an article in which a specialist in nutrition summed up, in a few words, one of the reasons behind the growing phenomenon of obesity: "The main problem is the lack of physical activity, especially in children." A year later, in 2003, the Puerto Rican legislature enacted Law No. 83, which proclaimed November as the "Month of Guidance on and Prevention, Control, and Reduction of Obesity."[71]

The problem of the divorce between cuisine and dietetics—and the tensions and ambiguities which it in turn produces between health and indulgence—is deeper and more complex and multifaceted than might be apparent on the surface. In the sphere of indulgence, the problem is spurred by flights of desire and by the practice—shaped by individual taste—of realizing freewheeling pleasures, comfort, and security through displaying excessive behaviors toward food. Other ramifications of the problem are associated with the abundance of food, in a context in which attitudes and comportment that develop around food habits and practices are potentially still conditioned by what Montanari calls the culture of fear of famine, which enveloped a wide swath of daily life as recently as five decades ago. As I noted earlier, it is still common to hear the expressions "nothing's lost if you've already eaten," or "if it's going to waste, best to eat it" in the context of opulent feasts and banquets.

This syndrome comes into sharp focus in the studies carried out by the Department of Work and Human Resources in 2002, which demonstrate that families place a higher degree of importance on the purchase of food and beverages (50.4 percent) than on other goods and services. The studies also indicate that this tendency has been on the rise since 1977 (when 30.2 percent of families assigned the highest importance to the acquisition of food and beverages).

This development is extremely important, because it contradicts the thesis—always invoked with respect to industrialized countries—that as income levels rise and living standards improve, the amount of money expended on food, relative to other purchases, decreases. Further blurring the picture is that, with respect to food, the consumer price index has been curving upward since 1995.[72]

However, Puerto Rico's current food culture may also be conditioned by the weakening of certain normative factors that have guided and regulated food and dietary practices throughout the island's postconquest history. The element of individual choice and the relative freedom which a greater variety of food has promoted, as well as the power of the market to mold snack and convenience food cultures, can open spaces for behaviors toward food and food consumption that bring enjoyment and pleasure, but also indulgence. Just as such behaviors were practiced during those times on the island when a great majority of the population indulged in an orgy of eating because some long-awaited food became momentarily available, so can they occur today within social spheres in which protocols, normative guidelines, and a sense of watchful propriety are only loosely applied. Yet today conditions are very different—an indulgent practice toward food (or "gorging oneself") is not contingent, as it once was, on the fleeting, momentary abundance of food.

The increase in the number and variety of products has been channeled to consumers through several avenues that promote consumption, one of which is the big-box hipermercado,[73] where one can find the traditional rice and beans, viandas, and ingredients to make sofrito, as well as cases holding roast chickens, compartments with cold cuts of different types of meat, semi-prepared meals, meals that reflect cuisines from around the globe, and even full-fledged sushi bars. The stratagem of positioning cases of semi-prepared food at the entrance of the hipermercados, or of food that can be taken home and instantly prepared or heated up, is followed to kindle two of the senses felt most acutely in stimulating the appetite: sight and smell. Asked about the changed layout of the new Grande hipermercado in the municipality of Dorado, the owner of the successful Grande chain, Atilano Cordero Badillo, explained that he decided to move the fruit and vegetable stands away from their usual spot at the entrance of his markets because research indicated that customers generally came in both hungry for something to eat and with less time in which to make their purchases. Therefore, he went on to say, "one enters going past a deli and a bakery, and so the first thing that a customer notices is the smell of bread and BBQ chicken."[74]

The varied, never-ending offer of articles containing some element of added value, and presented by the food industry as "new" (easy to open and store, ready to be cooked or for carry-out, added flavor, different texture, the authentic product of some country or region), helps induce customers toward indulging themselves. For example, in 1998, Pueblo International, the parent company of the Pueblo Extra hipermercado chain, announced that in the space of only three years it had increased its new product lines from 14,000 to 60,000.[75] Contemporary Puerto Rican society thus confronts a veritable cornucopia of products within a global hipermercado, a range of choice which before 1950 would have been inconceivable to people as they went about stocking the pantry and deciding what to eat for the three meals of the day. Indeed, a study carried out in 2001 demonstrated that consumers preferred to make their food purchases in those establishments that offered the "greatest variety of products and brands."[76]

Indulgent food practices can also be fulfilled in other places and ways in which, as in the hipermercado, social norms and messages that would discourage or restrain us from gorging ourselves get diffused or attenuated: "fast food" outlets; the "casual diner"—where the food and meal are themselves a kind of show—"alone in the privacy of the kitchen," availing oneself of the microwave oven and of products that require little if any effort on our part; calling in orders for meals that can be delivered to one's doorstep, or opting for take-away, wonderfully characterized by Roy Wood as "dining out to dine in."[77]

In this context, a study conducted in 1996–97 by the marketing research and strategy firm Gaither International estimated that there were 1,595 fast food establishments in Puerto Rico, counting hamburger franchises, casual diners, Chinese restaurants, outlets offering criolla fast food, and shops selling broiled chicken and pork to take away.[78] These figures, and all those that follow from the Gaither study, will doubtless have escalated considerably since they were first compiled.

Whatever the precise numbers, the proliferation of fast food restaurants, especially of Burger King and McDonald's—which between them had 275 locations in 2003—is a rather anomalous occurrence in a limited geographical space like that of Puerto Rico.[79] Gaither calculated that Burger King and McDonald's (with 165 and 110 locations, respectively) captured 32 percent of the market for meals consumed outside the home.[80] Burger King had 17.9 percent of this share, and McDonald's, 14.9 percent. The remaining 68 percent was spread, in descending order, among Chinese restaurants (14.6 percent), outlets—including lechoneras—providing Puerto Rican fast food (9.6 percent), Kentucky Fried Chicken outlets (9.5 percent), Church's outlets (5.1 percent), and so on, with the Domino's Pizza chain at the bottom (3 percent).[81]

According to Gaither's findings, hamburgers were the preferred type of food (35.8 percent), followed by chicken (19.8 percent), Chinese fare (14.6 percent), and local, Puerto Rican offerings (9.5 percent).[82] The most striking part of the study, however, was its discovery that every day in 1997, on average 184,000 families ate at least one of their meals outside the home, in one of the aforementioned establishments. One can extrapolate, then, that at the close of the twentieth century in Puerto Rico, approximately 404,000 people ate one of their daily meals in such eateries.

Fischler sees this phenomenon as a function of the amount of time that people wish to spend eating, in relation to the total amount of organized productive time available to them. The stance we take toward food is now dictated by the latter, whereas in the past, the reverse was true—our food habits and practices structured our use of productive time and other activities.[83]

Is Fischler's the likely scenario in contemporary Puerto Rico, above all when the rate of unemployment is so high—13.2 percent as of 2008–9?[84] Or do Gaither's figures reflect the powerful imprint, the spreading oil slick, of fast food, which is becoming almost the only option for eating outside the home in the context of a fragile employment market and rising food prices? As part of its study, Gaither International calculated that, out of a sample group of 1,200 individuals, 30 percent ordered food at least three times per month that they had delivered either to their home or their place of work, and 52 percent purchased their food at least six times a month via the "self-service" offered by fast food restaurants.[85]

Another study, carried out in 2001 by the company Professional Market Research, determined that out of its sample group of 650 persons interviewed, 25 percent breakfasted in fast food establishments. 71 percent ate lunch in them, and 36 percent frequented them for dinner.[86] The lunch figure is especially important, because in Puerto Rico this meal continues to be the biggest meal of the day, yet—as we shall see—the nutritional value of fast food is not particularly high.

The appearance of fast food outlets in the United States dates to 1940, and by the 1950s, they were mushrooming across the country, as the automobile exerted an ever greater influence on the rhythms of American life and the interstate highway system began to expand.[87] The first fast food franchise to open in Puerto Rico was Tastee Freeze Carrol's, specializing in hamburgers and ice cream, at the end of the 1950s.[88] Burger King followed in 1963,[89] and McDonald's in 1967.[90] Their marketing strategy in this period was aimed at attracting a largely teenage clientele, but since the 1980s—a decade that marketing experts have labeled "the decade of the child consumer"—it has focused on a younger population, a trend especially pronounced in fast food restaurants whose main offering consists of hamburgers.[91] By means of this strategy, marketers discovered that the young are the best sales people in the world, since the goal of child-directed advertising is crystal clear: just give the child a specific reason to consume the product. From that point on, the child becomes the messenger, stubbornly importuning her parents to give in to her demand.[92]

Along with the hamburgers and French fries, and interwoven with all this salesmanship and maneuvering, are other "hooks" designed to pull the child in: the invention of mascots as visual identifiers of the fast food chains, the installation of enclosed and outdoor playgrounds attached to the restaurants, special offers of cakes and sweets to celebrate birthdays, putting the food inside a little box or paper bag, designed for children, with the company's logo on it (e.g., McDonald's "Happy Meals"), and giving away little action and other hero-heroine figures inspired by Hollywood movies whose fetishlike appeal often lasts only until the release of the next blockbuster film.

Not surprisingly, the rapid expansion of the fast food industry has been reflected in the growth of its advertising budget. In 1996, for example, the company Publish Records Inc. noted that McDonald's allocated $4.8 million for television advertising between January and August 1995. It likewise determined that fast food outlets and other restaurants using the same general business model invested more dollars, $22.4 million, in television advertising than any other industry.[93] In 2000, Burger King, McDonald's, and Wendy's alone spent more than $26.6 million on advertising (via radio, print, and broadcast and cable television), an increase of 17 percent to their advertising outlay during the prior year.[94] Subsequently, it was reported that Wendy's expended $5 million on advertising in Puerto Rico.[95]

In the world of marketing and advertising, the term "fast food" now covers other establishments that specialize in dispensing food to the customer quickly and efficiently (pseudo- Chinese restaurants; "casual diners" such as Ponderosa, Denny's, Sizzler, or pizzerias like Pizza Hut, Domino's, and Sbarro; and restaurants or outlets, like Pollo Tropical or Martin's Barbecue, offering local fare). As in the more classic fast food outlets, there is no practice in these of food or dishes being served in any set order or of any protocol about how people should consume their meals. On the contrary, for present-day Puerto Ricans, and for the advertising industry, fast food outlets—in their expanded form—are thought of as practical destinations where informality reigns. Many people patronize them to fit a meal into a busy schedule, a problem that seems to afflict Puerto Rican women especially. Indeed, Gaither International's 1997 study found that 74 percent of women consumed meals in or from fast food establishments, versus only 18 percent of men.[96] In addition, it estimated that 64 percent of the families eating in fast food restaurants had between three and five members, which in turn meant that on a daily basis about 11,000 people—many of them children—who depended on their family for at least part of their food intake were consuming fast food. Moreover, the effective rate was pushed even higher, since 11 percent of families—a relatively high percentage—had six or more members. The day of the week when the greatest number of families frequented fast food establishments was Friday, known in Puerto Rico as "social Friday." In Puerto Rican households most observant of the traditional division of domestic responsibilities and work, this was the day on which wives were relieved of the obligation to cook for their husbands, who went out to drink with their friends while the rest of the family stayed at home.

In today's environment, fast food outlets and restaurants serve as places where social identity—especially for preadolescents and adolescents—is experienced, confirmed, and reinforced. Marketers understand that this is the stage of life at which people are least wedded to tradition as a whole, and to a rigid table etiquette in particular. The fast food culture, with its freewheeling atmosphere, pop music, lack of such amenities as table coverings or formal dishware, and a menu and prices tailored to the tastes and budgets of the young, mirrors and plays into this informality.

If fast food restaurants, however, have the virtue of enabling housewives to eat a quick meal and to avoid the problem of cooking for their family when time is so squeezed, while also serving as a social meeting ground for preteens and teenagers working out their identity, such convenience and amity carry a price, one that is measured out—as all the messages about observing a good diet make clear—in the nutritional shortcomings of fast food.

One of the more glaring aspects of present-day Puerto Rican society is adult and child obesity, increasingly attributed by medical research and findings to the intemperate growth in the consumption of fast food.[97] This phenomenon helped inspire a campaign, known as *Salud te recomienda*, launched in 2003 by the Department of Health, one of whose elements was to get "special labeling put on nutritive foods, low in fat content and high in fiber, which are sold in supermarkets and fast food restaurants."[98] While the department understood that the fast food outlets were not the only cause of the rise in obesity, its campaign placed a major emphasis on them, especially in light of their strategy of "supersizing" their portions without either raising prices substantially or reducing profits.[99]

Faced with this tactic, the Health Department sought the cooperation of the managers of fast food franchises in its informational campaign, even as the franchises played down the little food value contained in their "supersized" meals—considering them to be just special "offers"—and placed the responsibility for the growing phenomenon of obesity squarely on the shoulders of their customers, who were the ones who decided what and how much to eat.[100] In a certain sense, the *Salud te recomienda* campaign can be understood as a concession on the part of the Health Department that fast food has become embedded, a fait accompli, in the food culture of Puerto Rico.

Whereas in 1966 only 6 percent of Puerto Rican children and youth were obese, in 1996–97 this figure had risen to 20 percent,[101] and in 1997, fast food was regularly consumed by 12 percent of the under-twenty-four population, a figure that has undoubtedly gone up.[102] Around March 2003, the Health Department put the number of diabetics in Puerto Rico at 300,000 and classified 65 percent of the island's population as obese.[103]

In light of these statistics and trends, fast food franchise managers have tried to craft a more nutritionally attractive image, above all as a way of appealing to parents who want their children to eat a healthy diet. This concern, too, partly explains why in recent years newspapers have run a supplement, purchased by the marketing directors of the fast food franchises, devoted to profiling the practical advantages of their outlets. The supplements are full of corporate messaging about how these establishments help keep the rushed, modern family on a more even keel, sugarcoated with advice from nutritionists about how to combine quick and healthy eating in one or another fast food outlet.[104]

In Puerto Rico today, the act of overeating or of stuffing oneself is shadowed or accompanied by the idea that the body has a "practical," or "use," value, from which it follows that physical upkeep—at least among certain social groupings—is increasingly seen as both a personal responsibility and a wider social obligation. Similarly, gorging oneself is understood in a negative light insofar as there has come into existence, through forces external to the individual, a "cartography" of the human body as it presents itself in the public domain: the shapeless, overweight body violates our notion of the aesthetic; it poses a threat to Puerto Ricans as the cause-and-effect relationship between overeating and obesity sinks in. The obese body signifies a loss of order and may identify a person as self-indulgent and physically inactive, undisciplined, and prey to the seductions of plenty, or to what Giovanna Huyke, one of the island's most experienced professional chefs, refers to as "the food temptation."[105]

The negative value placed on the obese body is intensified to the extent that our outlook reflects a central idea of Ulrich Beck's regarding contemporary society, namely, that it exerts pressure on individuals to "perceive themselves as at least partly shaping themselves and the conditions of their lives" and that "life's events are ascribed not mainly to 'alien' causes, but to aspects of the individual (decisions, non-decisions, omissions, capacities, incapacities, achievements, compromises, defeats)."[106] The impersonal stares and reactions that the obese receive from people and institutions can thus be read, by them, as the sign of personal failure on their part. Hence, too, the ideal of the slender body—so highly valued among certain social sectors and often viewed as a mark of class and cultural difference—can, through the reverse practice of denying oneself food, lead to the same feelings of failure.[107]

Although many people find themselves unable to fulfill the ideal—the figures on obesity demonstrate as much—the validation of the model of the slender body in part accounts for the huge number of people walking and jogging in San Juan's Central Park on Monday afternoons, as well as for the annual expenditure of $101.3 million, $42.1 million, and $35.6 million, respectively, on diets, gym memberships or exercise equipment, and weight loss medications.[108] The recent popularity of the drug Ephedrine, taken to burn off fat and produce weight loss, is yet another sign of the desire to achieve the ideal, even though this diet pill, in extreme cases, can result in death.[109]

The power of the ideal of the slender body is also reflected in two current social-nutritional problems that, though affecting hundreds of Puerto Ricans, male and female, but especially young upper-middle-class women, have been little studied in Puerto Rico[110]: anorexia nervosa and bulimia.

The Puerto Rican *atracador* or *atracadora* (male or female glutton) is someone who, hiding behind the excuse of the plenitude and variety of food, desires to—and can—give license to his or her liberties with food. Yet the failure of this person to exercise discipline in the arena of eating—as contemporary discussion seems to characterize the problem—is not entirely self-inflicted; some external forces are also at work: work and office schedules, the division of domestic labor, the force and pressure of the market, the initiatives pushed by agroindustry and food advertising, and even the persistence of the old fear of hunger, manifested in the practice of devoting a large portion of the family budget to food purchases in the face of a growing insecurity about jobs.

Excessive overeating, fed by the desire to justify or lend approval to taking liberties with food, yet driven also by forces external to the individual, leads to what dieticians call nutritional disorders, or the lack of control that people exhibit over what it is they should eat, whether selected by themselves or given to them.

A recent study highlights that one of the giants of the food industry,

ConAgra, in its eagerness to exploit the quirks of human food behavior, has discovered that people eat more when they carry away a package that exerts some individual appeal for them. This finding has underlined the strategy of designing products that, more and more, have a personalized quality to them. In addition, however, the industry's marketing logic has also been to boost the volume of food contained in packages by 10 percent without imposing any price increase. As a result, personalized food containers and packages cause people to eat more without overtly proposing to them that they do so. When selecting and purchasing a little box or package of food, the consumer thinks that he is making a decision about what to eat that is rooted in its cost, or added value, but he is also eating a larger quantity of food without the faintest idea that he is doing so.[111]

The tensions that play out between health, on the one hand, and indulgence, on the other, have also strengthened the case, among some islanders, for vegetarianism. Although vegetarianism in Puerto Rico is tied to religious beliefs or to new ethical concerns about the relationship between nature and society (involving debates about such issues as the genetic modification of food, environmental destruction, the industrial exploitation of agriculture, and food additives), its practice is also connected to the introduction of medically driven dietary regimens, as nutritional disorders begin to affect the health of thousands of Puerto Ricans.[112]

The ambivalent tendencies produce even greater tensions, because the person who adopts a carefully regimented diet has to struggle as well with a food culture centered on products that nutritional science and teachings consider overly heavy and conducive of gaining weight. Put another way, in the attempt to find a more favorable relationship between human beings and the food they eat, nutritional science has opposed the traditional diet, "pedagogizing" that diets based on high intakes of rice and beans cause obesity.

Within these cross-currents, rice—some 89.9 pounds of which were consumed on a per capita basis in Puerto Rico in 2010—together with beans, viandas, and sweet confections, all of which have been at the core of the island's food culture, are now counted as dangerous to one's health if they are eaten indiscriminately.[113] As a by-product of this insight, the meaning that these foods always carried, by way of family life, social conviviality, a feeling of bounteousness and a wider sense of identity and connectedness, is likewise subject to doubt.

All in all, however, on the level of individual food practices and behaviors, the preference for these traditional products survives intact, despite the more questioning environment. Although in a general way in contemporary Puerto Rico dietetics and the cultivation of cooking and food find themselves at opposite poles, the tensions that have come to the fore between health and indulgence seem to have opened a new window onto traditional foods and past culinary practices and repertoires, effecting new ways of relating to them, while still permitting them to be visualized as restorative, healthy, and expressive of the bonds of family.

ECONOMY AND OSTENTATION
There are and doubtless will continue to be different perspectives on what consumption is and what dimensions it takes in the realms of individuals and groups. But can consumption continue to be understood in the simple sense of "who buys what in order to survive"? Would it not be better to think of consumption as a complex of practices inherent to different groups (ethnic, gender, age, professional, class) that mold and at the same time are molded by an economy that becomes increasingly cultural in nature, since it uses every type and kind of persuasive power to create images and offer its products, employing the ubiquity of commercial design and illustration, displays and shows, multimedia advertising, and systems of distribution.[114]

The consumption of food will express and transmit new social values when, as the chief springboard to change, and as has been happening in Puerto Rico, the act of eating starts to be perceived and carried out in ways that are very different from those which prevailed three generations ago. The earlier ways were fundamentally shaped, as Warde puts it, by the "matter of survival in the face of unequally distributed resources."[115] Today, "eating and the preparation of food"—free of the tyranny of routine, and holding the possibility of experiencing great variety—are practices that can express social currents and lifestyles, cultural differences, freedom and individualism, group identities and loyalty, as well as personal tastes and preferences and the assertion of control over one's own body.

Nonetheless, in contemporary Puerto Rico, as in many other parts of the world, eating and the preparation of food still depend to a great extent on a person's economic station, the simple truth of which is born out, however abundant food supplies might be, by persistent inequalities in food customs and practices.

The recognition of this fact is important, because it sheds light on two

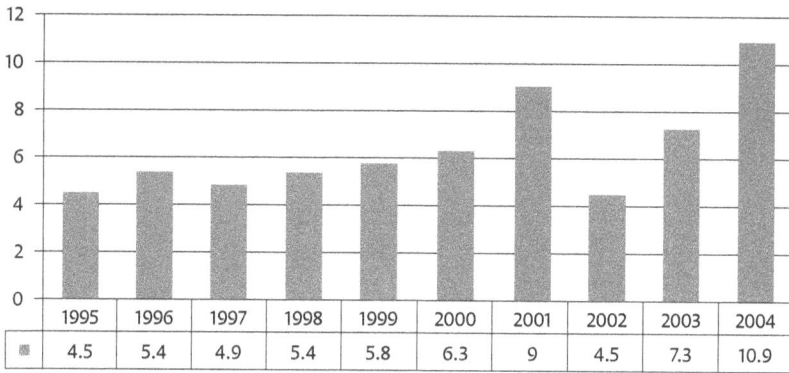

	1995	1996	1997	1998	1999	2000	2001	2002	2003	2004
▦	4.5	5.4	4.9	5.4	5.8	6.3	9	4.5	7.3	10.9

FIGURE 7.1 Consumer price index, annual percentage change

Source: Departamento del Trabajo y Recursos Humanos, *Índice de precios al consumidor,*
up to May 2004.

points made by Warde, both of which currently apply to Puerto Rico: first, that the preference for traditional core foods has not been erased; and second, that the food products selected by the poor and less advantaged tend not only to be the more economical but also—in broad terms—the least healthy; that is, they are the highest in salt, additives, fat content, carbohydrates (polished rice, white bread, preprepared pastries and desserts), and sugar.

In Puerto Rico, consumers spend 50 percent of their income on food, which—among other things—demonstrates that the culture of the fear of hunger is still alive, possibly revitalized by the rise in food prices that has occurred in recent years in the context of a highly fragile job market.[116] As shown in figure 7.1, the consumer price index has risen sharply during the past decade.

What is especially noteworthy in this rise, however, is that at the close of the twentieth century, food and beverage prices climbed at an unusually fast rate, while salaries changed little, as shown by the figures in figure 7.2.

The situation is made still worse when one considers that the purchasing power of the dollar has also declined; it is now only worth 52 cents today relative to a full 100 cent value in 1984, while the monthly cost of food has continued to go up. There are regions in Puerto Rico where in 1998 the monthly outlay for food, for a family composed of one child of preschool age and his two parents, ranged between $320 in areas with the most expensive prices and $213 in those with the cheapest.[117] According to the Labor Department, the pattern remains unchanged. Between August

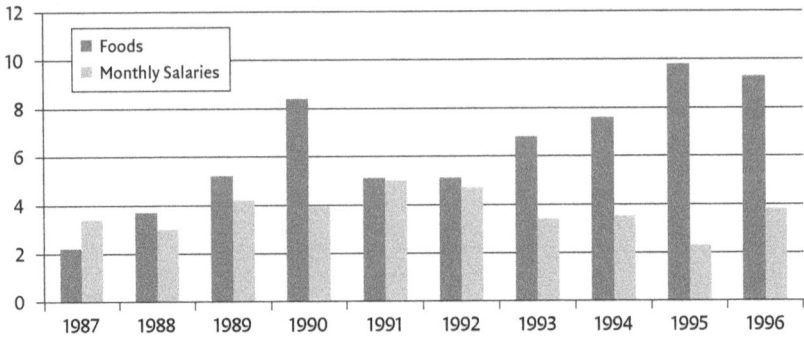

FIGURE 7.2 Percentage increase in food costs and salaries, 1987–1996
Source: Departamento del Trabajo y Recursos Humanos; El Nuevo Día, 15 February 1998

2001 and August 2002, the cost of food rose by 15.9 percent.[118] More recent studies indicate that food costs have inflated still higher, skyrocketing by 32 percent between 2002 and 2011.[119]

Moreover, if one bores down to the level of individual food products, the picture is even more telling. It is fruits and fresh vegetables that now, on a relative basis, cost consumers the most (+31.3 percent), that is, the very products that, in all the dietary messaging, symbolize a healthy lifestyle and form the base of a new nutritional pyramid.[120] This price trend contrasts to the cost of cereals and bakery goods (sugary products and complex carbohydrates derived from rice, pastas, and white bread), which has remained essentially unchanged in comparison to earlier years (+0.5 percent). The price of meat, poultry, and fish (which, as nutritionists have informed us, are the primary source of harmful lipids) has actually declined—by 7.4 percent in 2001 and by 0.5 percent in 2002.

Equally interesting, from the standpoint of potential health consequences, is that the cost of food consumed outside the home has increased by only 1.3 percent, while food products purchased for consumption in the home have gone up 16.1 percent.[121] The rise in the cost of fresh food used in home cooking might well have intensified the practice followed by some of eating more than one of their daily meals in a diner or fast food restaurant, as well as causing consumers to place a greater emphasis on less costly foods, tinned goods, and prepared and microwaveable meals and products.[122]

In the face of these conditions, lower and medium-income groups have had little choice but to opt for a diet that is affordable. Around 1998, purchasing a selection of twenty-five perishable items cost between $31.27 and $32.36. For families with more than two school-age children and an average yearly income of less than $32,892 (the average family income in Puerto Rico in 1999), an expenditure in this amount for fresh foods would be painful to absorb.[123]

The gap, and stress, is even greater for families with infants. Indeed, in 2002, a psychologist estimated that families spent $1,082 on baby food alone during an infant's first year of growth. Considering that the child will continue to live at home until (at least) his or her eighteenth birthday, the overall expense (food, clothing, recreation, transportation, and so on) of raising this person to young adulthood may go as high as $121,230.[124] Little wonder that a woman who teaches school, and earns $1,200 per month, had the following comment: "I can't give myself the luxury any more [from one month to the next] of making a big purchase, I have to limit myself, instead, to buying the necessities, or waiting for the specials."[125]

The teacher's practice is becoming the norm for a great many Puerto Rican families, the number is put at 509,339, who depend on the government's Nutritional Assistance Program (PAN), which covers about 1,078,822 individuals.[126] And it becomes all the more common as PAN's beneficiaries are compelled, by means of an electronic debiting system, to expend 75 percent of their food benefits on products deemed essential to the preparation of a so-called basic meal—in other words, on the cheapest grocery and other items.[127]

This requirement reveals the rather bitter irony that accompanies the present-day abundance of food. If before inequality lay in the access to and distribution of a limited quantity of food resources, today it turns on who has access to the best, most nutritious products, within the overall cornucopia of food, and who does not.

In terms of both health and symbolic representations, the abundant supplies of food are distributed very unequally among the population. What is most costly and refined, best for one's health, and most aesthetically and stylistically pleasing still belongs to those who make the greatest show of their wealth. To be sure, one hears it uttered that money is not everything, that taste—in the sense of "good taste," as something formed by education, travel, nutritional savvy and a knowledge of cooking, and so on—also counts. Yet both casual observation and sophisticated gastronomic talk make it clear that money and status, understood as symbols of class, still have their way.

The various upscale cuisines grouped under the rubric "nouvelle" offer the best proof of this fact. These cuisines emphasize a discriminating palate, exotic ingredients, small portions, and a stylish arrangement and presentation of food.[128] Nouvelle cuisine dishes are defined by fresh food and natural flavors; light, delicate sauces; and expensive vegetables, all of which stand in contrast to food that is heavy, starchy, and prepared according to the traditions of older ways of Puerto Rican cooking. As has been pointed out, the different styles of nouvelle cuisine depart even further from the traditional by their symbolic rejection of the utilitarian, conscious display of subtle tastes and flavors, and greater concern with the aesthetics of nutrition than with its efficiencies. Whatever form it takes, nouvelle cuisine is meant to be experienced and enjoyed in an unhurried, leisurely way.

Thus the gastronomic panorama is anything but one-dimensional. On the one hand, the sheer variety of food available in supermarkets, groceries, and restaurants offers everyone the opportunity to enjoy a richer, more expansive and inventive diet; yet at the same time this range of choice, this newfound abundance—if viewed in terms of the realistic prospect of having access to healthy, light, and costly food—is simply not open to a great many. So, while the variety exists, we need to be tempered in our celebration of it.

The differences that, historically, separated one segment of the population from another, insofar as attitudes and actions toward eating and preparing meals are concerned, are still very much in force. Indeed, as traditional ingredients and long-favored cuisine still make their presence felt, they put a new face on non-traditional cuisines and food practices. Moreover, they have helped convince some restaurateurs to bring back traditional dishes and ways of cooking, so that these now exist side by side with the contemporary cuisines shaped by abundance, variety, and a refined culinary aesthetic. Some restaurants exemplifying this trend are Ajili Mójili, in San Juan's El Condado district; Las Vegas, opened by the chef Alfredo Ayala in the tropical forest of El Yunque; La Habichuela Colorá, in Guaynabo; La Jaquita Baya and La Casita Blanca, in Santurce; and La Fonda de Ángelo, in the southern municipality of Santa Isabel.[129]

CONVENIENCE AND CARE

In contrast to how life once was, time today plays a major role in shaping and determining our food habits and practices. The differences that we observe between contemporary and past food cultures result as much from this consideration as from any other. Since cooking and eating are activities that transcend matters of nutrition and the body, time becomes the factor of greatest uncertainty when we prepare to cook or consume a meal.

This last section of the chapter addresses "convenience" in the sense in which Gofton and Ness define the popular perception of "convenience food."[130] In using the term "care," or the expression "taking great care," I have in mind the emotional resonances and qualities of learning and instruction that surround eating and cooking as an activity that helps create and sustain a home or a family and enables it to carry on over generations.[131]

On occasion we vacillate between convenience and a more discriminating, appealing choice of food because time is lacking or because, though we have the time, we prefer to spend it on something other than cooking or consuming a long, leisurely meal.

This hesitation is also tied to other factors affecting the circumstances in which eating and preparing meals take place today, but of all of them, time plays the determining role. In present circumstances, unlike in earlier eras, shopping for food and stocking the pantry do not simply eat up blocks of our time but often require that we travel from one place to another.

As the nature and configuration of work in the home have changed, together with the personal interrelationships that define it, the task of acquiring food and other provisions, which before was carried out by the domestic help, now falls on the shoulders of the female head of the household. The number of women classified as housewives is estimated at 1,250,000, a figure that exceeds the number of women who work outside the home. In a recent study, Zuleika Vidal Rodríguez, a professor at the University of Puerto Rico, explains that while women may have achieved certain types of socio-professional success, "many of them get married and go back to being at home [and] others continue studying, but remain in the house."[132] She concludes by stating: "The expectation is still there that a woman studies so she can eventually work, should a separation occur or should her husband not be able to take care of her. . . . The romantic notion still exists in Puerto Rico that if I meet a man who can take care of me, I will stay at home [underlined in the original]."[133]

Although the relations that govern the division of domestic labor have changed to some extent, making the purchases, doing the cooking, caring for the children, and fulfilling other domestic chores and duties are still viewed as a woman's responsibility in Puerto Rico.[134] Inevitably, the time spent performing all these tasks cuts down on the time that can be spent in provisioning a household, and thus on the time that can be devoted to acquiring food and to organizing, cooking, and serving meals (the "instrumental" and "technical" tasks, according to Warde) on the part of the 489,000 Puerto Rican women, or 35 percent of the island's workforce, who hold down jobs.[135]

To be fair, it could be argued that the time expended in cooking and shopping can be compensated for by the specialization in food products, that is, by the availability of boxed and packaged food, semi-prepared and readymade meals, and by orders sent in via the Web; as well as by advances in kitchen and household technology that simplify and expedite the preparation, serving, and disposal of food. These advances are certainly real, but their blessings are not unmitigated.

Interestingly, while buying a shopping cart full of food on a single trip to the market appears to be in decline, everything seems to indicate that the total amount of time devoted to purchasing food has increased, as the practice of making purchases more than once a week has similarly increased. In the urban business environment in which we live today, this implies driving in a car to the large commercial centers and malls located along the roads and streets bearing the highest volume of traffic.

The extension in "travel time" would seem to make little sense if the increase in the number of establishments selling food, island-wide, is also taken into account. As indicated in studies carried out by the Administración de Fomento Comercial (Commerce Department), there were approximately 1,222 outlets in Puerto Rico selling food products in 1997, or one market, corner grocery, or other food-selling enterprise for each three square miles of land.[136] The agency's estimate can be seen as corroboration of the improved access that people have to food sellers and suppliers, which presumably helps streamline the whole business of provisioning their homes and apartments. But now, unlike in earlier years, the way of getting to one of them is almost without exception by driving.

Traffic density in Puerto Rico has also grown prodigiously, and generally without any centralized coordination and control, during the past twenty years. The most recent studies made by the Department of Transportation and Public Works put the estimated number of cars on a mile of roadway at 146, and at 4,286 for each square mile of the island's streets and roads. These figures earn Puerto Rico the dubious distinction of having the highest density of automobile traffic in the world.[137] While trip and driving patterns can vary considerably from one person to another, the overall effect of these conditions is to increase the amount of "shopping time" relative to the amount of "cookery time."

In 1998, Atilano Cordero Badillo, the owner of the Grande hipermercado chain, noted, with regard to the tempo of shopping in his stores, that "customers are increasingly in a hurry. In fact, marketing studies indicate that the average consumer spends barely twenty-one minutes shopping."[138]

All of these factors—the press of time, the crowded roadways, the ease of acquiring packaged and take-away meals, and so on—help explain the appearance and success of another modern phenomenon: the stocking and sale of comestibles and convenience food by stores whose main line of business has nothing to do with food in the traditional sense.[139] Likewise, supermarkets have expanded the range of services they offer with respect to convenience food. A study conducted in 1998 by the trade association for the food distribution and marketing industry in Puerto Rico found, in a sample group of 209 supermarkets, that 63 had a deli service, 54 had cafeterias, and 108 had bakeries.[140]

Another study, carried out in 2001 by the firm Professional Market Research, found that out of nine variables, respondents ranked the "closeness to [their] home" of the supermarket in which they shopped as third from the top in importance.[141] The study also found that the two services most in need of improvement, from the respondents' point of view, were the "bagging service" at the checkout registers and "parking." Inadequate service in these two areas increases the amount of "shopping time" to the detriment of time spent on other domestic work and activities, among them cooking and consuming meals.

At the same time, however, the introduction of appliances and cooking accessories made possible by late-twentieth-century technological advances can substantially reduce the amount of time needed to complete certain tasks in the kitchen. A prime example is the microwave oven. Yet the containers and plasticware that we use to cook and warm up fast food in the microwave can also put us wrong, leave us with the sense that we have shortchanged ourselves, nutritionally and otherwise, by not exercising greater care in the selection and preparation of what we eat. Indeed, we may be sufficiently disillusioned as to think that "microwavable" food hardly merits being called food at all, a worry that is built into the tension arising from the practice of eating convenience food.

Nor do other technological advances, like the food processor, necessarily eliminate basic instrumental tasks that have always been with us, such as selecting, cleaning, and peeling the skin off certain foods. In addition, for the housewife who is looking for the best, most authentic results, a time-saving accessory like the rice cooker has little value, since it cannot produce rice as it really ought to be, *pega'o*, that is, having the slightly burnt scrapings that stick to the bottom of the rice after it is cooked in a shallow pan, the traditional way. Much new kitchen gadgetry and appliances also require that they be professionally installed and put into operation, cleaned in a certain way, and periodically serviced by a technician.

In this sense, the popularity of appliances like the food processor, dishwasher, and microwave oven, while highly effective in their own way, may also highlight the sense of disjunction that results from the loss of time that is given to the culinary experience overall, even as less time has to be spent on some of its "instrumental" aspects, such as shopping for provisions, preparing them to be cooked, and cleaning up after the meal.

Under these conditions, Puerto Ricans—and above all the working mother—find themselves party to one of the most salient aspects of contemporary food practices and culture: the erosion of the rich emotional content and meaning they once carried, a focal point of which, in the past, was the capacity that cooking, and the preparation of sweets in particular, always had to foster feelings of companionship and bonds of affection between people. To be sure, social theorists are of the opinion that allocations of time—whether decreased or not—are simply incapable in themselves of revealing the emotional dimensions of domestic work, and they further believe that should one sphere of domestic work experience a decrease in the amount of time it requires, others may well not.[142]

In the tension that envelops the two poles of convenience and care, the former seems to be interwoven with the latter. In contrast to the oppositions of health and indulgence and economy and extravagance, in which we can observe a clear, unambiguous division, the factor of convenience can be deployed to help realize its opposite; that is, at times people will opt for some element of convenience—such as purchasing a semi-prepared item of food from a store close at hand—without jettisoning the hope or expectation that their meticulousness, love, respect, or care will be on display when they sit down to share it.

Although it proves very difficult to tell which tendency exerts the greater force, we can see from simply looking around us that bound up with the act of eating a meal and with activities related to it (going out to dine, or gathering as a family around the table at home, or eating in the group atmosphere of school, hospital, and factory cafeterias) there is a conscious desire to please, to maintain social solidarity and ties of friendship, to use the business of cooking and consuming food to interact on a personal level, and to carry on an idea both of family as a positive institution and of what "food," properly understood, truly is.

The discussions and discourse that accompany the state-funded nutritional assistance program, administered through the Department of the Family, are an excellent example of this latter-most wish and objective. Within the program as it exists today, the notion of a carefully crafted and balanced diet is crystallized in the idea of the "family" as a bastion of social stability. In this discourse, "basic," as opposed to convenience food, is used as a prong by which to teach PAN's beneficiaries about a particular type of family life. In this sense, PAN's objectives are very similar to the home economics proposals put forward in the first half of the twentieth century, whereby traditional foods, when prepared in new ways and utilized correctly, would contribute to solidifying the family as a social institution.

This idea was also operative in the policy adopted in 2002 by the Department of Education to replace the "junk food" (comida chatarra) served or available in school cafeterias with traditional foods. The proposal culminated in 2004 with the adoption of a set of formal guidelines, the Guía de política pública para la venta de alimentos en las escuelas (Public Policy Guide for the Sale of Food in the Schools).[143] The new guidelines represented an attempt to juggle the menus of the school dining halls, so that students would be offered complete meals, while ridding the schools of the vending machines that dispensed items that failed to meet even minimal nutritional standards. Through all the discussions that led to the new policy, and embedded in the policy itself, ran the conviction that balanced meals containing nutritive foods helped produce the ideal home and family.

In like fashion, the proposals developed by the Department of the Family and by the advocates of a reformed school breakfast and lunch menu, as well as the advertising of the agro-food industry, with its references to the special flavors or secrets of home cooking (" homemade," for example, or "with grandmother's or mother's taste and touch"),[144] demonstrate that in Puerto Rico there are still certain traditional understandings and meanings, strongly held and valued among the members of different generations and social classes, about what qualifies as food in the proper sense of the term.

Despite the lack of studies on the topic, this observation illustrates that a consensus exists in Puerto Rico in the sense that "cooking," or producing a meal, is a culinary action that has to involve one or several of the following elements: be done at home with fresh ingredients (nothing premade); be deemed healthy and not sparing in quantity (this holds when eating outside the home as well); have a recognizable taste and flavor (recall a mother's or grandmother's special seasoning or secret recipe); use products with which the diner is familiar; ensure that everything is cooked in a way that is known, never unknown; that all items and dishes are brought to the table hot; and finally, that the meal be consumed in the company of one's family or of close friends in a family-like atmosphere. At present, just as in the past, the notion of preparing food remains closely tied to the desire to see society successfully carry on, from one generation to the next, within a set of ideal (or idealized) parameters.

Thus, in the face of many countervailing circumstances and conditions, together with the tendency to opt for convenience over care and the evident push by the state, and by state interests, for a society respecting and upholding certain ideals, the emotional resonances, comradeship, and transmission of knowledge and skills that have always surrounded cooking and food remain in force.

Although one would need to conduct more research to gauge the depth of its influence, the way in which adults use mealtimes both to instruct children in proper dining-table etiquette and to educate and socialize them more generally seems to indicate that the tradition of care still persists.

On this matter, paraphrasing Fischler, the geographers David Bell and Gill Valentine point out that "the home dining table" is a place that not only safeguards children's health but also helps form their personalities. Children are taught, at table, how to prepare and cook different foods, what is appropriate to eat under various circumstances, and what it is to have good manners and to behave accordingly: Simple things—the correct type of cutlery and place settings to use, the stricture against chewing with one's mouth open, and the need to sit up and not slouch—are taught and learned.[145] As Bell and Valentine note, these lessons begin from the very moment certain words and expressions like "I beg your pardon," "please," "thank you," and "excuse me" are first heard and repeated, together with such exclamations of approval, over different tastes and flavors, as "yummy, how delicious!"[146] In addition, they reflect on how the kitchen plays a wider, non-traditional role as a social and educational space. Children use the kitchen as a place in which to do their homework, describe what they liked or did not like about the day, and to sit and gab with their friends. In this way, the kitchen has become a communication zone, a point of contact through the day, and the meals that are taken there provide the family a special time in which to be together, to be a single unit, and to give parents the chance to hear about and take measure of their children's lives. Amid the constant intrusion of convenience food, the pull of personal freedom and stylized social behavior, and of "McDonaldization" and the shrinking of time given to eating, one still observes in Puerto Rico attitudes and practices toward food aimed at preserving part of an older way of life, by means of gestures and actions that signal affection, care, warmth, and the passing on of customs and tradition.

Nonetheless, these cannot escape the tensions produced by the dualism of convenience versus care. The strain between the two comes to life in the newspaper piece about food and eating, "Cuando vamos a comer en familia" (When We Go Out to Eat as a Family), by the veteran Puerto Rican chef Giovanna Huyke.[147] Huyke paints a picture of the essential features of this tension, which for many Puerto Ricans turn into a daily dilemma.

The story she recounts unfolded from the 1997 remodeling of her kitchen, which forced her to feed and arrange meals for her children outside the familiar confines of home. This disruption meant, of course, that decisions had to be made about where to eat. Under the circumstances, Huyke could simply have opted for convenience food. In her role as a working mother, however, she decided that the family's meals should be taken in an atmosphere that reproduced, as much as possible, the feeling and setting of their home and both its close-knit and instructive parent-to-child relationships. In her words: "I have always wanted to give the best to my children, and am very conscious that what is best is always what takes place at home, or if not that, something very much like that." Thus, for Huyke, the requirement of eating outside "prompted a search for which restaurants near my house could be stand-ins for what I needed while the new kitchen was being constructed."

Here we see the first tension appearing, in the understanding that meals served at home, around the dining table, form the ideal way in which to communicate with and instruct children, and that the interactions that occur during mealtimes in the home setting are difficult to manage in another location, even one like a family restaurant. For this reason Huyke set herself the task of finding restaurants that "[fulfilled] the basic rules, so we could enjoy ourselves when we went out to eat with our children." These rules were perfectly straightforward: the restaurants had to have types of food and dishes on their menu that Huyke's children were familiar with, and they had to offer a "warm and relaxed," that is, family, "atmosphere."

Huyke's account does not dismiss the fact that going out to eat presents an opportunity to "expose your children to other kinds of food," an activity that helps broaden their outlook and enlarge their knowledge of the world. However, she puts a premium on food and meals that the family knows and with which it readily identifies. Further on, in her dual role as professional chef and mother, Huyke notes that there are not many restaurants that "duplicate that day in and day out," meaning by "that" the family's own food habits and preferences and the emotional, educational, and social exchanges they embody and represent.

She concludes her eminently sensible report prognosticating that, for a number of families in present-day Puerto Rico, the time devoted in the home to matters of food and eating is steadily decreasing and that therefore the factor of convenience is intruding on a daily basis in a way that contravenes and undermines cooking and eating in the home as a vehicle for teaching and learning proper behavior and for building warm, close family relationships. If in fact there are periods of leisure time that could be devoted to preparing and consuming meals at home, families prefer to use them to pursue other ways of socializing their children and teaching them about life. To quote Huyke again: "In the world in which we live, where the father and mother often work, not all of us can cook every day, [and] for others of us, what happens is that we like to have fun with our children on the weekend."

As her parting words, Huyke implores working mothers, whatever the circumstances, to follow the culinary practices not of convenience but of care (eating as a family), even though the social environment of Puerto Rico no longer makes it easy to do so. In closing out her columns and her television broadcasts, this consummate professional chef sums it up by saying: "My signature goodbye is always: Let's cook. Today I bid goodbye with: Let's eat well [even] when we can't cook, but be a family by hook or by crook."

8 | Yesterday, Today, Tomorrow

Even more than words or speech, food serves as a bridge
between different cultures when culinary systems open themselves to all sorts of new influences, inventions, and exchange.

—MASSIMO MONTANARI, *La cocina: Lugar de la identidad y
del intercambio*, 2003

The foodstuffs that can be classified as basic to the diet and gastronomy of
Puerto Rico were also central to many other regional food cultures across
the globe prior to 1500. Their appearance in Puerto Rico, and in the Caribbean more broadly, resulted from such factors as the movement of people
and plants from the Old World to the new, the conquerors' failure to reproduce their commonplace foodscape in the new environment, the effect
of closely held religious beliefs, the necessity to feed enslaved Africans on
their journey as human cargo, and the decision by passengers to include
known foods in their baggage and aboard ships because of their fear of
hunger in an unknown world. Some food—salted cod is a prime example—was introduced to the island for commercial reasons; other foods,
like plantains, yams, and rice, found an ideal natural environment in the
Caribbean, prospering as essential crops and everyday food to our own day.
Still others, like wild and unbranded cattle and swine, found refuge in the
forests and outlying mountainous regions. In time, all of this once-foreign
food blended with the island's native food—corn, cassava, tannier, sweet
potatoes, beans, chili peppers, annatto, coriander leaves, and a wide variety
of fruits—to furnish a major part of the daily diet.

Still, while they formed the pillars of Puerto Rican cookery and were as
familiar to most islanders as the ground on which they stood, the manner
in which people thought about them and the possibility that they would
turn up on the dinner table was sharply differentiated by inherited tastes,
class distinctions, and economic and cultural considerations. In the case of

fresh meat, economic considerations had been paramount; for bread made with cassava flour, the critical factors were inherited tastes, which affected Iberian immigrants in particular, food expectations, and the inability to maintain a constant supply of imported wheat for making bread. With plantains and the majority of tuberous viandas, the distinctions of social class came into focus, as these products—while considered essential to the daily diet—had always been looked down on as being the food of the poor.

Corn ground into flour, which in the form of *guanime* (see glossary) had been central to the diet of the island's indigenous inhabitants, was for centuries a major component of what sustained the rural mestizo population, and it was likewise valued by many peninsular immigrants for its ability to be turned into bread. The most durable preparation of all, *funche*, was until quite recently viewed by the upper and better-placed sectors as being nothing more than the food of "blacks" and of rural and urban lower-class elements.

The most sharply defined distinctions operated with respect to meat. On this score, the two basic meat products—pork and beef—carried opposed meanings. Pork was considered a cruder type of meat, one that was consumed as prey on a more occasional basis, as part of festivities and celebrations, though on another level the majority of the population viewed pigs in a positive light, as a domestic animal that could be raised easily, reproduced in large numbers, and provided much-needed fat for cooking and other purposes. Beef, in contrast, was associated with a more urban, refined environment.

Whereas meat—from wild cattle as well as wild pigs—was available to a great many islanders during the first two and a half centuries that followed the Spanish conquest, starting at the end of the eighteenth century, the possibility of obtaining fresh meat steadily receded for three broad segments of the population: settlers living far away from towns and cities, the urban poor, and those—such as plantation slaves—who were forced to live on a regulated diet. For many, fresh meat ceased to be an option altogether, and along the radically opposed poles of the diet, it took on two distinct meanings, becoming emblematic of two distinct states—abundance and scarcity.

Bound up with the contingencies that surrounded the acquisition of fresh meat was the appearance of salted cod. Already a familiar food to Spaniards, salted cod was initially introduced as an item of food that preserved well during days that called for fasting from meat. The impact of the

Portuguese, Spanish, and later English fleets that worked the fishing beds of the Atlantic cod subsequently transformed salted cod from an inexpensive fish consumed for Lenten meals into the most practical and nutritional food for soldiers and slaves.

During the nineteenth century, the consumption of salted cod spread to the entire population, but on the tables of humbler families it became a peripheral food, used to add flavor to other products and to complement the otherwise scarce protein-rich nutrients available to the poorest segments of the population. While the amount and quality of salted cod used by people, and the way in which they prepared it, necessarily depended on their economic resources, starting at the end of the nineteenth century and gaining greater force between 1900 and 1940, salted cod became linked not only to a simple and traditional cuisine and style of cooking but also, and more keenly, to the meager diet imposed by poverty, misfortune, and social exclusion.

Rice and beans also served as staple food items. A local, unpolished rice (*arroz criollo*, or creole rice), developed and tended by African slaves, was successfully adapted throughout the seventeenth century to the wetlands of the island's coastal regions. By around 1776, some 2 million pounds of this rice were being harvested, and various ways of preparing it had become common among the population. As they did with other types of food, people found different ways of using this rice. In the homes of the wealthiest families, it was treated as an accompaniment, while for people at the opposite end of the economic spectrum it became a core food and came to symbolize food security.

In the nineteenth century, imported polished rice—clearer in appearance and smaller-grained—began to complement supplies of locally grown rice. This intermixing, which proceeded very slowly and gradually, caused a devaluing of local varieties and a growing preference for the smaller grain. The trend away from local rice was aided by two factors: the large-scale development of a successor crop, sugarcane, in these same coastal areas, and the force of the island's import market, both of which occurred within the framework of a colonial system of commercial relationships, initially maintained with the Spanish metropolis and later with the United States. The short-grained, polished rice was imported via the markets of three countries, Spain, England, and Germany, to which were later added a fourth—the United States. During the twentieth century, sugar monocropping did away with the few rice fields that remained in the coastal wetlands.

Other factors helping to erode the older preference for (or at least reliance on) creole rice were the problems encountered in cleaning off its outer skin; its more opaque appearance; the roughness of its kernels, which increased its cooking time; and the difficulty experienced in getting it moist and soft.

The rejection of local rice varieties, and the consequent spread of imported varieties, gathered pace in the first decades of the twentieth century. This development had serious health implications, because the polished rice imported from abroad was stripped of all its nutrients while being subjected to a high-tech milling process. Toward the beginning of the 1950s, in the face of an implacable preference for polished rice, specialists in nutritional science decided that the best line of attack was to fortify it to reduce the possibility that people would succumb to illnesses brought on by or connected to the consumption of rice lacking in nutrients. Even today, in its most common variety, polished rice remains the preferred rice of Puerto Ricans, although not even a single kernel of it is produced on Puerto Rican soil.

Beans, indigenous to the island and one of the foods eaten by its native population, likewise came to be a common dietary item, though they were not held in very high regard by visitors to Puerto Rico from early colonial times onward. The original varieties of beans seem to have been mixed without any criteria of selection, and over time their yields grew smaller. In any event, the beans *del país* (native to the island) had to compete, during the Spanish era, with the garbanzo bean and then later, under the U.S. territorial administration, with the dry red kidney bean. The capacity of the latter to preserve well, its ability to soak and soften quickly and to thicken up broths and soups, and its flavor and size, helped make it a favorite vis-à-vis other types of beans, including imported pink and white beans.

Originally served as separate items of food, rice and beans came to be treated as a single dish at the end of the eighteenth century. Toward the end of the 1850s, when a recipe for preparing beans appeared in the first published Puerto Rican cookbook, it was recommended that they be accompanied by local white rice. One can surmise, then, that around the middle of the nineteenth century, as the system of slavery became further institutionalized on the island and as other groups in society fell into chronic poverty, a typical way of consuming rice and beans was solidified: the two were prepared separately but then mixed together in the same bowl once people were ready to eat them. The liquid or broth that came out of the pot or stew in which the beans had been cooked was added to the rice to give it a richer flavor.

This custom of combining them was practiced, in one variation or another, by all social classes, and new cookbooks published in the early twentieth century followed the same indications. At the beginning of the 1930s, a chemist, Luis Torres Díaz, in undertaking a study of the nutritional value of the Puerto Rican diet, wrote vis-à-vis the ubiquitous combination of rice and beans: "It is the pan cotidianum of the poor people and it is always present on the menu of the rich."[1]

In broad terms, the different foods I have profiled came to form a substantial part of the general diet on the island, even though, within some social groups and according to some understandings, they were thought of as food that was either inadequate, or alien, or "infra dig." The unequal material circumstances of the population, the near permanence of a society that placed high value on maintaining a separation—literal and figurative—among social groups and classes, and the persistence of a colonial food market reinforced such notions.

Puerto Rican cuisine and foodways—that is, the use of certain common types of food, spices, and seasoning and of recurrent methods of cooking, the frequent preparation of the same meals and dishes, and the expression of informed opinions about them—were shaped by three principal factors: first, the interplay between the culinary knowledge and experience of the island's indigenous population and the desire on the part of the first waves of Spanish settlers to duplicate a familiar gastronomy in an unfamiliar land, under conditions of food insecurity; second, the development of constricted, homogenous dietary systems as a means of feeding hundreds of thousands of African slaves and large contingents of soldiers who arrived on the island between the seventeenth and nineteenth centuries and were later integrated into Puerto Rican society; and third, the basic human impulse to survive and reproduce in a context marked by simplicity, routine, and convention. In contrast to how we approach and conceive of it today, cooking (as a daily practice that transforms foodstuffs into meals so we can go on living) was an activity impelled primarily by basic physiological needs. It was circumscribed, for a long period of time, by the material circumstances of a rural population tied to the production cycles of small-scale agriculture, a system of farming that enjoyed scant possibilities of expanding against the weight and power of a monocultural export market.

It was similarly hemmed in by the priorities of a highly homogeneous food import market.

As recently as sixty years ago, Puerto Rico—in colloquial terms—was a land of "poor cuisine." The great majority cooked and prepared meals with what the immediate environment offered, what grew right under one's own gaze, using utensils fashioned at home out of the materials that nature provided. People ate ample portions of a narrow range of food, following recipes passed by word of mouth, or learned through observation and imitation, or jotted on pieces of paper, employing such limited understanding of nutrition as existed. Puerto Rican cuisine was the expression of the urge to survive; until the second half of the twentieth century, it relied on the types of food and techniques of preparation that I have described in these pages. Now, in the midst of an abundance of food, the advances made by agroindustry, and high-end food distribution and merchandising, cooking on the island, in all of its dimensions, is in a state of transition.

Can we also claim that, prior to 1950, Puerto Rican food practices were— for some—in line with the most elaborate, sophisticated models, employing food that was alien to the island's ecology and environment, and re-creating recipes from abroad by using products received via the import market? Ultimately, was a non-native haute cuisine practiced on the island? I fear that it was.

A taste for exotic foods and for the most intricate ways of preparing and presenting them had always been present, and those with the interest and means did everything possible to participate in this worldly food culture. In practice, however, such "sensibilities" were manifested only sporadically and were confined to certain groups. Evidence of their imprint dates to the earliest years of Spanish colonization and is seen above all in the practices followed by members of the ecclesiastical and military elite. Salient examples include the food (e.g., olives, marzipan, sweet wine, quince paste) and the cooking and tableware that Bishop Alonso Manso brought with him from Spain; Damián López de Haro's dismissive attitude concerning the island's native foodstuffs; the array of china and utensils found on the tables of some of the colony's governors; the wine cellar of the ill-fated pirate Miguel Henríquez; the vigilance shown by the municipal council of San Juan toward protecting casks of wine (albeit watered down); the observations of the monk Iñigo Abad y Lasierra regarding the tastes of the colony's wealthiest residents; the importation onto the island of fine food products as recorded in the nineteenth-century *Balanzas Mercantiles*; the three nineteenth-century editions of the cookbook El *cocinero puertorriqueño*, which contained more than just Puerto Rican recipes; the frequent banquets held in honor of the island's captains general; and references made during the nineteenth century to different restaurants in San Juan.

Still, as Jean-Louis Flandrin has pointed out, the cultivation of taste was one thing; necessity, or the fulfillment of basic needs, another.[2] In Puerto Rico, "necessity"—governed by what the local environment could effectively produce—was the norm. It was driven by a homogenous colonial food market and marked by a system of social relationships in which the work of cooking and preparing meals was—in almost all contexts—not in the hands of professionals but, instead, was entrusted to the intuitions and specialized knowledge of people, almost always slaves, who related to specific items of food and to what, of these, the land was capable of yielding. This set of factors acted as a brake on the development of a visible and persistent haute cuisine.

Starting in the mid-nineteenth century, influenced by the experiences of Puerto Rican students living in Europe; the opening of new markets, those of the Lesser Antilles especially; the solidifying of a creole bourgeoisie attentive to change and to foreign fashions; and the cosmopolitanism that some of the island's cities were beginning to acquire, the cultivation of a haute cuisine free of local content began to gain limited momentum. Nonetheless, its contribution to Puerto Rican food culture would remain quite circumscribed, until it could transcend a narrow band of social activities, celebratory events, and ceremonial representations, both public and private.

This constraint was brought vividly to life at a dinner hosted in 1898 by a well-to-do family of hacendados, to which a North American, William Dinwiddie, was invited. The centerpiece of the meal was meat, a clear indicator of wealth and privileged social status. It is noteworthy, however, that the menu for that night also included *gandinga* (stewed pork entrails), sweet potatoes, rice, and—for dessert—guava paste, cheese, and coconut with unrefined brown sugar.[3] It was this style of local haute cuisine—humble in nature, generous in quantity, resonant of a rural ambience, and born more of intuition or the inspiration of the moment than of studious planning and reflection—which emerged at this time.

As already indicated, the landscape of diet and cooking in Puerto Rico has been radically reshaped during the past fifty years. As such, it merits asking two questions: Is the food that was previously consumed still being consumed? That is, are the food products that formed the traditional core of the Puerto Rican diet still present to the same degree in our current food culture? And, if around these particular foods and the culinary practices developed along with them there evolved a powerful attachment that helps define people as Puerto Rican—a fact seemingly confirmed in the replies furnished by the people profiled at the beginning of the book—can these food-based referents, which are taken as marks of national and cultural identity, survive today in a less fixed and stable environment? Can the contemporary food culture countenance the profile of "other" Puerto Ricans?

The food products that were historically cooked and consumed on the island have lost the organic function shaping and molding them years ago. While statistical data show only a gradual decline in the consumption of such historic items as rice, beans, and tuberous viandas, the products that lay at the heart of the old stock of foods have ceased to be understood in present-day Puerto Rico as "food" in the direct, immediate sense of that which is needed, fundamentally, to reproduce human life.

Traditional food habits and practices, and the meals consumed by individuals and families alike, have similarly ceased to be understood as routine and obligatory activities of daily life and have, instead, become optional and discretionary in nature. If certain types of food and recipes still carry the stamp of day-to-day routine and convention, this faithfulness to past tradition is due to the slow pace at which food and culinary tastes tend to change. They leave traces of the familiar with us, but not a sense of robust survival. The historic relationship we have with them, and the taste formed by sheer necessity, still underpin Puerto Rican food practices, but in the mode of "conscious coexistence" with the elements of variety and abundance.

If the loss of the old organic function exerted by food and cooking is by now a reality, there are other spheres of food culture that have begun to exhibit new profiles that are open to being more fully defined and fleshed out in the coming years. One such example involves the place and relative importance of certain foods in the composition of meals overall. Some historic foods have come to occupy a distinctly second tier, as is the case with viandas, which once were a central component of meals but now are treated more as a side dish; other dishes, such as the more humble preparations made with corn flour (*marota, marifinga,* and *funche;* see glossary for the first two) have been eliminated from the common repertoire altogether; and still other types of food are now consumed less frequently, as is occurring, for example, with beans. These changes extend as well as to the number of times certain foods and dishes are consumed in the course of a day. For example, the combination of rice and beans used to be a fixture on the menu and was even served for breakfast, whereas today it tends to be consumed just once per day, at lunchtime, when the main meal of the day is taken.

Time-honored culinary rules have also been bent and interpreted more freely to prepare dishes that are represented as or considered to be traditional. For example, the texture, color, and flavor of *pasteles* have all changed as new ways of grating plantains and green bananas have come into play, artificial coloring and ingredients to bring out flavor are added, or the boiling is done in a microwave oven. Moreover, pastel has acquired an entirely new function: now, at any time of the year, families will be seen hawking pastel as a way of generating additional income, rather than waiting until the end of the year to prepare it, as one of the dishes invariably eaten at home during the Christmas holidays.

By the same token, where various manual skills grounded in old foodways once played a key role in the preparation of traditional dishes, they are disappearing from the scene today, made obsolete by agroindustry and its arsenal of processing techniques. Increasingly, grating and peeling, kneading, careful slicing and cutting, boiling over a slow heat, preparing *sofrito*, roasting pork on a spit over hot coals, and confecting traditional sweets form part of a lost art of the kitchen.

The changed landscape of Puerto Rican culinary practice is reflected in the current paradigm that governs cooking and cuisine. Foods and activities formerly accepted as part of an inevitable routine are now viewed as voluntary in nature, dictated not by necessity but by personal preference and choice. While declarations such as "today I feel like cooking the Puerto Rican way" or "I'm up for a dish of rice with beans stewed with pig's feet" clearly attest to inherited tastes and culinary sensibilities, they do so in a wider, more fluid context of conscious, deliberate choice, of the desire to evoke memories of particular tastes and flavors. Such old-style, native dishes—when ordered in a restaurant or cooked at home—may indeed be familiar to Puerto Ricans, but not any longer as part of the fabric of daily life. It is this latter distinction that suggests that the present is a time of transition, a period in which traditional food and dishes—set against the great abundance of food overall—are seen as items of special value which run the risk of being lost. Hence they become part of the island's cultural patrimony.

The introduction and mixing of non-Caribbean dishes into the menus of restaurants specializing in native cuisine likewise illustrates the changing face of Puerto Rican cookery. A prime example is lasagna, which—accompanied by rice and beans or, alternatively, by *tostones* (fried green plantains), has become a central component of the lunch plate in many traditional eateries. Similarly, macaroni—typically known as *coditos* (elbow macaroni)—is now the invariable accompaniment to the glazed Virginia ham served in the same type of restaurant. Like French fries, macaroni is sometimes used as a substitute for rice and beans. Edgardo Rodríguez Juliá observed the same phenomenon in El Jibarito, an old San Juan restaurant prized for its native cuisine, where the daily lunch plate included cordon bleu, accompanied by tostones, viandas, or a portion of rice and beans.

Another notable example of this trend is that of roast turkey, which has been given the name *pavochón*, because it is seasoned and cooked in the same way as the *lechón*, or pig roasted on a spit over coals. Christmas Eve dinners, in fact, will often feature turkey as a substitute for roast pig. A similar process involves fish by-products—marinated "surimi," for example, which has gradually come to replace *serenata de bacalao*, or salted codfish salad, as a dish consumed during Lent. The same effect is achieved when once-unfamiliar ingredients or food are incorporated into the preparation of traditional dishes, as has happened, for example, with the tostones now served with a topping of caviar in the most stylish restaurants.

The most basic food products and most deeply rooted dietary practices have thus not been impervious to change and refashioning. Moreover, what at times is defined and identified as the essence of Puerto Rican food or cooking is not always shared and passed on in the same way, nor do some Puerto Ricans necessarily inherit any of this tradition. Luis Rafael Sánchez nicely captures this checkered culinary inheritance when, in his *Elogio de la fritura*, he notes that fried salted cod, a venerable dish that served to tamp down the hunger pangs so often felt by the poorest Puerto Ricans, today goes under the name *bacalaito* and appears as part of the "finger foods" served at the most stylish banquets.

Furthermore, certain foodstuffs, dishes, and styles of cooking that, over time, have come to be seen as central to the very notion of "Puerto Rican culture" have not always existed on the island. Salted cod is standing proof of this fact, introduced as it was between the end of the seventeenth and the beginning of the nineteenth century, in a food context that was problematic for certain sectors of the population. Other examples of this grafting of a new product onto the older culinary tradition are "corned beef," which—though not appearing on the island until fairly recently—is nonetheless considered as authentic Puerto Rican cuisine; or the Carmela-brand tinned sausages, which turn up once per week in the *fondas* as part of the customary dish of rice and sausages or sausage stew; or even sofrito, which—now made according to a more or less standardized formula only after a long process of experimentation—is acclaimed as the ne plus ultra of what characterizes the unique taste of Puerto Rican cooking.

In the midst of all these changes and anomalies, however, certain elements in the island's culinary history have remained constant and coherent. Experienced in a generally uniform way by the majority of the population, they have helped shape the idea of stability and permanence that is a cornerstone of the newfound desire to define a particular type and style of food and cooking as Puerto Rican.

The longevity enjoyed by certain products in the island's agriculture and in its food import market formed one of these elements. During a period of nearly four hundred years, these were the only products that either proved successful within the local agro-ecological environment or were fed into the pipeline of the colonial food market. As a result, they turned up—repeatedly and monotonously—in the dishes and meals cooked by the majority of the island's population. Moreover, this element changed in very slow increments.

Hence, in the midst of the current abundance and variety of food, these products retain their familiarity and come to stand for durability and permanence. They have nothing of the provisional or fleeting about them; on the contrary, they have helped shape a collective memory of the palate, an emotional response that evokes a world of food practices and habits and calls up experiences associated with particular flavors, textures, colors, food shortages, survival strategies, festivals, religious rules, and pleasures and displeasures.

The future possibilities of this "palate" can be foreseen in the ideas advanced by Claude Fischler: "There exists a moment of transition, not of an oral tradition to a written and bookish tradition, but to a situation that is compounded, indeterminate, open to all manner of transformation. It involves a process of individual relearning. Through trial and error, each person must retrace the whole road, integrating multiple strands and blocs of information: family memories, diverse written sources, information obtained from those closest to one. Very divergent culinary influences . . . can coexist in this nebulous haze of information. This individual relearning, then, is the opportunity to effect an integration composed of culinary elements from outside local tradition . . . a syncretic mixture."[4]

What we encounter, then, is a state of "suspension," that—examined from Fischler's point of view—entails fusion, indeterminacy, a syncretic intermixing. For Puerto Rico, the best example of this process will be found in the 2001 recipe book *Cocina desde mi pueblo*, which brings together most of the home preparations featured between 1997 and 2000 on "Nobody Cooks Like Mama"—a segment of the popular television show *Desde mi pueblo*. In addition to its collection of traditional home-style recipes, the publication also re-creates a number of very old dishes. Moreover, it takes ingredients that are new to Puerto Rican cooking or that were unknown in earlier times and incorporates them into traditional preparations. It also invents entirely new, personalized dishes using food long present in Puerto Rican cuisine. A second cookbook, *Puerto Rico: La gran cocina del Caribe*, which appeared in 2004, is also richly illustrative of this blending of the old and the new. Its recipes combine traditional items with new ingredients to produce novel dishes, such as curried pastel of cassava stuffed with land crabs, accompanied by a red pepper sauce and chutney composed of mango and papaya; or *piononos* (see glossary) containing lamb, and fettuccini with pigeon peas.[5]

There are other factors at play that lead one to think that both traditional foodstuffs and older ways of cooking them are still a persistent part of the Puerto Rican culinary scene, in the midst of the tremendous contemporary variety of food and the many possibilities for change it opens up. Here we see a clear example of Fischler's "state of suspension."

One such factor is the contribution made by immigrants, from neighboring islands, whose repertoire of dishes is grounded in food that has likewise been at the heart of Puerto Rican gastronomic history, but whose societies have not experienced the changes that took place in Puerto Rico between 1950 and 2000.

This is the case, for example, with Cuban and Dominican diet and foodways, transmitted to Puerto Rico by thousands of immigrants who have come to fill an important place among the island's population.[6] According to Sidney Mintz, before it is national, cooking is regional in character. It is thus to be expected that Puerto Rican cuisine falls into a state of "suspension," aided both by the demand that Dominicans and Cubans place on local food markets and by the significant degree to which they influence the meals and menus found in various eating places, doubtless furthered in this regard by many Puerto Ricans. Neither the food they use nor the ways in which they prepare it differ substantially from what Puerto Ricans themselves are accustomed to.

The clearest way to understand how Caribbean immigrants further the process of suspension is to recognize that in the Commonwealth of Puerto Rico, unlike elsewhere, no ethnic confrontation with Cubans or Dominicans has occurred, in which the element of cooking has served, even minimally, as the basis on which to exclude or reject either community. One can find no evidence, for example, of a move to reject *mangú* (a Dominican mashed plantain dish) or *congrí* (a Cuban rice and beans dish) because they belong to the gastronomy of immigrant populations. If there was some time lag before these dishes became familiar to the Puerto Rican palate, it was not due to any dislike of their taste or appearance but to a lack of knowledge about how to prepare them.

Another factor in the mix is the recognition, by agroindustry and by those responsible for food advertising, that the idiosyncrasies of food practices and consumption change very slowly. Thus, for these stakeholders, there is ample scope for profit in catering to what strikes a familiar chord in Puerto Rican cooking or in artificially adding some element of tradition in the midst of the great variety of food products.[7]

Fischler notes that another point worth investigating is the inverse tendency brought on by the effect of cultivating upscale tastes; that is, the tendency that results from the practice by those social groups historically tied to cuisines and habits born of necessity to distance themselves from these in order to opt for variety and for what is mass produced. In this dynamic, the food that was consumed out of necessity reappears in the tastes of other social sectors as something of special value, because some element redolent of tradition gets added to it, such as a hard-to-come-by ingredient, an antiquated, laborious method of preparation (soaking dry beans instead of using canned beans), or a cooking technique tied to a specific region. A telling example is La Jaquita Baya, a trendy restaurant that recently opened in the upscale San Juan neighborhood of Miramar. Its owner, the young chef Xavier Pacheco, has branded the restaurant with the slogan "Como lo hacían las abuelas" (grandma's style). The menu features such old-style preparations as *habichuelas guisadas ablandadas* (soaked stewed beans), funche with coconut milk and fresh coriander leaves, guanimes, *arroz con dulce* (rice pudding), *alboronía de bacalao con apio* (salted codfish with arracacha), and gandinga.[8] Invested with some such quality, the food that was once eaten purely out of necessity is turned into a kind of museum piece, or historical curiosity, by those fleeing from abundance, massification, and homogeneity. At times, it becomes an object of remembrance, a souvenir that carries with it memories and emotions.

Still other factors can be tied to the "fixation" that Puerto Ricans of a certain age, or from certain social groups, have with particular types of food and culinary practices and traditions. On this score, some 585,071 Puerto Ricans, or 15.4 percent of the island's population, are above the age of sixty. This generational component developed its food tastes and its culinary leanings and skills when hunger was still a serious threat and Puerto Rican food culture was far more homogeneous. Since tastes tend to change very slowly, one would have to countenance the possible "suspension" effect that such gradualism causes and that finds expression in the coexistence of traditional foodways with the more recent condition of abundance and new ways of cooking and of structuring the diet. In addition to these factors, there is the role played by food assistance programs. To bring food to the table, some 28 percent of the island's population depends almost exclusively on state subsidies. In the most recent period, however, the state's policy of nutritional assistance has narrowed the range of food that can be purchased, restricting it to the types of food that are considered most basic in putting together a meal. It is possible, under these circumstances, that this quite substantial portion of the population will find that much of its diet consists of traditional foodstuffs.

Finally, it appears that the inclination to identify oneself as Puerto Rican through the agency of food and the practices and comportment that historically surrounded it enable one to lay claim to the mantle of the "authentic Puerto Rican," because—paradoxically—this archetype has lost the relationship to the past that previously gave it life. The distinctive food-related connections that nurtured the maxim "tell me what you eat and I will tell you who you are" have today begun to split off and unravel.

It is certain that the combination of new influences and experiences—acting as they necessarily do on the accumulated body of traditional food habits and practices—will not result in a complete leveling down, until Puerto Ricans reach the point of asking themselves who they are, as in effect Fischler would so radically have it, in speculating whether the just-cited maxim "reflects . . . a truth not only biological, not only social, but also symbolic and subjective," such that the contemporary diner—confused and perplexed by anomie and diversity—comes to ask himself who he is.[9]

Rather, the effect of these present-day influences and culinary displacements is that the referents of the maxim get redefined, re-created, reshaped—even invented anew. In the future, then, making parboiled viandas a regular part of one's diet will not signify a lack of variety, or a cuisine of deprivation, or a reliance on eating a certain food out of sheer necessity, but, instead, will reflect a very different set of influences, in which ethical, political, and personal health concerns play a key role. For example, the decision to consume boiled viandas may represent a response to the deforestation occurring in Central America as the result of so much land being given over to raising cattle for beef, or it may express a person's belief that the body's biochemical system is ultimately cared for better by eating a healthy proportion of vegetables and other non-meat products. Within this process of redefinition, having to eat much the same food day after day, or having to eat food with a high fat content, will no longer indicate a diet formed by sheer necessity. Rather, it will signify unequal access to the cornucopia of the global supermarket, where the distinctive and the lean equate the expensive.

Similarly, being slender will not mean that one is nutritionally deprived or that one suffers from hunger; nor, conversely, will being plump mean that one is in the bloom of good health. These referents will indicate, on the one hand, that there are Puerto Ricans who choose to eat meagerly because, for cosmetic or health reasons, or both, they want to be on the thin side; or, on the other, that the abundance of food leads many people—unsure and ill-informed as they are about diet and nutrition—to indulge voluntarily and accept their body as is.

In the years ahead, taking meals outside the home will continue to shape people's diets and eating habits in comparison to the circumstances of earlier periods. By the same token, family and home life, and the passing down of customs associated with them, are no longer identified so closely with the feelings of warmth and affection that traditionally emanated from the kitchen. That experience, and those functions, will increasingly take place in family restaurants, diners, fast food establishments, food courts, and at food festivals. This change, of course, could undermine people's abilities to judge and distinguish between a high-quality cuisine that is carefully prepared and one of low quality that lacks variety and is mediocre at best. Indeed, the loss of the power to make such judgments and distinctions can already be observed.

In like fashion, as information about gastronomy spreads and becomes a global phenomenon, other food referents will serve to refract the sense that one occupies and belongs to an exclusive, self-contained geographic space. And finally, as the geographers David Bell and Gill Valentine suggest, all of these referents will serve to nurture new axioms with new referents, grounded in "Puerto Ricanness" to be sure, but also replete with other identities (socio-professional, or those based on gender, religious affiliation, sexual orientation, and age), as, for example, "tell me where you eat and I will tell you who you are," or "tell me how you think and I will tell you what you eat," or "tell me when you eat and I will tell you who you are."

All these new currents and elements will run parallel with the preservation of some of the features of traditional culinary practice and with the recognition that to invent and celebrate culinary traditions (as will happen with today's candidates, such as *pincho* [spicy pork kabobs sold by street vendors], *tripleta* [a baguette sandwich, also sold on the street and called the triple because it is filled with pork, chicken, and Italian sausage, along with chili peppers, onions, ketchup and whatever else the vendor can offer], pavochón, spaghetti with chicken, or *alcapurrias* [see glossary] filled with corned beef) is not to nod stubbornly toward the past but to honor a more complex reality, the reality that—before inserting themselves into gastronomic history as traditions—repertoires of food and diet travel a considerable distance and get defined, shaped, and remade by a host of influences and factors imposed from both within and without. They come to be what they are not in some static, frozen way but because they are exposed and receptive to constant change.

Selected Glossary

Achiote (Bixa orellana): A seed produced by the achiote tree, native to the tropical belt of the Americas. The word is of Mexican origin (*achiotle*), although the scientific term, *bija*, derives from Arawak. There are two varieties of the seed, red and yellow, with the latter being more highly valued, because—containing 2 percent more coloring—it produces a brighter, more luxuriant sheen. For its ability to add color and flavor, achiote is indispensable to a great many Puerto Rican and Caribbean dishes (it is known as *rocou* in the French Antilles). Its continued use through the colonial period to the contemporary era was facilitated by the central role that saffron and palm oil played in the food and cooking of Andalusian immigrants and of Africans, respectively. In earlier times, the seeds were sautéed in lard to color the fat and lend both flavor and coloring to what was cooked. Their constant use was also indicative of the presence, during that time, of the *achiotera*, a type of sieve employed for straining the colored fat, which was then reserved for other uses. In testimony to its popularity among both Puerto Ricans and people of the Caribbean more widely, agroindustry has made achiote available in combination with other flavoring supplements, such as garlic powder and dehydrated *recao*. In much home as well as commercial cooking, however, it is being replaced by a product known as *Bijol*, demonstrating the capacity of agroindustry to weave in appeals to the native elements of the island's cuisine.

Alboronía or Boronía: In Puerto Rico, a stew made with *chayote* (*Sechium edule*) and scrambled eggs. Analogous to the Andalusian dish of the same name, which is made with eggplant.

Alcapurria: A type of fritter or turnover made with plantain, cassava, or tannier dough, or a combination of these, to which fat colored with annatto and salt is added. Using one's hands and a spoon, the dough is spread onto plantain leaves or the leaves from the sea grape tree, or—as is done today by city dwellers or the less tradition-minded—onto waxed paper. A filling of well-seasoned ground meat or stewed land crabs is also added and the leaves are folded into the desired shape. In the most authentic fry stands and other such establishments found along the island's northeast coast, the frying is done in lard. To many Puerto Ricans, alcapurrias top the list of the food served by the *freidurías.* Making them well calls for careful judgment and a good eye, above all in the grating by hand of the viandas, so that the dough is light, not dense, as well as in adding the coloring and getting the right degree of heat for frying, which is critical for producing alcapurrias that are crisp and crunchy, like those served up in the freidurías in the seaside town of Piñones, near San Juan. Although no one in Puerto Rico has managed to pinpoint its origin, the alcapurria clearly points in the direction of Middle Eastern cookery, being closely akin to the *kibbi.* Alternatively, the word "alcapurria" could be connected to the figurative use of the word *al-kappára,* derived from *aljamiada,* as found in Andalusian vernacular. According to the lexicographer Antonio Medina Molera, the word *alcaparrón*—the fruit of the caper plant—is used figuratively in Andalusian popular speech to indicate the penis of a male child.

Alfajor: A sweet that, though taking its name from the popular Christmas sweets of Medina Sidonia, in Andalusia, is completely different in appearance and basic ingredients. In Puerto Rico, it has a flattened rather than cylindrical shape, and the base is composed not of ground almonds but of ground cassava, to which is added sugarcane syrup—instead of honey—cinnamon, anise, pepper, and cloves. The ingredients are mixed together and heated, then allowed to cool, after which the mixture is cut into pieces. In the popular confectionary of the coastal regions other ingredients, such as grated coconut, are also used. Although from the mid-nineteenth century on, the alfajor appeared in almost all Puerto Rican cookbooks, it is a rarity today.

Alfeñique: From the Arabic *al-finig,* a confection that shares its name with the Mexican alfeñiques, or Day of the Dead sugar skulls, but is prepared very differently. The custom in Puerto Rico is to make this sweet with unrefined brown sugar, water, lemon drops—vinegar is sometimes used—cream of tartar, and essence of peppermint. The ingredients are combined and heated until they become a thick syrup. When the syrup is thick enough to be shaped with one's fingers, it is poured into a shallow dish and stretched out. Before it hardens, pieces are removed and molded into little figures. If white sugar has been used, the alfeñiques are painted with different colors. This confection is no longer made in Puerto Rico.

Almojábanas: From the Arabic *al-mnuyabana*, meaning *torta*, in this case a fritter or bun, made of wheat flour and usually filled with cheese, and still a popular item in some Andalusian homes. In Puerto Rico, by contrast, the almojábana is prepared with either rice meal or the finely ground rice agroindustry has made available. Eggs, milk, butter, and cheese are added to the rice meal to make a dough that is fried in lard. Today, almojábanas are rarely cooked at home, though the most tradition-minded do occasionally prepare them as appetizers or as food on which to nibble. The difference between the Puerto Rican almojábana and its Andalusian forebear demonstrates the adjustment forced on it by a tropical environment. Wheat never prospered in Puerto Rico; it was a scarce commodity on the island, carefully husbanded and hidden away by import merchants during the period of Spanish colonial rule. There are still street vendors in contemporary Puerto Rico who sell almojábanas—made of rice meal, of course—during the morning hours in the municipalities of Humacao and Caguas, on the eastern end of the island, as people love to have them as accompaniments to the coffee they take at breakfast. Almojábanas are also popular in Colombia, where they are made with cornmeal.

Almuerzo: During the period of Spanish rule, the almuerzo was a morning snack, taken before ten o'clock. It preceded the *comida*, the workday's principal meal, which was generally consumed after the noontime hour. With the introduction of the U.S. dietary regimen, in which the "luncheon" was eaten considerably earlier, between the hours of eleven and twelve, the word "almuerzo" came to designate what had previously been the comida. Eventually, as things evolved in practice, *almorzar*, or to have lunch, meant that one ate the main meal of the day between 11:00 AM and 1:00 PM. The comida came to be known as the early evening meal, taken between 5:00 and 6:00 PM. This arrangement, which replaced the old colonial model, is still in force today, and it explains why, for many Europeans who live on or visit the island, lunch in Puerto Rico comes too early in the day. Over time, the almuerzo varied in accordance with individual social and material circumstance, but for the majority of families, it included rice, stewed beans and seasonings (salted cod or salted beef), a stew made from viandas, or salted cod, viandas and cornmeal, and—as a dessert—some tinned fruit and coffee. At one time, when the majority of the working population (free or slave) was employed in agriculture, the almuerzo was eaten on the work site itself, amid the cane fields of the great coastal plantations or the coffee plantations that dotted the central mountain range. As a rule, it was carried in lunch pails by a boy known as the *almuercero* or by the wives or daughters of the workers. Eating in this way (informally on the ground, with only a modicum of cutlery) strongly influenced table etiquette and the manner in which food was served in bowls, with all parts of the meal served together. In the homes of the most well-to-do families, of course, the almuerzo could consist of several dishes brought to the table at the same time, with rice and beans a near constant on the menu.

Amogolla'o: Apocope of the word *mogolla*, which in one of its usages signifies something done badly, something executed with a lack of care or in haste. In Puerto Rico, the word is used adjectively, to characterize rice that comes out sticky and lumpy because the person making it has miscalculated the cooking time or been negligent in measuring the amount of rice and water needed. In Puerto Rican food culture, one expects that the rice will always turn out light and fluffy.

Apastela'o: Apocope of the word *pastel*. It is used adjectively to describe a mixed rice dish that includes some of the ingredients of pastel (pork, chickpeas, peppers, occasionally raisins) and is covered with either green banana (*Musa paradisiaca*) or plantain (*Musa cavendishi*) leaves. This treatment gives it its name, apastela'o, since—as with pastel dough— the casserole-like mixture is covered with leaves and has similar ingredients. Where traditional flavors and methods of preparation are most closely imitated, the dish includes a strong *sofrito* (seasoning sauce) containing a heavy portion of fresh coriander. Some people also add cumin, tomato sauce, and achiote. The pieces of meat and accompanying ingredients are arranged over the sofrito; water is added to make a broth, into which the rice is put. A short-grained rice, rice "japónica," is normally used. The mixture is boiled in a deep cauldron, over wood embers, and covered with leaves. When the dish is almost fully cooked, it is seasoned with grated green plantain. Although apastela'o constitutes a meal in itself, it is sometimes garnished with pieces of pork crackling. The effect of the heat on the plantain leaves gives the dish one of its special qualities—a subtle flavoring of pastel. The rice comes out *pega'o*, with encrusted scrapings at the bottom, but is otherwise loose and not at all lumpy. Associated with festivities and celebrations, apastela'o is frequently made during the Christmas season or for family and community parties.

Asopao: The name is given to various soupy preparations of rice, which have been a mainstay in Puerto Rican rice cuisine. By and large, the dish is made with chicken, but dried codfish, pigeon peas, and meat can also be used. At one time, asopa'o played a key role in social and community life as a dish that was served at receptions, farewells, and family celebrations, or to mark rites of passage. It may have originated in poverty and necessity—people with little food at hand could bring a relatively substantial dish to the table. A strong sofrito is added to flavor the broth in which rice will be cooked. So that the dish does not come out lumpy and sticky, custom dictates that for each measure of rice, there should be four measures of liquid.

Burén: Arawak word for the flat clay griddle on which cassava cakes and other doughy food items wrapped in plantain leaves were cooked. The burén has fallen out of use, replaced by iron griddles.

Catibía: Arawak word, designating the stringy, fibrous residue left after grating cassava. Called *paja de la yuca* (straw from the cassava) in Loiza, catibía generally refers to the finer residue; the thicker variant is called *cosubey*.

Cazuela: Literally, earthenware. One of the vianda-based sweet desserts, made with mashed sweet potatoes (*Ipomoea batatas*) and pumpkin (*Cucúrbitae pepo*) first boiled in salted water. Depending on individual taste, some people also include tannier, mashed ripe plantains, and rice meal or wheat flour. A whipped egg, coconut milk, and—from time to time—shaved coconut are added to the mixture, which is seasoned with sugar and ginger, a pinch of cinnamon and powdered cloves, and a splash of sweet wine. The entire mixture is poured into a casserole or pudding pan (in the past a glazed earthenware dish was used) and baked. Over time, the dessert acquired any number of variations, but its main ingredient is sweet potato, without which it cannot merit the name "cazuela." To come out correctly and to be properly enjoyed, the mashed sweet potatoes and pumpkin must be strained to remove any fibers. As prepared and baked in the traditional fashion, in an earthenware dish, cazuela reflected the flair and ingenuity, and the items available to them, of the cooks who were employed by well-to-do families. The procedures (boiling and mashing the viandas) used in preparing the dish ultimately trace back to the African culinary heritage. Although a mid-nineteenth cookbook, El cocinero puertorriqueño, has no recipe specifically for cazuela, it included one similar to it (bocado de batata), but the latter omits any other viandas, such as pumpkin, which would give the dish more texture and consistency. The first recipe for cazuela proper appears in the 1914 cooking manual Home Making. From that point on, a Puerto Rican cookbook without a recipe for the dish will rarely be encountered. Yet, as with other sweet desserts that have viandas as their base, cazuela has increasingly become a kind of "culinary museum piece," cooked only occasionally in the home and appreciated all the more for this reason.

Chicharrón: Name given both to small portions of pork that retain some of their fat and are fried until coming out slightly burnt and crisp, and to hard, crusty pieces of pork skin fried in their own fat. In Puerto Rican gastronomy, the first type of chicharrón is enjoyed above all during the Christmas season, as a finger food or an item on which to snack, accompanied by boiled green bananas (Musa sapientum or Musa cavendishi) or yams. The latter version is an essential ingredient in the fried green plantain (Musa paradisiaca) mixture used in making mofongo.

Ciguatera: Indigenous word for the food poisoning caused by ingesting fish that have eaten toxic algae and other dinoflagellates that adhere to the coral reefs in the Caribbean Sea. Ciguatera has also been recorded along the coasts of the Gulf of Mexico and among islands in the Pacific Ocean. The toxicity is common in the larger fish that consume families of smaller fish living around the reefs of Puerto Rico's fishing grounds. The incidence of poisoning in the species of large fish increases in the wake of hurricanes, which strike the Caribbean between June and November and stir up the seabed. There is no symptom of toxicity that discloses the presence of ciguatera in these fish, nor any scientific means of detecting it, so it is not associated with fish that have decomposed or lost their freshness. Thus to the human eye fish infected by ciguatera appear perfectly fresh and healthy. The toxins, on the other hand, are thermosetting and persist through any drying, salting, and marinating process. Human poisoning via ciguatera is therefore unpredictable. Anglers' wisdom has it that two ways—fallible, alas—exist to detect ciguatera: the discoloring of metals, such as copper or silver, that occurs after inserting them into a fish's flesh; and the absence of flies swarming around the viscera removed from the fish. The symptoms of poisoning appear during the first six hours after eating the flesh of an infected fish, although they can sometimes overtake one in as few as fifteen minutes. Ciguatera manifests itself in more than seventy-five ways. These include hallucinations, memory loss, and nausea, and even death in 1 percent of cases. The desire to avoid such poisoning contributed to the adoption, by slave owners, of a rigid use of salted cod and other salted fish on Lenten days, when eating fish was well-nigh obligatory.

Colmado: The name given in Puerto Rico to small retail stores and corner groceries that are theoretically in business to sell comestibles but also stock many other kinds of dry goods. Elsewhere in the Caribbean, they are known as *pulperías,* or—in the case of Cuba—as *bodegas.* The word, which is an adjective, was applied to these modest stores because of the colorful array of items stocked to the very top of their shelves. In the past, they formed part of the cluster of buildings situated around the town or village marketplace, or at the crossroads of rural districts, visited by a regular clientele from the surrounding area. In contrast to the centrally located markets, which sold fresh edibles, the colmados were distinguished by their concentration of tinned products and preserved food. A store whose owner could wear two faces in the community—that of the benevolent protector or of the mean-spirited miser—the colmado was a social institution, a place for engaging in friendly chitchat, exchanging local news and gossip, and buying needed items on credit. With the development of the impersonal, suburban hipermercado and its model of stocking everything under the sun, the colmado is fast disappearing.

Corned Beef: A type of cold, canned meat that has nothing in common with the corned beef or brisket popular in Anglo-Saxon, and especially Irish, cookery. The adjective "corned" derives from the custom of preserving the brisket by lacing it with coarse salt ("corns" of salt). Unlike both fresh British and U.S. corned beef and the high-quality tinned variety, which comes from the lean meat of young cattle and is free of cartilage and excess fat, the corned beef consumed in Puerto Rico is an industrial derivative, produced from marginal cuts and trimmings of beef (*carne de canal*), including cow's tongue. It is vacuum-packed, having been pressure-cooked and preserved with copious amounts of salt and fat. Some 8 million pounds of this corned beef are imported annually into Puerto Rico, the largest share coming from Brazil, followed by Uruguay and Argentina. Its prominent place in the island's culinary history may be traced back to the jerked or salt-cured beef that was imported from Argentina in the nineteenth century as an inexpensive source of protein for the meals given to slaves. With the development of agroindustry and the mass production of tinned food, corned beef began slowly to replace jerked or cured beef, although the latter can still be found in supermarkets. During the 1930s and 1940s, when the state began to offer food assistance, mainly in the form of processed and canned products, and the school dining hall program fully took shape, partly to combat protein deficiencies by offering canned meats, corned beef took its central place in the diet of the majority of Puerto Ricans. The corned beef used in Puerto Rico is not the type known as hash, which contains potatoes and is a popular item in the diets of the less economically well-off in the southern states of the United States. In Puerto Rican cookery, it is made by preparing a moist sofrito, to which is added tomato sauce, and by then blending the shredded corned beef into this mixture. The dish is dressed up with other ingredients (sweet corn, green beans, or fried potatoes). The end product is a stew, invariably accompanied by white rice and fried ripe plantains. In *fondas* and in the restaurants serving home-style cuisine, it is rare not to find the dish on the menu at least once per week.

Dita: Arawak word designating a bowl or other vessel carved from the higuera, or fig, tree (*Ficus carica*). The word was also applied to bowls of various sizes, used for cooking and other domestic purposes, carved from coconuts, once the coconut palm (*Cocus nucifera*)—first brought from the Cape Verde islands in 1549—had succeeded in spreading across the island. Until well into the twentieth century, the dita was the only object of its kind found in poor households, and it has become enshrined as an emblem of once-needy times. Made and decorated now by skilled artisans, the dita has essentially turned into a collectible that is sold in the many food fairs held on the island.

Frangollo: Pertains to the low-end plantain gastronomy. Erroneously thought by many people to be a preparation having much in common with *marifinga*, *marota*, and *funche*. Frangollo is a dry sweet confection based on green plantains that are first chopped into fine strips and then ground up. In earlier eras this base was blended into a thick syrup, to which toasted peanuts were added. It closely resembled a sweet made with almonds and coconut that is still sold along the island's coasts.

Friquitín: The name given to a small establishment or informal eatery (what in the United States might be called a "hole in the wall"), made out of very simple, poor building materials, that specializes—almost exclusively—in selling fried food. Family-run, without any set hours of operation, the best known friquitines are located on the portion of the Atlantic coast that extends from the municipality of Carolina, at the northern end of the island, to the municipality of Luquillo, on the northeastern end. Although it might sell other types of food and drinks, to think about going to a friquitín in Puerto Rico is to think about eating fried items (above all alcapurrias and *bacalaítos*). The word may possibly be a corruption of *guariquitén*, an Arawak term that refers to the house or place where cassava cakes were prepared. The rather tacky, ramshackle character of so many friquitines has caused the name to be applied to a range of businesses—including the offices of physicians, attorneys, and other professionals—that lack any hint of luxury and whose services are administered on the fly.

Gandul (Cajanus cajans): A protein-heavy legume that appears to have been domesticated in either India or Africa and was first introduced in the Caribbean in the eighteenth century, together with the breadfruit tree (*Artocarpus altilis*). The latter was brought to Jamaica in 1794 to complement the rations given to slaves when the sugar plantation economy was expanding rapidly. Able to thrive in dry soil, the gandul bush can produce consecutive harvests for up to five years, and the longer the maturation period of the seed, the higher its protein content. In earlier times, the gandul, or pigeon pea, was harvested between December and January, hence its appearance in rice dishes during the Christmas season, such as the popular rice with pigeon peas and pork.

Gofio: A word from the language of the Guanches, the original inhabitants of the Canary Islands, and preserved by their descendants. According to the linguist M. Álvarez Nazario, the word in old Canarian Spanish referred to a flour obtained from some type of roasted grain (corn in Grand Canary, wheat in Tenerife and Gomera, and wheat and chickpeas in Fuenteventura and Lanzarote), which was kneaded into a dough with either water and salt (*gofio ar puño*) or honey or cane syrup, or—alternatively—diluted in broth or milk. In Puerto Rico gofio turned into something else; it refers to cornmeal that is roasted and ground into a powder, to which sugar and milled sesame seeds are then added. That is also how it is known in Cuba and Santo Domingo. It was formerly consumed in Puerto Rico because of its energy-giving properties; today, however, it is sold in little cones as a candied sweet. It is rarely made in the home and is only sold in sweet shops that specialize in traditional desserts and sweetmeats.

Guanime: An Arawak word, referring to a cornmeal preparation to which is added coconut milk, water, sugar, and anise. In times past, for the poorer segment of the population, sugar was a replacement for cane syrup. To make guanime, the seasoned dough is wrapped in banana or plantain leaves. These are formed into a tubular shape, tied at the ends, and boiled in salted water. Thus prepared and cooked, guanimes turn out exceedingly sweet, for which reason they are always made as an accompaniment to salted codfish. One only finds them made in the simplest, most tradition-bound homes. Outside of domestic kitchens, some people still prepare them on weekends; they are for sale, at random locations, to persons driving along Puerto Rico's southeastern coastal highway.

Juey: Arawak word for the land crab (*Cardisoma guanhumi*), a crustacean which lives on land and returns periodically to the sea to reproduce. Prior to the Spanish conquest, the land crab was a common dietary item among the indigenous inhabitants of the Caribbean. It can be found in coastal areas ranging from Florida to Brazil and is still regularly eaten by people living on the islands of the Caribbean. In Puerto Rico, however, it is now an endangered species, because urban development along the coasts is destroying its habitat. A kind of gastronomic subculture, with its own terminology, grew up around the juey, embracing both the ways for capturing it (either *de cueva*, grabbing it out of the hole it digs and burrows into, or *de corrida*, when it is running about, during the mating season, when there are heavy rains and its burrows are flooded); the instruments used in this process, an *hacho* (a flaming resinous log) or a powerful flashlight that immobilizes it and a *garabato*, or stick with a hook attached at its tip; the actions taken to trap these creatures (*emboquillarlos*—maneuvering the hook so as to hang the claws and stringing them with lianas), and, last of all, fattening them up (*engordarlos*) by feeding them corn and chopped coconut. The most well-known and popular dishes utilizing land crab meat, which is very difficult to extract, are *arroz con jueyes*, *salmorejo de jueyes* (a land crab stew), and the artisanal creation called *jueyes al carapacho* (crab meat baked in the shell). The meat of the land crab is also used as a filling in alcapurrias and *piononos*.

Majarete: A sweet creamed confection that came out of the island's traditional use of corn. Although today the name applies to a similar creamy dish made with rice flour, Puerto Rico's first cookbook has it prepared with corn grated from young sweet cobs, from which one obtains a milky paste. The paste was then pressed through a fine cloth or strainer and the milk extracted. Rich in starch, the milky paste gave the majarete its texture and consistency. Depending on what other resources were at hand, sugar, cinnamon, cloves, or anise were added to the milk. The mixture was cooked in a pan over moderate heat, stirred until it formed into a thick cream, after which it was poured into individual dishes, allowed to cool, and sprinkled with cinnamon powder. By the middle of the twentieth century, cookbooks called for it to be made with rice flour, though at times one can find it prepared in the original way, with corn.

Marota: One of a range of dishes based on corn that formed part of the diet of the poor. Made with cornmeal, in the style of *funche*, marota called for using water to thicken up the porridge-like mixture, into which small amounts of many other fatty, tasty foods were variously incorporated. The dish was also called *marifinga*, and the two—though referred to differently—were essentially alike. The way each version came out, the slight differences in the final product, depended on who was cooking it and what ingredients she had before her. For this reason, higher or official gastronomy excludes the two as recipes in their own right. In contrast to *mazamorra*, which was a recognized dessert, marifinga and marota were heavy concoctions, food designed to fill one's stomach.

Matrimonio: Colloquial term for the combination of white rice and stewed beans, especially red beans. Because each was invariably served with the other as part of a meal, the combination came to be known, with much irony, as a "matrimonio" (married couple).

Mazamorra: A dessert, originally of the poor, made with cornmeal, sugar or syrup, aromatic flavorings that vary from recipe to recipe, and different types of milk. Some more recent cookbooks recommend using sweet corn grated off the cob, but the traditional version used cornmeal, which gave the dessert its name, derived from the helpings of cheap cake given to passengers making the voyage to America. The same item was given to prisoners in jails, from which came the custom of sometimes hearing the word used in reference to prison cells.

McDonalización: A neologism, credited to the North American sociologist George Ritzer, referring to the "system of rationalization" employed by the popular hamburger outlet. Although the term has a clear referent, Ritzer, in his book entitled *The McDonaldization of Society: An Investigation into the Changing Character of Contemporary Social Life*, notes that it was adopted because it sounded more attractive than "Burger Kingization," "Seven Elevenization," "Fuddruckerization," . . . or "Nutri/Systematization." The term thus refers to more than just the McDonald's chain. Rather, it is a metaphor, inspired by the system of rationalization used by fast food companies to refer to "a process through which the principles that govern the operation of fast food restaurants have increasingly come to dominate wider aspects of both U.S. society and the rest of the world." While the term today is often used to mean the spread of McDonald's outlets across the world, I use it to mean an unchanging food or dietary regimen, a condition that for all intents and purposes arises from the process of McDonaldization.

Melao: Apocope of the word *melado*, or syrup. In Puerto Rico and the Antilles more widely it refers to sugarcane syrup. Mela'o is the syrupy liquid obtained from the evaporation of the *guarapo*, or juice from sugarcane. In the preindustrial system of sugar production, mela'o was collected from the troughs or receptacles in which the sugar was deposited to bleed it, that is, to eliminate any excess liquid or impurities from it, for which reason it was also called *miel de purga*. Recovered by means of decantation in guttered canals made of bamboo or wood, mela'o was sold as an inexpensive sweetener or used to fatten up cattle or to moisten the food given to slaves. In an economy in which sugar, whether white or unrefined brown, was a lucrative export product, mela'o served as a substitute for sugar in the poorest households.

Mixta: Colloquial term referring to the combination of white rice with red beans, accompanied by a hearty side dish of stewed beef, or beefsteak marinated in onions, vinegar, oregano, salt, and pepper cooked in a skillet (*bisté encebollado*). In the preindustrial period, and even today in certain areas of the capital city, those frequented by workers in particular, mixta is a meal of rice and beans accompanied exclusively by stewed meat from the shank of an animal. In current parlance, it has come to stand for any meal that is considered native to the island, though it must include rice and beans. From the word mixta has come the verb *mixturar*, which in low-end Puerto Rican cookery refers to rice and beans that can be accompanied by any other food, with canned meat being a favorite.

Pega'o: The crusty residue that adheres to the bottom of the pan or pot in which rice has been cooked. Rice will more commonly turn out with this layer if the fat used is lard and if the rice is cooked more vertically than horizontally. The weight of the rice pushes it downward in a pot that is deep rather than wide. The grains of rice at the very bottom of the pot thus come into contact with the fat, leaving them *requemados*, or browned and singed. Although at one time this part of the rice was not especially valued, today it is taken as a measure of success in getting the rice just right—pega'o but not burnt. Although this way of cooking rice can be done with mixed rice dishes, the preference is to prepare pega'o using white rice. The custom in Puerto is to combine this part of the rice with the broth from cooked beans. In some countries of the Caribbean and of Central America, such as Cuba, Colombia, Costa Rica, and Nicaragua, it is called *raspa*.

Pilón: A large mortar and pestle. This utensil has many uses in Puerto Rican and Caribbean cookery, one of which is to mash the slices of fried or boiled plantains forming the basis of Puerto Rican mofongo, Dominican mangú, or Cuban fufu. The mortar is also used as a mold, to give a concave shape to mofongo and to facilitate its being filled with meat, shell fish, or stock of some kind. When slave society still existed on the island, there were pilones of enormous size—bearing little resemblance to the mortars found in people's homes today—for mashing the starchy tubers and root vegetables used in preparing the community meals served to plantation slaves. Invariably, a much smaller pilón was also used for crushing the various ingredients that went into making sofrito. The historic relationship between the pilón and sofrito explains why the former has become an emblem in all of the advertisements for readymade sofrito, even though kitchens now have food processors to do the work once done by the mortar and pestle. Pilón also refers to a candied sweet made in the style of a sugarloaf, but with a cylindrical or conical shape, to which sesame seeds are added.

Pionono: A preparation, based on ripe plantains, that is on the verge of disappearing today. It belongs to the gastronomy of the island's coastal regions, the northeast coast above all. To make pionono, one cuts a ripe plantain in long slices. These are folded into a rounded shape and closed up at the ends. The hollow center is filled with ground meat, well cooked, and seasoned. The filled plantains are then basted with a mixture of thick flour, water, and beaten egg, and fried in a skillet on both sides. The name of this dish may have passed over to Puerto Rico from a wafer-thin sponge cake that was soaked in sweet liquor, rolled to take the form of a cylinder, and then topped with a special cream produced in the Province of Granada, in Spain. As the story goes, it was created in the nineteenth century by Ceferino Ysla, a pastry chef in the city of Granada, in honor of Pope Pius IX, a great partisan of confectionery.

Recao or Culantro: (Eryngium foetidum) An herb that grows wild on the island, including on the undeveloped land around housing estates. Having a pungent flavor and earthy smell, culantro—coriander in English—seems to have been native to the humid, tropical zones of Central America. The eighteenth-century botanical manual of Sesé classifies the herb as one used exclusively for culinary purposes. It may by this time have become a standard ingredient in sofrito. Like many other items found in Puerto Rican cookery, the herb is also used extensively throughout the Caribbean, reaffirming the regional character of Puerto Rican cuisine. Some common names for recao or culantro in the Caribbean are shado beni (Trinidad), chadron benee (Dominica), fitweed (Guyana), and coulante

(Haiti). The practice in Puerto Rico is to use a moderate amount of this herb, since its highly pungent flavor can ruin any dish, even sofrito.

Salchichas: These are agroindustrial products that have nothing in common with European sausages. Rather, they are a processed, canned food, composed of meat by-products (from cows, swine, poultry, or even some combination of these). As with corned beef, the introduction of these products into the Puerto Rican diet resulted from the growth and development of agroindustry, in the period following the Second World War, as well as the implementation of state food assistance and school lunch programs. One sees them most commonly either stewed and eaten separately or in the form of *arroz con salchichas* (yellow rice mixed with salchichas).

Serenata: A dish composed of boneless, desalted codfish alongside hot chilies, pimientos, tomatoes, coriander leaves, onions, and boiled eggs that are cut into slices for decoration. The dish, dressed with vinegar and olive oil, has its origins in old Lenten prescriptions. At present, the more traditional fondas serve it on Wednesdays and Fridays—a reminder of days of abstinence called for in the church's traditional liturgical calendar. The name "serenata" comes both from the rich coloring which its various ingredients give to it and from its association with the meaning of a serenata, or folk music played at night in the open air to court a woman or to celebrate someone's birthday. Serenata is always accompanied by viandas.

Sopón: A soup thickened with rice. It differs some from *asopao* in being a much drier dish, with a heavier amount of rice, which is its dominant feature. Sopón originated when the island's poor had few options in their diet. In some of the island's regional cuisine, there are versions of sopón in which salted codfish, or pigeon peas and plantain, are the central ingredient.

Sorullos, Sorullitos: Another in the line of preparations based on corn. Sorullos are cylindrical fritters made with cornmeal. The ingredients in the dough vary, depending on the intended meal or snack. Normally, the bigger sorullos—which tend to be eaten for breakfast—are prepared with a little salt, sugar, a pinch of anise, and perhaps some coconut milk. The sorullos that are served as appetizers or as accompaniments are smaller and thinner, and their dough also includes cheese.

Tiempo Muerto: An expression used to describe the six-month seasonal work stoppage affecting workers in the sugarcane fields. When the sugar latifundium was at its zenith, at the end of the 1930s, tiempo muerto, or dead time, could extend from the end of June into the first weeks of February, when the cycle of harvesting the sugar began again. This period of downtime could mean unemployment for 120,000 workers in a total workforce estimated at 273,875. Some workers were accustomed to migrating to the tobacco and coffee-growing zones as a way of mitigating the effects of the stoppage. In terms of food and dietary options, tiempo muerto was the time of year in which field hands and their families depended most on what they could grow in their own home gardens. Unfortunately, however, it was also the period of lowest food production in the agricultural calendar (with the possible exception of fruit trees and citrus products). At bottom, tiempo muerto was synonymous with the absence of income, purchases made on credit in little country restaurants and stores, and the fear of looming hunger.

Notes

ABBREVIATIONS

ACSJBPR Actas del Cabildo de San Juan Bautista de Puerto Rico
  AGPR Archivo General de Puerto Rico
  CIHBM Centro de Investigación Histórica, Universidad de Puerto Rico,
         Balanzas Mercantiles
  DRHPR Documentos de la Real Hacienda de Puerto Rico

FOREWORD

1 A small quibble here: one wishes for a chapter on drinks—rum, *guarapo* (a sugarcane or pineapple-based drink containing herbs), *mabí* (a spiced fermented beverage made with bark from the mavi tree), coffee!
2 Otto Bauer, *La cuestión de las nacionalidades y la social democracia* (Mexico City: Siglo XXI, 1979).
3 Gervasio García, "La nación antillana: ¿Historia o ficción?," *Revista* (San Juan), no. 16 (2005): 43.
4 José Luis González, *El país de cuatro pisos* (San Juan: Huracán, 1980).
5 Ángel G. Quintero Rivera, *¡Salsa, sabor y control! Sociología de la música "tropical,"* (Mexico City: Siglo XXI, 1998).

INTRODUCTION

1 A tag applied, sarcastically, to the thinking and program of those among the island's political class, and to Puerto Ricans in general, who favor full statehood for the island, naively believing—in the view of their critics—that through negotiations with the U.S. Congress, Puerto Rico can become the fifty-first state of the union without having to accept an "English only" policy or adopt such markers of mainland identity as the U.S. national anthem or flag. The term "jíbaro" itself refers to someone from the island's mountainous heartland who embodies its traditional, rustic way of life.
2 For these and other interviews of people in politics and the sports and entertainment worlds in Puerto Rico, see the 1999 Sunday editions of the San Juan newspaper, *El Nuevo Día*.
3 García Arnaíz, "La alimentación," 15–38.

4 Montanari, "La cocina," 11–15.

5 Ibid., 11.

6 For theoretical envisionings of the food-nation relationship, see Bell and Valentine, *Consuming Geographies*, 165–83; as well as Cook and Crang, "The World on a Plate," 131–53; and Appadurai, "How to Make a National Cuisine," 3–24; Mintz, *Tasting Food*, in particular the chapter "Cuisine: High and Low or Not at All," and the same author's "Eating Communities," 19–34. For studies specifically related to the Caribbean and Central America that take this relationship as a point of departure, see Higman, "Cookbooks," 77–95; Pilcher, "Tamales or Timbales," 193–216; Dawdy, "La comida mambisa," 45–80; and Wilk, "Food and Nationalism," 67–87.

7 Fischler, *El (h)omnívoro*, 77.

8 Montanari, "Historia," 24–25.

9 Harris, *Good to Eat*, 13–18.

10 The notion of a "complement" food is Fischler's. See his *El (h)omnívoro*, 156 and passim. It involves newly introduced foods that take their place beside food which has, to that point, played a central role in a society's agriculture and diet (for example, the plantain or the *ñame* [yam] next to tannier, rice next to corn, the African bean next to indigenous beans, etc.) The "complement" foods are added to the older food and eventually come to play a strictly dietary role, without ever substituting for or displacing the earlier-established food. The process continues; other important foods subsequently arrive and play the same role, although they are not discussed in depth in this work. I am referring to *malanga* (another name for tannier), *panapén* (breadfruit), *gandul* (pigeon pea), and *quimbombó* (okra).

11 The notion of a "supplement" food is likewise Fischler's. See ibid. It refers to food to which something happens that enables it to fulfill a new role or, better put, a different function. As a rule, Fischler points out, food that evolves into a "supplement" does so in the context of intense interethnic contact or mixing, a phenomenon that has characterized Puerto Rico throughout its history. At an early stage in its appearance, the supplement gets linked to a similar food, as with salted cod and herring, for example, taking their place next to fresh fish. Eventually, the supplement either replaces its predecessor as a basic food or it gets adopted as the food associated with specific new culinary functions—for example, the fulfillment of Lenten rituals or the imperative faced by certain groups, such as slaves, prisoners, and soldiers, to feed themselves or be fed on low cost diets.

12 On this point and on the system of food consumption in societies reliant on subsistence agriculture, see Martin Bruegel's comments regarding Mintz's thesis with respect to the notion of "matrix," in *Food and Foodways: Explorations in the History and Culture of Human Nourishment* 7, no. 2 (1997): 140–41. Clearly, this matrix is being (and has been) restructured based on the flexibilities existing within different food and dietary complexes. For example, in the composition of a plate of food, proteins are not now considered "fringe," as they were

before when they served the "companion" function of heightening flavor and taste. They are fulfilling the role of a new core, with other nutritional components, in both a symbolic and directly sensory way. Meat is a major player in various guises. In this movement, tubers (viandas) have been pushed out of the core to occupy a marginal place, in the process becoming more of a secondary food source. They are seen today as an accompaniment to certain meals. In like fashion, rice—corn has disappeared in toto—has slipped off onto the fringe, all but taking on the role of a garnish, albeit one that is ever-present. As a key part of the meal, however, it is receding further and further into the background. For their part, legumes are no longer protein-bearing complements but simply food that one expects to be part of a meal.

13 Mennell, "Divergences," 278–86.

14 Fischler, El (h)omnívoro, 34.

15 Lévi-Strauss, Mitológicas I, 11–13.

16 Mintz, Tasting Food, 97–98.

17 Ibid., 40–42.

18 Ibid., 96.

19 Ibid., 40 and passim.

20 Ibid., 98.

21 Higman, "Cookbooks," 77–95. In turn, Higman's essay drew inspiration from the discussion spawned by two important studies published by anthropologists in the post-1986 period: Jack Goody's Cooking, Cuisine and Class: A Study in Comparative Sociology (Cambridge: Cambridge University Press, 1982) and Arjun Appadurai's "How to Make a National Cuisine: Cookbooks in Contemporary India" (1988). For additional, recently published studies relating to Central America and the Caribbean, see note 6. Higman's Jamaican Food: History, Biology, Culture (Mona: University of the West Indies Press, 2008), is a still newer addition to the literature.

22 Piero Camporesi, The Anatomy of the Senses: Natural Symbols in Medieval and Early Modern Italy (Cambridge: Polity Press, 1994); Camporesi, Bread of Dreams; Gian-Paolo Biasin, Flavors of Modernity: Food and the Novel (Princeton: Princeton University Press, 1993); Geet Jan van Gelder, Of Dishes and Discourse: Classical Arabic Literary Representations of Food (Richmond, Surrey: Curzon, 2000). See also Montanari, The Culture of Food; Manton, Fed Up: Food and Culture; A Reader, ed. Carole Counihan and Penny Van Esterik (London: Routledge, 1997); Alan Beardsworth and Teresa Keil, Sociology on the Menu: An Invitation to the Study of Food and Society (London: Routledge, 1997); and Peter Atkins and Ian B. Bowler, Food in Society: Economy, Culture, Geography (London: Arnold, 2001).

23 With the notable exception of the historians and researchers who grouped themselves around Jean-Louis Flandrin and Massimo Montanari in Europe and Warren Belasco in the United States. See Storia dell'alimentazione, ed. Massimo Montanari and Jean-Louis Flandrin (Rome: Laterza, 1997), translated into English as Food: A Culinary History; From Antiquity to the Present, trans. Clarisa Botsford et al. (New York: Columbia University Press, 1999); El mundo en la

cocina, comp. Massimo Montanari; and *Food Nations: Selling Taste in Consumer Societies*, ed. Belasco and Scranton.

24 Belasco, "Food Matters," 6.

25 Montanari, "Historia, alimentación," 25.

26 Ibid.

27 Dawdy, "La comida mambisa," 48.

28 Montanari, *The Culture of Food*, 171.

CHAPTER 1

1 "Empieza hoy el nuevo sistema de uso del PAN," *El Nuevo Día*, 1 September 2001, 4.

2 *Documentos de la Real Hacienda de Puerto Rico, 1511–1519*, comp. Aurelio Tanodi (Río Piedras: Centro de Investigaciones Históricas de la Universidad de Puerto Rico, 1971) 1:212, 241, 263–64, 271. Hereafter referred to as DRHPR.

3 Ibid., 212. The first shipment registered for Puerto Rico, totaling only twenty-five pounds, was brought by the sailor Ruy Díaz in November 1513.

4 Ibid., 271. Alonso Manso was born in 1460 in the community of Becerril de Campos, in the region of Palencia. Nominated as a bishop on 8 May 1512, he was officially consecrated in Seville, in September 1512, to preside over the first Catholic diocese established in the New World, on the island of San Juan Bautista de Puerto Rico. He arrived on the island on 25 December 1513. Sometime between 1515 and 1519 he journeyed back to Salamanca, but he later returned to the island and served as bishop until his death, in 1540.

5 "Carta del obispo de Puerto Rico Don Fray Damián López de Haro a Juan Diez de la Calle, con una relación muy curiosa de su viaje y otras cosas," 1644, reproduced in Fernández Méndez, *Crónicas*, 159–69.

6 Johnston, *Staple Food*, 172–75; Linares, "African Rice."

7 Lewicki, *West African Food*, 22–24; Carney, "The Role of African Rice," 527.

8 Johnston, *Staple Food*, 172–75. In using the term "displacement," Johnston is not equating it with "substitution." Instead, he is referring to an inversion of the importance of the "original" food and to a "complementary" adoption of the new food.

9 Alegría, "Notas," 58–79.

10 Mintz, *Tasting Food*, 39.

11 Carney, "The Role of African Rice," 530.

12 Ibid., 526. See also Khoo et al., *El gran libro del arroz*, 12.

13 For more on the varieties of rice which over time got established in Puerto Rico, see Correa, "El cultivo," 28–36; Hernández, "El cultivo," 282–85; and Cadilla de Martínez, "Breves apuntes," n.p.

14 Abad y Lasierra, "Diario del Viaje," n.p. Entry for 2 August 1772, corresponding to his visit to the community of Cangrejos: "Almost all of its inhabitants are negroes, who having been able to free themselves from the slavery in which they previously lived, have received lands in these parts which, although sandy,

are amenable to growing cassava, beans, sweet potatoes and other vegetables and fruits which they supply to the city. . . . Part of the terrain is flooded, they plant rice on it when the water level drops." On 8 August, having arrived in Loíza—a community located in the north not far from Cangrejos and with a similarly high concentration of people of African extraction—Abad y Lasierra noted: "On the flat lands there are some lagoons, formed out of the slopes of the mountains, where they concentrate rice, they plant it in the dry season and when the rains arrive, the rice has already shot up, they cut it when its ripe, and it produces a second spike, and then a third. I have seen the same thing in other communities on the island, so with only a single planting they get three harvests."

15 Abad y Lasierra, Historia geográfica, 162.
16 From the 8 August entry of Abad y Lasierra's "Diario del Viaje."
17 Ibid.
18 López Tuero, Cultivos, 11.
19 Allston Pringle, A Woman Rice Planter, 12–13.
20 Ibid.
21 "Rice: Morphology and Growth," http//www.riceweb.org/Plant.htm. See also Khoo et al., El gran libro del arroz, 26.
22 López Tuero, Cultivos perfeccionados, 17.
23 "Rice: Morphology and Growth."
24 López Tuero, Cultivos, 17.
25 El cocinero puertorriqueño, 120. Discrepancies exist regarding the precise date of the first edition of El cocinero. The book appears to have been reprinted twice after its initial publication. In his prologue to a 1971 facsimile edition of the book, the librarian Emilio M. Colón gives 1859 as the year when it first appeared, under the imprint of Imprenta de Acosta. Subsequently, Berta Cabanillas, in her pathbreaking and still unduplicated history of food in Puerto Rico, assigns 1849 as the date of first publication. Colón's case seems to be stronger. He cites Manuel María Sama's Bibliografía puertorriqueña of 1887, which included the first listing of El cocinero, dating its publication to 1859. See the introduction to Colón, El cocinero; Cabanillas, El puertorriqueño, 336; and Sama, Bibliografía, 22. In March 2002, I confirmed that the library of the University of Catalunya, in Barcelona, holds a copy of the original, bearing the date 1859.
26 El cocinero, 120.
27 Abad y Lasierra, Historia geográfica, 186.
28 El cocinero, 120–21.
29 Roberts, "Nutrition," 299.
30 Ferguson, Home Making, 35; Dooley, The Puerto Rican, 78.
31 For more on sofrito, see chapter 2.
32 Méndez Quiñones, "El cuento," 30. Ever intent on representing the traditions of poor campesinos, Puerto Rican costumbrista writers were wont to re-create dishes that did not necessarily accord with campesino tastes in food. As Gian-Paolo Biasin has noted, the use of food in literature carries figurative meanings

and serves to connect the story's narrators, the world that surrounds them, and other social sectors. See Biasin, *Flavors*, 16–17.

33 Alonso, *El jíbaro*, 29. *Costumbrismo* was a literary genre, tied to nineteenth-century romanticism, that focused on depicting local customs and traditions.

34 Méndez Quiñones, *El cuento*, 30.

35 Ferguson, *Home Making*, 162.

36 Alonso, *El jíbaro*, 77.

37 Iglesias, *El derrumbe*, 14.

38 The recipe given in Dooley, *The Puerto Rican*, 64, is the only one describing the preparation of pastel de arroz.

39 The recipes for "*Sopa de arroz, Sopa de arroz a la Trinitaria,* and *Sopa de arroz de ajiaco de monte,*" in *El cocinero*, 16–17.

40 Ibid., 196. *El cocinero* uses the neologism *pudinera* for this bowl.

41 Ibid., 244.

42 Redon et al., *Delicias*, 440–41. The *Libro de cocina*, written by Ruperto de Nola, a Catalan by birth, appeared in Spain in ten separate editions between 1520 and 1527. While Juan de la Mata's *Arte de repostería*, published in Madrid in 1741, lists the dish in the index, the recipe does not appear in the book itself. On the other hand, fifty cookbooks were published in France between 1480 and 1799, twenty-nine of them between 1714 and 1799 alone. It is therefore more plausible that *El cocinero* took its recipe from a French source. See Iranzo, *Libro de cocina*, 47; de la Mata, *Arte*; and Hayman and Hayman, "Printing the Kitchen," 394.

43 Redon et al., *Delicias*, 25.

44 Dooley, *The Puerto Rican*, 165.

45 Cabanillas et al., *Cocine a gusto*, 275; Valldejuli, *Cocina criolla*, 423. "Majarete de harina de arroz" requires some clarification, since the oldest recipe for majarete, which in fact appears in *El cocinero puertorriqueño*, calls for using young corn scraped off the cob, which was passed back and forth over a sieve to eliminate the starchy part. By contrast, Cabanillas and Valldejuli give the name "majarete" to a preparation made not with the pieces of young corn but with rice meal. If one consults historical cookbooks, the majarete of Cabanillas and Valldejuli is intrinsically a manjar blanco, since its basis is rice meal. In the recipe given in 1948 by Dooley—appearing two years before Cabanillas's and six years before Valldejuli's—the difference between the two is spelled out: manjar blanco is made with rice meal and majarete with corn. In many parts of contemporary Puerto Rico, however, the rice-based confection is called majarete. For the majarete recipe in *El cocinero*, see page 256 of that cookbook. See page 165 of Dooley's book for the distinction that she makes between the two recipes.

46 Cabanillas, *Cocine a gusto*, 275; Valldejuli, *Cocina criolla*, 422. It is only Valldejuli who recommends orange tree leaves.

47 See the notes made by Coll y Toste to Alejandro Tapia's autobiography, *Mis me-*

morias o San Juan como lo encontré y como lo dejo (New York: DeLaisne y Rosseboro, 1927), 54.

48 Ferguson, *Home Making*, 139, Cabanillas et al., *Cocine a gusto*, 238; Valldejuli, *Cocina criolla*, 340.

49 Cabanillas, *El folklore*, 28.

50 Fischler, *El (h)omnívoro*, 95–98.

51 In 1976, when rice growing in Puerto Rico had ceded the ground to imported short-grain, polished rice, the Agricultural Experiment Station tried to revive local production, with the purpose both of lessening dependence on imported rice and of stimulating the production in Puerto Rico of a more nutritive rice. Long grain rice, or "parboiled" rice, falls into this category. The station conducted a study of consumers' (all of them women) preferences when cooking and eating rice. Among other findings, the agency discovered that expectations about how to cook and eat the cereal were quite inflexible. Among them: that the rice stay "grainy," that it be a central and large part of the meal, that some type of fat be added during its preparation to make it tasty, and that it even come out pega'o. These expectations, which still hold just before it is eaten, do not apply with such force to other foods. See Rodríguez de Zapata, *Aceptación por el consumidor*, 9.

52 Some examples of rice allowances are: in 1765, four ounces daily for those condemned to forced labor on military fortifications; in 1767, three ounces daily for professional soldiers quartered in El Morro; in 1826, four ounces daily for plantation slaves; in 1843, six ounces daily for the slaves on the plantation of Don José Martínez; in 1848, two portions daily for the mentally ill and other inmates of the Casa de Beneficencia; in 1857, according to the inmates of the Real Cárcel of San Juan, "every day the food consists of rice and beans in the morning, and rice and garbanzos in the afternoon"; in 1873, in the same jail, the allotment became nine pounds on Tuesdays and Saturdays for each group of twenty-five inmates (or approximately 6.8 ounces per inmate), twelve pounds (approximately 8 ounces per inmate) on Mondays and Thursdays, and twelve pounds again on Wednesdays, Fridays, and Sundays. Between 1862 and 1864, the soldiers en route to the war in the Dominican Republic were allotted five ounces daily. The same amount was given to sick soldiers aboard war ships; at the beginning of the twentieth century, eight pounds of raw rice was allotted to each group of forty children enrolled in the school cafeteria programs established in urban areas (an amount that equaled some 3.2 ounces per child per day, a considerable quantity when one considers the limited intake of younger children). In rural school dining halls, rice was provided three days of the week: white rice on Mondays, stewed rice containing beans on Tuesdays, and a rice casserole, with either pieces of sausage (smoked or otherwise) or salted cod on Thursdays. See López Cantos, "La vida," 149; Barrios Román, *Antropología*, 111; "Reglamento," *Boletín histórico*, 10:262–73; "Sumaria averiguación . . . Don José Martínez Díaz," reproduced from documents in the Fondo

de los Gobernadores Españoles, Archivo General de Puerto Rico [hereafter cited as AGPR], in *Anales de investigación histórica*, 80–83. I am indebted to Fernando Picó for showing me this document. See also Rivera Rivera, *El estado*, 194; Picó, *El día*, 85–87; Government of Porto Rico, *Manual del comedor*, 9.

53 Reference here is to the use of fatback, lard, dried or jerked beef, smoked sausages, salted cod, pig's feet, or ham. The complaint made in 1857 by the inmates of the Real Cárcel de San Juan that the food they received every day—invariably composed of rice and beans in the morning and rice and garbanzos in the afternoon—"is usually uncooked and badly seasoned" (meaning that it lacked fat and tasty flavorings and was thus insipid on the tongue) highlights the centrality of the practice. Cited in Picó, *El día*, 87. The recipes for white rice and stewed rice included in the 1929 *Manual del comedor escolar* lead to the same conclusion: eight pounds of white rice calls for three-quarters of a pound of fat; rice mixed with beans, fatback, and ham, or stewed rice, call for three-quarters of a pound of fat, sausage, ham, and salted cod. See *Manual del comedor*.

54 López Tuero, *Arroz y cacao*, chap. 3 in particular, 13–16; Correa, "El cultivo," 28–36; Hernández, "El cultivo," 282–85; and Cadilla de Martínez, "Breves apuntes."

55 Centro de Investigaciones Históricas, Universidad de Puerto Rico, *Balanzas Mercantiles*, 1850 (cited hereafter as CIHBM).

56 Ormaechea, "Memoria acerca," 226 and passim.

57 Abad, *Puerto Rico*, 211–12 and 227–28. By 1897, in fact, rice took up only 2 percent of land devoted to growing food crops. See Cabanillas, *El puertorriqueño*, 300.

58 Torres de Alba, "Testamentos," 64–108; González, "Pintueles," 96–107; Carroll, *Report*, 48.

59 In the last decades of the nineteenth century, the majority of rice imported by local commercial interests came from the British and German colonies in Asia. Spain, until the middle of the century a key supplier—with rice from Valencia especially notable—fell to third place during the 1890s. See Hitchcock, *Trade*, 84. Two factors drove the lower volume of imports of rice from Spain, to Cuba as well as to Puerto Rico. First, the inability of rice growers in Valencia to satisfy the enormous demand for rice that was building for two reasons: population growth, and a newfound taste for polished rice (although rice from Valencia was polished, it was not as refined as that produced in English and German mills); and second, rice growers in Valencia consistently stood fast against importing unprocessed rice to Spain from India and the Philippines and then having it processed in Catalan mills for reexport to the Caribbean colonies. On this interesting point of contention, which demonstrates the advantages that accrued to rice growers in Valencia from a Caribbean diet that focused—all through the nineteenth century—on rice primarily as a source of carbohydrates, see Molins, *Las admisiones*.

60 López Tuero, *La reforma*, 24–25. Córdoba, *Memorias*, 5:409–10. The island's population was estimated at 358,836 and 953,243 for 1834 and 1899, respectively.

61 On the negative trends in local rice cultivation during the first decades of the twentieth century, see the opinions expressed by the secretary of agriculture in Clark, *Porto Rico*, 492. On the geographic expansion of rice growing in the United States, see Departamento del Interior, *Cultivo de arroz*, and on the subject of its very rapid growth, see Brown, *Cómo aumentar*, 226.

62 AGPR, *Judicial, juicios verbales*. On 24 May 1891, Claudio Mora Y Ruíz, a businessman and resident of Viví Abajo, filed a claim, by means of oral argument, against Don José Frau, to recover the sum of forty-three pesos.

63 Lang and Morales Otero, "Health and Socio-economic Studies," 113–33.

64 Ramos and Bourne, *Rural Life*, 79.

65 Descartes et al., *Food Consumption*, 13.

66 Roberts and Stefani, *Patterns of Living*, 367.

67 Cooper, "Chinese Table Manners," 179–84.

68 On the distribution of seeds by the Puerto Rico Food Commission in 1917–18 and by the Department of Agriculture in 1924–25 and 1938, see Correa, "El cultivo," 28–30. The anecdote about farmers eating the seeds comes from Correa. On the ransacking of groceries and local shops, see AGPR, Fondo de la Policía, "Serie de querellas," specifically the folders dealing with incidents of rioting, breaking and entering, and thieving and shoplifting during 1933. For details and data on food importation during the First World War, see Puerto Rico Food Commission, *Informe*.

69 Quoted in U.S. War Food Administration, *Report of Operations*, 31. In point of fact, 262.6 million pounds of rice had been distributed in the year 1940–41. Allowing for population growth, this quantity was tantamount to the figures for 1925, when 165.5 million pounds were made available. See, among others, the following articles in the newspaper *El Mundo*: "Comercio de arroz no ha podido sustanciar demanda," 16 April 1942; "El gobernador proclama racionamiento de arroz," 17 June 1942; "Forma en que operará el racionamiento de arroz," 18 July 1942; "El fallo del arroz," 19 October 1942; "Sugestiones sobre la distribución de arroz," 25 November 1942; "Congelado el arroz para establecer el sistema de cuotas," 12 December 1942; and "Distribuirán 16 millones de libras de arroz el mes," 15 December 1942.

70 *Report of Operations*, 17.

71 Rodríguez Pacheco, "La siembra," 138.

72 Departamento de Agricultura, Oficina de Estadisticas y Estudios Económicos, *Consumo de alimentos en Puerto Rico*, 1950–51/1973/74, 2:38.

73 See Ashford, *Progreso*; Valle Sárraga, *Ideas*; Cook and Rivera, "Rice and Beans"; Torres Díaz, *A Preliminary Study*; Lang and Morales Otero, "Health and Socioeconomic Studies"; Roberts, "Nutrition," 298–304; Blanco, *Nutritional Studies*; Zeijo de Zayas, "El puertorriqueño."

74 Hernández, "El cultivo," 283.

75 The statistic is from a pamphlet authored by Roberts, *Mejor arroz*, 6.

76 Ibid.; and also Roberts, "Nutrition in Puerto Rico," 247.

77 Torres, "Consideraciones," 255–56. Biochemistry and nutritional science be-

lieved that the lack of thiamine was a possible cause of neurological imbalances, poor blood circulation, deficiencies in the digestive process, and lack of appetite. The chronic absence of niacin was linked to pellagra, a disease whose symptoms included dermatitis, diarrhea, and—in extreme cases—mental disorders. In Puerto Rico, pellagra was not then seen as a serious public health problem, though it was observed to occur with some regularity in children, for whom rice was a basic food and, in the period following breastfeeding, almost the only food.

78 Roberts, *Mejor arroz*, 6.

79 For Roberts's accomplishments in the field of nutrition in both the United States and Puerto Rico, see Levenstein, *Paradox of Plenty*, 65–66; Schierman and Hourd, *Notable*, 580–81; and Martin, "The Life Works," 299–302.

80 Comité de Nutrición, *Historia*, 5.

81 Rodríguez Pastor, *Nociones*.

82 Asenjo, "Composición química," 279–88.

83 Comité de Nutrición, *Historia*, 5.

84 See Rodríguez Pacheco, "La siembra," 6; García Pomales, "Política pública"; and Rodríguez de Zapata, *Aceptación*.

85 Sánchez Cappa, Luis, "Respaldan proyecto del senador Berríos sobre cultivo de arroz," El Mundo, 23 March 1973, 16. See also José Vicente Chandler et al. *Cultivo intensivo y perspectivas del arroz en Puerto Rico* (Río Piedras: Universidad de Puerto Rico, Colegio de Ciencias Agrícolas, 1977).

86 Clarence Beardsley, "Se fueron 30 millones en la siembra de arroz," El Mundo, 26 April, 1988, 18.

87 Departamento de Agricultura, Oficina de Estadísticas Agrícolas, *Consumo de alimentos en Puerto Rico (cosechas), 1979/80–1986/87*, 67; Departamento de Agricultura, Oficina de Estadísticas Agrícolas, *Consumo de alimentos en Puerto Rico (arroz total), 1975–2003*, Folder 17–59b1.

88 Estado Libre, *Anuario estadístico*, 322.

89 See Fischler, *El (h)omnívoro*, 198. Fischler notes a decline in France in the consumption of vegetables, and of cereals in particular. He goes so far as to assert: "Thus, foodstuffs wax and wane [in popularity] with the classes that consume them: the decline of the peasantry and later of the working class in part explains the decline of some of the characteristic foods once viewed as utterly necessary by them."

90 For example, "potatoes" in their several versions, but above all "French fries," as substitute choices for rice in the composition of a meal. Figures compiled by the Department of Agriculture show a remarkable increase in the annual per capita consumption of potatoes between 1975 and 2001: 1975, 9.71 pounds; 1985, 20.9 pounds; 1990, 70.2 pounds; 1995, 52.3 pounds; 2000, 72.3 pounds; and 2001, 73.6 pounds. Departamento de Agricultura, Oficina de Estadísticas Agrícolas, *Consumo de papas elaboradas, 1975–2001*, Folder 16–57b16.

91 For example, the per capita consumption of "converted" rice, while fluctuating, has reached 5.24 pounds (1993), when in 1975 it stood at 0.50. In 2000,

however, it was recorded as 1.46. The comparable figure for "whole rice" was 1.31 pounds in 2000. See, Estado Libre Asociado de Puerto Rico, Departamento de Agricultura, Oficina de Estadísticas Agrícolas, Arroz en proceso de cómputos, 1975–2000, Folder 1759b4.

92 "Supplemento de negocios," El Nuevo Día, 21 September 1997, 2.

93 Junta de Planificación, External. Similarly, the label on some "medium" rices—such as the Rico or El Mago brands, a three-pound package of which may sell for forty-nine cents—carries the statement that less than 4 percent of their contents contain "broken rice."

94 Ibid., "Shipments into Puerto Rico."

CHAPTER 2

1 Habichuelas—the red, pink, and black varieties—are included in the species Phaseolus vulgaris. They all belong to the family Leguminosae, or Fabaseae, and are grouped into the subfamily Papilionideae as the species Phaseolus vulgaris. See Vaughan and Geissler, The New Oxford Book, 40.

2 Fernández de Oviedo, Historia, 243.

3 Ibid., 244.

4 Cubero, "Traditional Varieties," 296.

5 Before the conquest, the island's Taíno population is estimated to have been 125,000. In Puerto Rico, as in the Antilles generally, mining for gold took place in riverbeds or in the surrounding grasslands, using the native population as draft labor, either granted outright and permanently to conquistadores or parceled out to them for specific projects and tasks. The encomienda, which at bottom was a form of slavery with a veneer of legality, distorted and undermined a major part of Taíno social and economic organization, by forcibly diverting the Indians into (primarily) the gold-mining enterprise. There is no better way of comprehending the level of exploitation than to read book 6, chapter 8 of Oviedo, who—in his desire to record and impress the reader with the organizational logic and efficiency of the Spanish mission—lays bare its inhumanity. Some authors estimate that more than 5,000 Indians could have been parceled out in a single year to extract gold, and as many as 600 were, at times, assigned as labor to a single conquistador. See Oviedo, Historia, 161; Brau, La colonización, 257–58; and Moscoso, Sociedad, 34 and 98.

6 Thus the royal instructions issued in July 1514: "I am informed that one of the reasons, understandably, why these parts are not settled and why those going into them do not stay, is for lack of houses and things they should be given . . . and it seems that it would help greatly to mandate that each resident of the island to whom fifty Indians are granted as labor should be obliged to have and keep on hold eight thousand loads and this more or less should be their distribution, because it is believed that with it there will be a safe reserve so that the Indians can be well maintained and everything will not have to be transported in as is now done." See Murga Sanz, Historia documental, 2:90.

7 The description that Oviedo gives of how the work of mining gold was arranged leaves the impression that its organization did not affect levels of food production. However, though he grants that on farms not far from the Indian miners there were female Indians who had remained in "the countryside making bread and other provisions . . . and . . . there are women constantly cooking for them, making bread and wine (made from corn or cassava), and others who take food to those laboring in the fields or mines," he also acknowledges that it was mainly Indian women who were employed in the task of washing the gold. He further notes that each gold-washing tray required the involvement of five people. It is well known that in the division of work in Taíno society, it was the women who were in charge of planting and of gathering and cooking food. Thus the allocation of thousands of Indian women into the operation of washing the gold must necessarily have diverted much attention from agriculture and the task of gathering edible foodstuffs. Oviedo, Historia, 244.

8 DRHPR, "Relaciones de navíos de 1512 a 1513," 140–273.

9 See "Relación de precios a que se acuerda por los oficiales de su Alteza que se venda el pan de su alteza que se traído y trajere de la isla de Mona que está a cargo del factor Baltasar de Castro," in Cabanillas, El puertorriqueño, 382–84.

10 It has been estimated that during the island's peak years of mining activity, out of the total number of Indians forced into the work of extracting gold, as many as one third may have been Indian women.

11 DRHPR, 301–6.

12 Bartolomé de las Casas recalls a time when, because of scarcity of food from the land, people "used up a lot of bread and wine," and he also recalls that "it happened that five had to purge themselves with a hen's egg and a kettle of cooked garbanzos." The uncertainty about food supplies was reflected in the promulgation of several royal ordinances during this early period, in which the importance to the colony of ensuring the cultivation and provision of "basic foodstuffs" was emphasized. See, among others, "Instrucciones enviadas al repartidor de indios Sancho Velásquez," 4 April 1514, reproduced in Murga Sanz, Historia documental, 2:90–91; and "Provisiones de Don Fernando el Católico y Doña Juana dando ordenanzas para remediar y ennoblecer a la población de la isla," ibid., 3:269, 271.

13 Alegría, "Notas sobre la procedencia," 63, 66. Alegría draws a distinction between Ladino slaves who arrived in San Juan from Seville between 1519 and 1521 (a total of 580) and the slaves who were brought directly from Africa, that is, from the small kingdoms extending from Senegal to Cape Verde, beginning in 1527.

14 Johnston, Staple Food, 172–75; Lewicki, West African Food, 54.

15 Lewicki, West African Food, 54.

16 Ca da Mosto, Relation, 30.

17 Cubero, "Traditional Varieties," 296.

18 Vaughan and Geissler, The New Oxford Book, 48; Lewicki, West African Food, 54.

19 "Ordenanzas hechas por el Cabildo, justicia y regimiento de esta ciudad de

San Juan de Puerto Rico pertenecientes al buen gobierno y aumento de la república," 11 September 1627, in Real Díaz, *Catálogo*, 281.

20 Harris, *Good to Eat*, 9–16.

21 Kaplan and Kaplan, "Phaseolus," 124–42.

22 Debouck, "Early Beans," 62–63.

23 Ibid.

24 De Grosourdy, *El médico*, 473–74. In fact, during the second decade of the twentieth century, on the tobacco plantations studied by a team from the Brookings Institution, the planting of beans averaged 2.1 acres within the total area that tobacco plantations of six or fewer acres devoted to the cultivation of *frutos menores*, or any crop other than sugarcane, coffee, or tobacco. The Brooking Institution's figures for the planting of beans in such areas on tobacco plantations were as follows: on plantations of 7 to 13 acres, 4.0; 14 to 20 acres, 4.2; 21 to 27 acres, 8.1; 28 to 34 acres, 4.3; 35 to 41 acres, 8.4; 42 to 63 acres, 9.6; and those larger than 64 acres, 24.4. Clark, *Puerto Rico*, 679.

25 González Ríos, "El mejoramiento," 140–42.

26 Abad y Lasierra, *Historia geográfica*, 163.

27 AGPR, Fondo de Hacienda, *Catastro de fincas rústicas*, 1888.

28 Córdoba, *Memorias*, 5:432; López Tuero, *La reforma*, 24–25.

29 "El cultivo de legumbres," 7.

30 Russell Perkins, *The Leguminosae*, 215–18.

31 In the evolution of stewed beans, the culinary traditions of Castile, Extremadura, and the Arab-Andalusian Mediterranean have all made worthy contributions. Each, for example, has called for cooking lentils and garbanzos in more or less similar ways: boiling them in a watery mixture and—depending on circumstances and religious precepts—adding portions of lard or lamb's fat as well as various vegetables. See Granja Santamaría, *La cocina*, 29; Huici, "La Cocina hispanomagrebí," 137–55; and Benavides Barajas, *Al-Andalus*, 55–58. See also the introduction to Cofradía Extremeña de Gastronomía, *Recetario*.

32 Mintz, *Tasting Food*, 40.

33 Sherman and Billing, "Darwinian Gastronomy," 453–63. Paul W. Sherman and Jennifer Billing, the coauthors of this highly original piece of research, posit that what in cookbooks generally falls into the category of spices actually derives from different shrubs and bushes, woody vines, trees, aromatic lichens, roots, seeds, and herbaceous plants. They insist as well that what cookbooks commonly call spices (seasonings, condiments, and fresh herbs) contain phytochemicals, that is, secondary compounds that evolve in spices and herbs as self-defense mechanisms against insects, funguses, pathogens, and bacteria. Once mixed with food, they act as antimicrobial shields, since many of them are thermosetting, that is, they survive even when subjected to high temperatures. According to Sherman and Billing, phytochemicals not only help protect food from rapid biodegradation but also reduce the possibilities of poisoning to human beings caused by the presence of bacteria in food. On these bases, the two—who examined 4,578 recipes based on meat,

obtained from ninety-three "traditional" cookbooks from thirty-six countries around the world—conclude that the heavy use of spices and herbs is more common in countries and regions with hot, humid climates, because the biodegradation of food, and of meat products in particular, was a recurrent problem before the invention of refrigeration. Although in the popular imagination the pronounced use of spices and herbs today is credited to the cultural idiosyncrasies of countries in this climatic belt, Sherman and Billings argue otherwise, claiming that it did not originate exclusively out of the desire to improve the palatability, taste, or color of food but, instead, also grew out of what they term "gastronomic Darwinism," that is, survival strategies. They further consider that the incorporation of new spices and herbs into old recipes was likely a response to environmental factors. New, unknown bacteria and funguses made their appearance; to combat these effectively, it was necessary to begin experimenting with new spices and herbs. The two researchers carried out laboratory studies on thirty spices to determine their antimicrobial properties and the degree to which they could repel bacteria, fungus, and the like. They discovered that the phytochemical concentration of all thirty was sufficient to kill or inhibit at least 25 percent of the bacteria to which they were subjected, and that 15 could achieve this result against 75 percent of the bacteria. Interestingly, they found that garlic, onions, and oregano inhibited or neutralized all of the bacteria to which they were subjected.

34 Ibid.

35 The prime example of the deep reservation over using certain ingredients in sofrito is the notable absence of recao (wild coriander) in the recipes for legume dishes contained in the nineteenth-century cookbook El cocinero puertorriqueño. The reservation persisted among some even though botanists had realized almost a century earlier than the use of this herb lay exclusively in the realm of cooking. The 1909 Puerto Rican Cookbook, compiled by North Americans, exhibited the same exaggerated sense of caution toward the use of garlic and onions in recipes for bean and pigeon pea dishes. For a detailed account of such reservations and exclusions in the preparation of beans and sofrito, see Ortíz Cuadra, "Somos," 63–65.

36 Oviedo, Historia, 236. See also Moscoso, Sociedad, 114–15.

37 Ramcharan, "Culantro," 506–9. A botanist, Ramcharan in fact believes that cilantro or recao is original to the New World tropics and Caribbean islands, pointing out that it is used extensively in the cuisine of Trinidad and Tobago, where it is called shado beni and bhandhania, in Dominica, where it is known as chadron benee, in Haiti, where it goes under the name of coulante, and in British Guyana, where it is referred to as fitweed. See also Mahbir, Medicinal and Edible.

38 Granja Santamaría, La cocina; Huici, La cocina hispanomagrebí; and Benavides Barajas, Al Andalus.

39 Villapol, "Hábitos alimentarios," 329. See also Bascom, "Yoruba Food," 42; and a second article by Bascom, "Yoruba Cooking," 124–25.

40 On the description of this sweet pepper in Murcia, see Muro Carratala, *Diccionario*, 2:709; and Gispert Cruels, " Las plantas," 213–30.

41 CIHBM, 1879.

42 Blanco Fernández et al., *Exploración botánica*, 275–76.

43 Long Solís, "El tomate," 215–37.

44 Mintz, *Tasting Food*, 40–44.

45 Hamm, *Puerto Rico*, 139.

46 See, for example, the recipes for "rice with bacalao" and "rice with chicken" compiled by the home economist Grace J. Ferguson, in her *Home Making*, 79 and 147.

47 Malaret, *Diccionario*, 482.

48 Hamm, *Puerto Rico*, 139.

49 Wilsey and Janer Vilá, *Vegetales tropicales*, 27.

50 Ibid. Around this time, the recipe for sofrito did appear in another publication, but it had nothing to do with cooking per se. It was a twenty-nine-page thesis entitled "A Preliminary Study of the Common Puerto Rican Diet," submitted in 1930 by Luis Torres, a student in the University of Puerto Rico's Chemistry Department. In calculating the nutritional value of the island's common diet, Torres found himself obliged to adjust his research methodology on discovering that a formula, or recipe, existed for a preparation—sofrito—that was added to stewed beans. Since earlier calculations had not taken this formula into account, Torres realized that he needed to do so, because it was always present in the preparation of beans. He therefore copied the following formula: for two cups of legumes use: ¼ cup of ham, ¼ cup of fatback, 1 spoonful of vegetable coloring (achiote?; paprika?), ½ cup of onions, ½ cup of capsicum, ½ cup of tomatoes, ½ clove of garlic, 1 teaspoonful of capers and 2 quarters of a liter of water. He gave this information in his thesis, 3.

51 Ortíz, *A Taste of Puerto Rico*, 16.

52 It is not by chance that the sofrito recipes in *Cocine a gusto* and *Cocina criolla* are used as introductions to the chapters devoted to beans. Cabanillas's recipe in the former is as follows: 2 ounces of fatback, 2 ounces of cured ham, 1 spoonful of lard, 1 chopped capsicum, 1 chopped tomato, 1 chopped onion, 1 crushed garlic, salt to taste. In *Cocina criolla*, Valldejuli includes three sofrito recipes; one that she calls basic sofrito, another that is called practical, and a third that is made in a blender. This last recipe can be interpreted as an attempt on her part to appeal to or accommodate a modern ethos, building in Puerto Rico and spreading into the home, according to which the mortar and pestle were viewed as archaic. The ingredients in Valldejuli's basic sofrito were: 1 spoonful of vegetable oil, 1 ounce of fatback, 1 strip of bacon (which she also recommends using in place of vegetable oil), 2 ounces of cured ham chopped into small pieces, 1 small onion, 1 green pepper, 3 sweet chili peppers, 3 leaves and 3 stems of fresh coriander, ¼ teaspoonful of dry oregano, 2 medium crushed cloves of garlic, 2 spoonfuls of tomato sauce, 2 spoonfuls of vegetable oil or

achiote paste. See Cabanillas, *Cocine a gusto*, 71; and Valldejuli, *Cocina criolla*, 337–39.

53 As evidence of this development, see among other references, "Ordenanzas hechas por el Cabildo, justicia y regimiento de esta ciudad de San Juan de Puerto Rico pertenecientes al buen gobierno y aumento de la república," 11 September 1627, in Real Díaz, *Catálogo de cartas*, 279; Abad y Lasierra, *Historia*, 163; "Directorio General que ha mandado formar el Sr. D. Miguel de Muesas," 22 March 1770, in Caro Costa, *Antología de lecturas*, 446–47; Córdoba, *Memorias*: 5: 432; De Grosourdy, *El médico*, 495–96; Stahl, *Estudios*, 1:263. For references in Stahl to the gandul, see 278–79; to fríjoles, 281; to the cimarrona bean, 282; to the parda bean, 282–83; and to white, yellow, red, black, and multicolored beans, 284.

54 Archivo Histórico Diocesano, Arquidiócesis de San Juan, Fondo Carmelitano, Serie "Cuenta y Data de las Monjas Carmelitas," figures for January 1862, February 1863, and May 1865.

55 Extrapolating from the numbers for 1862, when the Carmelite convent had twenty-two resident nuns as well as a priest and an accountant, who both doubtless took their meals with the nuns. See *Guías eclesiásticas*, 26–27.

56 The figure for 1832 is from Córdoba, *Memorias*, 4:432; for 1891, López Tuero, *La reforma*, 24–25.

57 Dávila Cox, *Este inmenso*, 185–88. On the role of Italy and Germany, see also CIHBM, 1869–1896.

58 See Hill and Noguera, *The Food Supply*, 5 and 8. As an indication of the sharp increase in local production, in 1937–38 the quantity of legumes produced in Puerto Rico was reported as 31,432,488 pounds, distributed thusly: dry beans, 15,359,350; pigeon peas, 8,666,938; fríjoles (black-eyed peas or snap beans), 3,748,200; and others, 3,658,000.

59 Ramos, *Rural Life*, 79–81.

60 Roberts and Stefani, *Patterns of Living*, 161 and 372.

61 Cited in the preface to Blanco, *Nutrition Studies*.

62 In their study of nutrition in Puerto Rico's rural areas, covering 1937, Rita Lang and Pablo Morales Otero found no purchases of fresh beans among 800 families during a weeklong period within four rural agricultural zones. On the other hand, they do cite purchases of up to 928 and 866 pounds of dry beans in coffee-growing and tobacco-growing country, respectively. Lang and Otero's complete food sample numbered 165 different foods. See Lang and Morales Otero, "Health and Socio-economic Studies," 113–33.

63 Clark, *Puerto Rico*, 439.

64 See González Ríos, "El mejoramiento," 140–42.

65 The food consumption study carried out in 1937–38, and published in 1940, showed that, in the main, Puerto Ricans obtained beans from what on the island is called a *colmado*, or grocery store. Known as *pulperías* in other countries, the colmados were stocked with imported processed, nonperishable (i.e., canned) foodstuffs, in contrast to markets, which as a rule sold fresh

products, locally produced. In addition to the colmado, other outlets included the municipal or city markets, the *ventorillo* (a small store, often located on the outskirts of a community, selling produce, fruit, groceries, and many other items), the *panadería* (bakery), the *revendón* (individual peddling fruit, vegetables, eggs, etc.), and others. The breakdown among these was: in San Juan, 98 percent of foodstuffs were acquired in colmados, in 22 other urban zones (that is, in the urban center of 22 municipalities on the island), 97 percent of foodstuffs were similarly acquired. In the rural parts of the island (meaning outside the urban centers of municipalities), 20 percent of food purchases were made by people traveling into the urban center; 75 percent of purchases were made in neighborhood (parish) colmados; and 5 percent of the food consumed was grown in family gardens and farm plots. See Descartes et al., *Food Consumption*, 72.

66 The calculations made by the chemist Conrado F. Asenjo, using the varieties available to him in 1953, yielded the following figures, in terms of the number of grams of protein contained in each 454-gram portion of edible legumes: dry soy, 158 grams; dry red, 104.9; dry peas, 108.1. See Asenjo, "Tabla de composición," 279–81.

67 Jaret, "Things Go Better," 32–35.

68 Ibid.

69 To wit, local medical knowledge at the end of the nineteenth century had invoked the gastric upset produced by legumes to justify its arguments—aimed at the upper classes—about acting prudently when eating them: "They are healthy in moderate quantity, but if not well cooked or if consumed to excess, they induce flatulence and are painfully difficult to digest." See Valle Atiles, *Cartilla*, 73. The botanist Russell Perkins echoed this conclusion, writing in her book: "In keeping with the abundance of legumes and their starchiness, they [beans] are very nutritive." Nevertheless, she immediately added that "they are also somewhat difficult to digest." Russell Perkins, *The Leguminosae*, 215.

70 Roberts, "Deficiencias," 259–65; Zeijo de Zayas, "El puertorriqueño," 256–79.

71 Zeijo de Zayas, "El puertorriqueño," 256–79.

72 González Ríos, "El mejoramiento," 141. "Borínquen" is the Hispanicized derivative of the Arawak word *borique*, the name given by the Taínos to the island of Puerto Rico.

73 Hill and Noguera, *The Food Supply*, 19.

74 Estado Libre Asociado de Puerto Rico, Departmento de Agricultura, Oficina de Estadísticas Agrícolas, *Consumo de alimentos*, 1975–2000, "Habichuelas Secas," Folder 2057 A15.

75 Hill and Noguera, *The Food Supply*, 5, 8, 19.

76 Departamento de Agricultura, Oficina de Estadísticas Agrícolas, *Consumo de alimentos en Puerto Rico*, 1979–80 – 1986–87, Publicación Oficial, October 1989, 41–42; and Commonwealth of Puerto Rico, *Department of Agriculture, Facts and Figures on Agriculture in Puerto Rico*, Office of Agricultural Statistics, 1996. See also Departamento de Agricultura de Puerto Rico, *Consumo de alimentos*, Folder

2057ª15, "Habichuelas secas," 1975–2001. A preliminary figure for 2003 is available at http//www.agricultura.gobierno.pr.

77 Ibid.

78 Ibid.

79 Departamento de Agricultura de Puerto Rico, *Consumo de alimentos*, Folder 2057ª15, "Habichuelas secas," 1975–2001. The figure is a preliminary estimate.

80 Fischler, *El (h)omnívoro*, 202. Goften and Ness have defined convenience food as follows: "The ease with which a product may be prepared, served, and eaten. Even this, of course, may involve different aspects—simplicity in the cooking process, or speedy cooking, or being able to cook a product without special utensils, or being able to serve without cooking, or without special tableware, or being able to use the product in combination with many different things, or being able to serve it to different sorts of people on different kinds of meal occasions. Convenience may involve a large number of other characteristics, however—ease of acquisition through being available at a large number of retail outlets, being easily stored and so available for use at any time, or suitable for use as a lap or TV meal." Cited in Warde, *Consumption, Food and Taste*, 133.

81 "Crece la popularidad de los productos light," *El Nuevo Día*, 22 September 1991, 108.

82 The proposal of the Department of Education and its secretary, César Rey, went even further in January, 2004, in establishing what were called *Nutritional Guides* to regulate the content of meals offered in school dining halls, the 3,200 food vending machines located in all elementary schools—kindergarten through sixth grade—and 75 percent of all middle schools and high schools belonging to the public education system. Although the proposal does evidence a latent concern over the problem of child obesity, what really stands out in it is a belief that traditional Puerto Rican food has more nutritional value. Of course, the combination of rice and beans was only one of the daily offerings, since the thinking behind the proposal was to offer variety and choices and "to get the student to understand that eating something of high nutritional value can be just as pleasing as eating something that is not." Nevertheless, there was a revalidation of the importance of the historic combination (of rice and beans) in the new approach. At present, Puerto Rico's public education system has 1,543 school dining halls in which 300,000 lunch trays are served daily. See Carmén Millán Pabón, "Aconseja a Rey el gremio de comedores escolares," *El Nuevo Día*, 7 October 2003; Camile Roldán Soto, "A mejorar la nutrición en las escuelas," *El Nuevo Día*, 28 January 2004; and Francisco Rodríguez Burns, "Comida chatarra fuera de las escuelas," *Primera Hora*, 28 January 2004.

83 *Noticiario Teleonce, Sección Arte y Cultura*, 22 February 2001. Olga Tañón is an impassioned Puerto Rican singer known as "the woman of fire." Although she has sung "tex-mex" ballads and pop, she owes her fame to *meringue*, a subgenre of tropical music that originated in the Dominican Republic.

84 For 1998–99, the volume of imported red kidney beans was calculated at 265,012,000 pounds and for black beans, only 10,679,000 pounds. In 2000–

2001, the figures were 125,778,000 and 13,140,000, respectively. Departamento de Agricultura, Oficina de Estadísticas Agrícolas, *Importación y exportación de legumbres secas y enlatadas*, Folder 20–35.

CHAPTER 3

1 Korsmeyer, *El sentido*, 213–14. See also Bryson, *Looking at the Overlooked*, 61–62.
2 See the interview conducted by the journalist Lupe Vázquez with the sales manager of Molinos de Puerto Rico regarding the introduction in the market of an extra-fine cornmeal called "La cremita," in *El Nuevo Día*, Sección "Por dentro," 22 March 2000.
3 Álvarez Nazario, *El elemento*, 264.
4 Oviedo, *Historia*, book 7, chap. 1, 228.
5 López Tuero, *Cultivos perfeccionados*, 3.
6 On how corn is propagated and grows, see Mangelsdorf, *Corn: Its Origin*; Hui, *Encyclopedia of Food*, 1:482–90; Toussaint-Samat, *History of Food*, 164–65; Ward, *Encyclopedia of Food*, 151–56; Vaughan and Geissler, *The New Oxford Book*, 6–7; and López Tuero, *Cultivos perfeccionados*, 1–5.
7 Oviedo, *Historia*, book 7, chap. 1, 227–28.
8 Ibid.
9 Ibid., 229.
10 The quotation is from Cabanillas, *El puertorriqueño*, 394–95.
11 "Real Cédula a los oficiales reales de la isla de San Juan de Puerto Rico para que lleven cuenta y razon [*sic*] de lo que se hubiere gastado y gastare en una estancia que el gobernador Antonio de Mosquera ha tomado pera sembrar maíz y plátanos," in ibid, 400.
12 "Relación del viaje," *Boletín* 5:49–70.
13 The chapter of the ordinances devoted to food products consists of seventeen regulations arranged in "descending numerical order by food." The hierarchical organization suggests a local adaptation by the *cabildo* of beliefs about food that the European aristocracy had formalized, between the fifteenth and sixteenth centuries, on the basis of different interpretations and classifications of the natural order of the world. According to Massimo Montanari, this belief system "described living beings, plants, and animals as links in a vertical chain or as rungs on a ladder. In either case, the value of each plant and each animal depended on the position it occupied in the chain or on the ladder." Of course, Montanari continued, "the higher the position, the greater the value, and vice versa." Needless to say, Montanari points out that the belief system also drew a parallel between food and society, that is, foodstuffs were also organized in accordance with the symbolic role they played in the very act of eating. On this plane, products capable of producing bread—understood as "sustenance," or food earned with the sweat of one's brow—were considered primary. Thus the first three foodstuffs listed in the ordinances are wheat flour, cassava, and corn—the three that can be "made into bread." After them, the remaining

foods in descending order are: meat products (beef and pork, the tripe from pigs and cattle, and domestically cured meats); fresh and salt-cured fish and turtles; oil or fat products (fat from cattle and pigs, oil); birds and related offshoots (hens, eggs and chickens); dairy products and sweeteners (cow's cheese, syrup, dark honey, white sugar); followed by the most ordinary food, or what were called *menudencias*—the most readily available food (rice, beans, yams); and last, garden produce. See Real Díaz, *Catálogo de cartas*, 279–81; and Montanari, *The Culture*, 88–89.

14 Abad y Lasierra, *Historia geográfica*, 165–67. Abad y Lasierra gives his figures in *arrobas*, a unit of weight varying between 24 and 36 pounds. I have used a conversion ratio of 25 pounds per arroba, since this is the weight most commonly used in documents from that period. Abad y Lasierra's production figure translated into at least 22 pounds of corn per person annually. The role of corn in the diet should not be underestimated, though it was frequently obscured by the frequent references to plantains.

15 Vaughan and Geissler, *The New Oxford Book*, 215.

16 "Reglamento sobre la educación, trato y ocupación que deben darle a los esclavos sus amos o mayordomos," 1825, in Coll y Toste, *Boletín*, 5:49–70; Moreno Fraginals, *El ingenio*, 3:57–58; AGPR, *Fondo de los Gobernadores Españoles en Puerto Rico*, "Sumaria averiguación instruida por orden de Su Excelencia por queja producida por cuatro siervos propiedad de Don José Martínez hacendado de Guaynabo," 1843, 80–83.

17 Lang and Morales Otero, "Health and Socio-economic Studies," 201. Lang and Morales, who carried out their fieldwork in 1937, discovered, in fact, that among 34,265 families studied, 9,403 (or 27.4 per cent) ate funche with salted codfish and viandas as a midday meal. See also Díaz Pacheco, *Consumo de alimentos*, 21; Hill and Noguera, *The Food Supply*, 19; and Descartes et al., *Food Consumption*, 55.

18 Brau, *Las clases jornaleras*, 45.

19 See Baralt, *La buena vista*, 53. According to Abad y Lasierra's account, the highest corn production at the end of the eighteenth century was in the municipalities of Ponce, San Germán, and Aguada, located in the southwestern part of the island. See Abad y Lasierra, *Historia geográfica*, 165–67. In the early 1850s, the farmer Juan Jardy, of the municipality of Sabana Grande, harvested 170,000 ears of corn annually. See "Memoria de la primera Feria," 1854, in *Boletín*, 178. And at the end of the nineteenth century, when commercially produced corn made available some 4.4 pounds per person annually (a total of 4,200,000 pounds, without counting the corn harvested by campesinos from their own plots), the extensive fields of corn planted along the road from Sabana Grande to San Germán, in the southwest, elicited the following observation by the North American writer Albert Gardner Robinson: "Before many of the houses immediately beside the roadway, mats were spread upon which corn, shelled from the cob, was drying in the sun. The whole place seemed reeking with corn. Bushels of it were thus drying in the bright sunshine. It hung in great

bunches from the rafters inside the little dwellings, and lay in piles upon the porches. In the fields it stood, some of young growth and some of ripened ears ready for gathering. Apparently, one might have boiled green corn upon his table, if he so wishes, every day of the year in Porto Rico." See Robinson, *The Porto Rico*, 94–95. The figures cited for the end of the nineteenth century are from López Tuero, *La reforma*, 24–25.

20 López Tuero, *Cultivos perfeccionados*, 21–23; Ward, *Encyclopedia of Food*, 151–56; Legrand, "El maíz," 25–30. See also Conde Millet, "El cultivo," 145; two articles by Riollano, "El cultivo de maíz," 78; and "Maíz y arroz," 382. For an account of similar manual operations as practiced in South Carolina by women of African ancestry, see Ferguson, *Uncommon Ground*, 98–99.

21 *El cocinero puertorriqueño*, recipe for "maíz finado criollo," 115.

22 "Carta del Obispo de Puerto Rico Don Fray Damián López de Haro," in Fernández Méndez, *Crónicas*, 159–69.

23 Gispert Cruels, "Las plantas," 213–30; Hernández Bernejo, "El papel," 225–78; and Johnston, *The Staple Food*, 172–75.

24 The island's population exceeded 44,883 inhabitants in 1765, and by 1802, it had increased to 163,414. During this same period, the African slave population increased from 5,0237 to 17,508. It is estimated that more than 2,000 Canary Islanders arrived in Puerto Rico between 1695 and 1750. See Díaz Soler, *Historia de la esclavitud*, 260–61; and Cifre de Loubriel, *La formación*, 36.

25 Álvarez Nazario, *El elemento*, 264.

26 Álvarez Nazario, "El vocabulario canario," 26–29; Cadilla de Martínez, "Del maíz," 291–95.

27 López Tuero, *Cultivos perfeccionados*, 21–23.

28 The first recipe for majarete appears in *El cocinero puertorriqueño*, and calls for using tender corn removed from a dozen cobs. Eliza Dooley's 1948 *Puerto Rican Cookbook* reproduced the recipe, copying it from Sarah Méndez, and substituting cornmeal as the base. After 1950, majarete recipes began to stipulate the use of rice flour as well. See *El cocinero*, 256; Dooley, *The Puerto Rican*, 166; Cabanillas et al., *Cocine a gusto*, 238; Valldejuli, *Cocina criolla*, 422; Busó de Casas, *777 aventuras*, 350; *Cocina desde mi pueblo*, 148. Mundo nuevo, which is mentioned in several nineteenth-century costumbrista texts, seems also to have been known, in the mid-twentieth century, as mazamorra. That is perhaps why, in editing the entry for mazamorra in the index to the 1950 edition of *Cocine a gusto*, Cabanillas put the name "mundo nuevo" in parentheses. See Cabanillas et al., *Cocine a gusto*, 254. The 1966 edition of the cookbook no longer includes this reference. Mundo nuevo also appears in Valldejuli, *Cocina criolla*, 401. In *Cocina desde mi pueblo* the dish is called mazamorra (148).

29 Conversation with Sandra Rodríguez, Humacao, Puerto Rico, 10 July 2001.

30 For example, in the Pantagruelian campesino dinner re-created in "El cuento del matrimonio," after he has described all the main dishes of the meal, Ramón Méndez Quiñones mentions majarete as one of the sweetmeats that was offered along with others, such as dulce de coco and mundo nuevo. The serving

of fruit preserves as a final plate is also instructive. Méndez Quiñones alludes to them in the form of a rhyming couplet, loosely translated as "And an orange paste / ground in a pilón / and custard apple and milk sweet / made of syrup and Señor Cleto." See Méndez Quiñones, "El cuento," in Pedreira, "La actualidad," 31. Likewise, in his essay entitled "El carnaval en las Antillas," Luis Bonafoux Quintero re-creates—for a Spanish readership—a carnivalesque party scene in what is possibly the home of a provincial family. At the party, a maiden, resting after dancing "deliriously," is courted by her partner with "sugar water mixed with wine, majarete [italicized in the original], rice with coconut and plantain pie." See Bonafoux Quintero's essay in Cautiño Jordán, La sátira, 100.

31 Caballero Balseiro, Bajo el vuelo, 35.

32 Dooley, The Puerto Rican, viii.

33 Dooley, for example, recalls the following interchange with Isabel when she wanted to replace the stove with a gas oven: "I recall when the gas was installed, Isabel refused to part with the old stove: 'But, Isabel, I should think you would like a new gas stove.' No, mistress, I'se prepared to meet my Jesus, but I ain't prepared to meet Him ahead of time!' So she went along with the old-fashioned equipment. I early gave up the idea of making innovations. Once, having been given a breadmixer, she gazed fascinated as it stirred the sponge. 'Knowledge is increasin'!' was her comment. But a few weeks later, her strong right hand was mixing the sponge. A rosebush was planted in the mixer." Ibid.

34 El cocinero puertorriqueño, 256.

35 Ibid.

36 Mauleón Benítez, El español, 83–85.

37 See El cocinero puertorriqueño, 199. The infiernillo was used by cooks and bakers who had stoves with enclosed ovens. It was a considerable challenge to execute this dish in a kitchen that had only an anafe (portable brazier) or a fogón de tres piedras, whereby the pot or cauldron simply rested on large stones, generally three stones in a roughly triangular arrangement, with a fire lit under the cooking vessel. It is important to note that the unnamed cook cites—though with reference to other pudding-like sweets—the alternative of baking in "an oven," a distinction that may be aimed at experienced pastry cooks working in local bakeries. On the development of methods of baking, see Muro Carratalá, Diccionario, 2:77–78. On the development of ovens, see Hardyment, From Mangle; Cowan Schwartz, More Work; and Du Vall, Domestic Technology.

38 El cocinero puertorriqueño, 256.

39 Bonafoux Quintero, "El carnaval," 100.

40 Ibid. In "El carnaval en las Antillas," Bonafoux Quintero portrays and celebrates a mestizo creole society that comes together during carnival largely free of race-based problems. Nevertheless, his fictionalized social world is marked by unmistakable dividing lines. During carnival, funche with salted codfish is presented as a gift, but Bonafoux Quintero has it given between couples of "color," who "give themselves over voluptuously to an orgiastic dance, called

merengue." In this way, he contrasts it, socially and culturally, to majarete and other dishes which white creole "niños" offer to "maidens" as a display of courteousness and discretion after finishing a dance. For their part, the young ladies of color—to whom their male counterparts offer funche with salted codfish—are represented as voluptuous, full of ardor, with heaving breasts. Through the gift of food, the young men of color manage to tamp down their erotic feelings. (My own interpretation here has been inspired by the ideas of the Puerto Rican sociologist Ángel Quintero Rivera.) With respect to the celebration of *mestizaje* as an overarching discourse or ideology that conceals the historical realities of racism, see Kutzinski, *Sugar's Secrets*, 5.

41 Álvarez Nazario, *El elemento*, 264.

42 Ibid.

43 Carreño, *Compendio*, 84–94.

44 Ortiz, "La cocina afrocubana," 421.

45 Álvarez Nazario, *El elemento*, 264. Nazario takes the reference from Fray Bernarde María de Cannecatim's *Colleciao de observacoes grammaticaes sobre sa lingua bunda ou angolese e Diccionario aberviado da lingua conguenza* (Lisbon, 1805). For the names of dishes made with starchy foodstuffs in some Yoruba communities, in particular the preparation known as *fufu* (which was the version of starch-based funche that predominated in Cuba), see two articles by Bascom, "Yoruba Food," 41–53; and "Yoruba Cooking," 125–35.

46 Between 1815 and 1840, the number of Africans introduced into Puerto Rico as esclavos bozales—that is, as slaves brought to Puerto Rico directly from Africa, or from Africa to other Caribbean islands with slavery and from there to Puerto Rico—has been very conservatively calculated as 60,000 to 80,000. See Scarano, *Sugar and Slavery*, 31; and the same author's *Puerto Rico: Cinco siglos*.

47 Messer, "Maize," 1:97–112.

48 Figures compiled between 1812 and 1832 by the memoirist Pedro Tomás de Córdoba give the number of harvested ears of corn as 38,298,000 in 1812; in 1813, 52,586,000; 1814, 51,637,500; 1817, 41,131,500; 1820, 32,345,000; and 1827, 37,737,000. If these figures are correct, they would translate into a total of 132.5 corncobs per inhabitant annually. A supply on this order would not have been a source of worry for very many hacendados, given the complementary role played by rice, plantains, and starchy foodstuffs that added some variety and volume to meals. See Córdoba, *Memorias*, 3:359–408.

49 AGPR, "Sumaria averiguación . . . Don José Martínez."

50 On the concept of a basic matrix or basket of food and the peripheral function of foodstuffs, see Martin Bruegel's comments to Sidney Mintz's thesis in *Food and Foodways: Explorations in the History and Culture of Human Nourishment* 7, no. 2 (1997): 140–41.

51 AGPR, "Sumaria averiguación . . . Don José Martínez." In 1943, it was calculated that a pound of cornmeal could provide 1,590 calories. See "Alimentación," 8. I am indebted to Mario Roche for this reference. Although the historian Maurice Aymard long ago warned about the methodological risks of calculating the

nutritional value of food between one era and another as though they were equivalent—this ignores bromatological changes and equates the minimal nutritional requirements of recent and past epochs when they in fact are not remotely the same—the 1,590 calorie figure may be quite accurate, especially as it pertains to food that antedated the advances made by agroindustry, and because the energy expended daily by the working classes may have varied little over the course of the nineteenth century and into the mid-twentieth. See Aymard, "Toward the History of Nutrition," 1–16.

52 Carroll, Report, 114.

53 Colombán Rosario, "The Porto Rican Peasant," 562. That, at least, would be the conclusion drawn from the central place it occupied in the lunches eaten by 359 campesino families in 1929, as discovered by Colombán Rosario while carrying out research in Puerto Rico's central mountain range following the 1928 San Felipe hurricane. At that time, 248 families ate funche as their midday meal, accompanied by salted cod, or rice, or viandas.

54 Government of Puerto Rico, Department of Education, Manual del comedor, 8.

55 Roberts and Stefani, Patterns of Living, 166.

56 Roberts's analysis showed that cornmeal was consumed once or more per day in 5.3 percent of the families under study. Twenty-one percent stated that they ate cornmeal several times each week. Ibid., 374. Roberts sampled 1,044 families.

57 A recorded interview with Epifania Estrada conducted by the students Luz and Ruilen García in Estrada's residence in Ceiba, April 1995. At that time, the interviewee was seventy-nine years old.

58 In 1994, as part of the requirements for a course on the history of Puerto Rico, I offered my students the option of writing a final paper based on the findings obtained from a questionnaire that dealt with different aspects of the history of diet and food consumption on the island. The survey was directed to women and, among other questions, asked them if they had ever obtained food from the Puerto Rico Emergency Relief Administration (PRERA), an assistance program put into operation, between 1933 and 1935, as part of the Federal Emergency Relief Act. Two students, Zulaika Díaz and Eliezer Santana, administered the questionnaire to women above the age of fifty in several municipalities lying in the eastern part of the island. A total of twenty-one questionnaires were completed. The instrument contained twenty-three questions, covering such matters as specificities of diet, the work involved in cooking and preparing meals, the range of experiences in domestic kitchens, and holiday and party meals. If the interviewees did not know how to write, the students copied down their responses. The questions dealing with state food assistance were: "Did you have the opportunity to obtain food from the PRERA? [If so], what type of food did you receive and how did you cook it?" It is important to note that since the end of the PRERA, all subsequent social assistance programs, most notably those directed at providing food assistance, have been called PRERA by the majority of their recipients.

59 Ramona Denis Madonado, born in Naguabo in 1927, spent her life as a house-

wife. In May 1994, when she answered the questionnaire, she was seventy-seven years old.

60 Born in 1938, Julia Acosta is a native of the greater San Juan Tejas de Humacao neighborhood. In February 1994, at the time she responded to the questionnaire, she was fifty-six years old. Her education went up to high school. She currently works as a cook in a restaurant.

61 Secundina Ortiz's written response was brief and to the point: "They provided corn, a strawlike rice, raisins, cornmeal, wheat flour, it was made into funche, bits of fried salted codfish." Secundina was born on 27 November 1923; her reply was received in March 1994. She is now retired, after working in school dining halls. At the time she completed the questionnaire, she was seventy-one years old. Another participant in the survey, Julia Díaz, likewise answered the question very succinctly: "Cornmeal. Funche. With water, and it affected me so badly that not even dogs could have eaten it, and I used to toss it out." Julia was born in Naunabo, in May 1924. When the interview was conducted she was working as a cook's assistant in the School Dining Hall Program. Her responses were received in March 1994.

62 Conversations with Víctor (Vitín) Medina Ortiz, 17 July 2001.

63 Ortíz, "La cocina," 421.

64 According to cookbooks containing recipes for it, mazamorra is very similar to mundo nuevo, in that the corn must be tender, with the kernels scraped off the cob and then squeezed to obtain the starchy content. It is a sweet dish, taking both sugar and syrup, as well as aromatic spices and *leches* that vary from recipe to recipe. Marota is a dish made with cornmeal, in the style of funche, except that water is used to thicken the porridge, to which are added numerous small amounts of other tasty, fatty items of food. It is also called marifinga. In broad terms, marota and marifinga were essentially the same, differing only in name. It all came down to the different touches applied by particular cooks. Hence in formal, written culinary terms these two dishes could not, properly speaking, be classified as recipes. In contrast to mazamorra, which was an authentic dessert, marifinga and marota were light meals of substance, eaten to satisfy one's appetite. The recipe for mazamorra is contained in Cabanillas, *Cocine a gusto*, 275; Lugo Lugo, *Las recetas*, 142; and *Cocina desde mi pueblo*, 148. Marota is mentioned in Quintero and Tolosa, *Recuerdos y recetas*, 175, but no actual recipe for it is given. Rather, the authors simply mention it, alongside marifinga and funche, in the context of discussing the food crisis that broke out during the Second World War. It is thought by many in Puerto Rico that *frangallo* is a related dish, but it is not. Frangollo is a dry sweet, with a green plantain base that is finely chopped and later ground up. The base is mixed into a squeezed syrup, to which are added toasted peanuts. This sweet was very similar to "almonds with coconut," which are still sold in coastal areas. See *El cocinero de los enfermos*.

65 Vergés and Soto, *Cocina desde mi pueblo*; Hernández, *Sabores de ayer*; and Lugo Lugo, *Las recetas*.

66 Ortíz, "La cocina," 88.

67 Camporesi, *The Magic Harvest*, chap. 5 ("Dietary Geography and Social History") in particular.

68 Departamento de Agricultura, Oficina de Estadísticas Agrícolas, *Consumo de alimentos en Puerto Rico: Cosechas, 1974–75/1982–83*, 18.

69 Descartes et al., *Food Consumption*, 57.

70 Departamento de Agricultura, *Consumo de alimentos . . . 1974–75/1982–83*.

71 Departamento de Agricultura, *Consumo de alimentos . . . 1975–2003*, "Cornmeal," Folder 1758b6.

72 In 1944, 106,614 *cuerdas* of corn (each cuerda equaled 3,929 square meters) were planted on the island, whereas the agricultural census for 1998 reported the figure as 1,376. Government of Puerto Rico, Department of Agriculture and Commerce, *Annual Book*, 74; and U.S. Bureau of the Census, *Census of Agriculture*, table 46, 104. A cuerda measures longitude and area. During Spanish colonial times, it was used as a measurement of parcels of agricultural land. After the Spanish-American War and the beginning of a new colonial era under the United States, it was readily adopted so as to minimize land ownership disputes.

73 Departamento de Agricultura, *Imports into Puerto Rico from [the] United States by Commodity*, fiscal year 1999.

74 On the tendency to nibble on snacks, see Bell and Valentine, *Consuming Geographies*, 61–62; and Warde, *Consumption*, 148.

75 Junta de Planificación, *External Trade Statistics*, 1999. From Spain came 88.4 percent of imported prepared baked goods, followed by those from Colombia, with a 21.2 percent share of the market.

76 Junta de Planficicación, *Imports into Puerto . . . United States*, fiscal year 2001.

77 "Goya Remains a Fixture of Puerto Rican Homecooking," *San Juan Star*, Food and Beverage Supplement, 31 July 1997.

CHAPTER 4

1 Departamento de Agricultura, Oficina de Estadísticas Agrícolas, *Consumo anual 1950/51–1973/74*, 25.

2 Kurlansky, *El bacalao*, 43.

3 United States Food and Drug Administration, Seafood Products Research Center, Center for Food Safety and Applied Nutrition, *Regulatory Fish Encyclopedia*, 2001, <http://www.//vn.cfsan.fda.gov>.

4 Ibid.

5 Kurlansky, *El bacalao*, 38, 46.

6 Ibid., 46–48. See also "Maricultura: Otra frontera de la pesca organizada," *El Nuevo Día*, "Revista Negocios," 15 July 2001, 15.

7 Kurlansky, *El bacalao*, 43. See also United States Food and Drug Administration, Seafood Products Research Center, *Regulatory Fish Encyclopedia*, 2001, <http://www.vn.cfsan.feda.gov>.

8 Toussaint-Samat, History of Food, 324.

9 Ibid.

10 Kurlansky, El bacalao, 39. See also Samat, History of Food, in particular the section entitled "Drying, Salting, and Smoking Fish: An Age Old Procedure," 323 and passim.

11 Fischler, El (h)omnívoro, 156.

12 Ibid.

13 Montanari, The Culture of Food, 78–82.

14 Ibid. As Montaneri makes clear, although cod was fished, salted, and consumed from the Middle Ages on, it lacked a market as prominent as that for the herring that was fished and distributed by members of the Hanseatic League. It was not until the final years of the fifteenth century, with the more frequent voyages to Newfoundland and the consequent discovery of its abundant supplies of cod, that salted cod began to edge out and replace herring as the fish consumed by the poorest elements of urban populations. This theme is also taken up by Toussaint-Samat, History of Food, 318–24; and, though quite superficially, by Kurlansky as well. See the latter's El bacalao, 30.

15 Kurlansky, El bacalao, 54.

16 For figures on both kinds of fish, see DRHPR.

17 González Turmo, Comida de rico, 128–29. See also Toussaint-Samat, History of Food, 322, who draws attention to sardine fishing in Moroccan waters.

18 Kurlansky, El bacalao, 72–73.

19 Innis, The Cod Fisheries, 34. See also Kurlansky, El bacalao, 29–30.

20 Innis, The Cod Fisheries, 38; Kurlansky, El bacalao, 54.

21 "Cargos contra el Licenciado Sáncho Velásquez, Juez de Residencia y Justicia Mayor de la Isla," in Murga Sanz, Historia documental, 2:98.

22 "El consejo de la Ciudad de San Juan entrega una instrucción de treinta y siete puntos o problemas que Juan de Castellanos, procurador, ha de presentar al Rey," 6 July 1534, in Murga Sanz, Historia documental, 1:131. See also the case of the 1536 excommunication of Dr. Velásquez, who was subjected to an auto-da-fé because "he, who is a hidalgo, had consumed meat during Lent," in Murga Sanz, Puerto Rico, 307.

23 "Maricultura: Otra frontera de la pesca organizada," El Nuevo Día, Sección "Por Dentro," 22 March 2000.

24 Ibid.

25 Real Díaz, Catálogo de cartas, 280.

26 Kurlansky, El bacalao, 61; Innis, The Cod Fisheries, 38, and chap. 6, "The Struggle against Monopoly," 53 and passim.

27 Various historians concur that once the Caribbean lost its importance as a mining area and that as the principal Andalusian commercial interests developed a maritime system for provisioning the New World, the number of ships crossing the Atlantic and anchoring in Caribbean ports declined noticeably. In the case of Puerto Rico, this trend apparently began in 1550. Scholars likewise agree that as strategies for ensuring the security of the fleet evolved,

the size of certain vessels steadily increased. This development further disadvantaged Puerto Rico, because ships' pilots, after offloading supplies in the western port of Aguada and San Juan's port in the north, had to navigate in a southerly direction, which meant fighting the currents of the Mona narrows. Given this problem, they increasingly chose to approach the Caribbean at the latitude of the islands near Barlovento, from which point they could head to other ports, such as Nombre Dios and Veracruz. This route was not only better from a navigational point of view but also better served merchants' interests, since the ships could take on new cargoes of precious metals while finding wealthier markets for Andalusian goods and products. In the seventeenth century, shipping traffic in the direction of the ports of San Juan and Santo Domingo became still riskier and more problematic, as vessels that had reached the Barlovento islands as part of the fleet had to break away and head alone in a west-northwest direction, without the protection of Spanish galleons, at a time when fear of attack by pirates was extremely high. According to Frank Moya Pons, the threat posed by piracy not only bolstered the size and security of fleets supplying the Caribbean but also discouraged merchants from establishing regular trade with the two islands. The numbers tell the story. During a period of almost a quarter of a century (1626–50), only eighteen ships reached the shores of Puerto Rico, a figure that dropped to a mere eight between 1651 and 1675. The best synthesis of this development is found in Fernando Picó's *Historia general*, 75–77.

28 López Cantos, *Historia*, 110–13. The records of fish imports examined by López Cantos specifically note them as being fish, not salted cod, and as coming from non-codfish regions, such as Tenerife and Cumaná.

29 Kirkland, *Historia económica*, 114; Innis, *The Cod Fisheries*, 189 and 301.

30 Morales Carrión, *Puerto Rico y la lucha*, 92.

31 Innis, *The Cod Fisheries*, 301.

32 López Cantos, "La vida cotidiana," 149.

33 Moreno Fraginals, *El ingenio*, 3:56–58. Guillermo Baralt has noted, in the case of one estate in Puerto Rico—Buena Vista—that of all the food furnished by its managers to the slaves, salted cod was the most important. See Baralt, *La buena vista*, 64–67.

34 "Reglamento para la educación, trato y ocupaciones que desean dar a los esclavos sus amos y mayordomos," 12 August 1826, in Coll y Toste, *Boletín histórico de Puerto Rico*, 10:262–73.

35 It should be emphasized that salted cod was not an unknown food to those Africans who were brought as slaves to the Caribbean islands in the eighteenth and nineteenth centuries. In the eighteenth century, for example, an active slave trade existed that was based on exchanging slaves from the west coast of Africa for salted cod that came from the Massachusetts Bay colony. See Kirkland, *Historia económica*, 113–14.

36 CIH, "BM," 1849.

37 Cabanillas, *El folklore*, 34. The saying is a play on the Spanish word for cow, *vaca*,

the pronunciation of which sounds almost the same as the first two syllables of the word "bacalao."

38 United States Food and Drug Administration, Seafood Products Research Center, Center for Food Safety and Applied Nutrition, *Regulatory Fish Encyclopedia*, 2001, <http://www.vn.cfsan.fda.gov>.

39 Innis, *The Cod Fisheries*, 53 and passim. See also Kurlansky, *El bacalao*, 58–62.

40 Kurlansky, *El bacalao*, 58–62.

41 Salted fish went under several names in seventeenth-century Spain. Cervantes alludes to this fact in the scene in which Don Quijote sallies forth to arm himself after the fashion of a knight. Having not yet breakfasted, the *manchego* arrives at the inn of an Andalusian, where the following takes place: "That day happened to be a Friday, and in all the inn there was nothing but a few nibbles of a fish which in Castile they call abadejo, in Andalucía bacallao, and in other parts curadillo, and in still others truchuela." A fish known by four names in seventeenth-century Spain indicates that people used the same name to refer to different types of fish. Cervantes, *Don Quijote de la Mancha*, chap.2, 44.

42 Kurlansky, *El bacalao*, 80–81.

43 Kirkland, *Historia económica*, 114. It was also referred to as "West Indies Cured." See Kurlansky, *El bacalao*, 80–81; and Walsh, "Untropical Fish."

44 CIH, *Balanzas Mercantiles*, 1897. Only 166,000 pounds were imported from Spain.

45 "Reglamento para la educación, trato y ocupaciones que deben dar a los esclavos sus amos y mayordomos," 12 August 1826, in Coll y Toste, *Boletín histórico de Puerto Rico* 10:262–73.

46 On this point, see Martin Breughel's earlier cited (introduction, note 12) review article in *Food and Foodways*.

47 See the chapter entitled "Meat."

48 The quoted material is from Cruz Monclova, *Historia de Puerto Rico*, 2, pt. 2:803 and passim. The observation made by the journalist writing in *La Razón*, that day laborers generally ate salted cod minus any oil, is important. The purpose of adding oil was to restore the soft dampness that the fish lost in the process of being cured, and thus to render it more palatable and tasty. And while desalting salted cod did restore some water content to it, the amount was minimal. As noted earlier, fresh salted cod is composed of 80 percent water. When dried and salted, this percentage drops to 14.20 percent. On this point, see Toussaint-Samat, *History of Food*, 324. See also Hui, *The Encyclopedia of Food Science*, 2:926–28. In the nineteenth century, the use of oil set apart the dishes eaten by the well-to-do from those consumed by the poor. Olive oil was far more costly than the more popular, more accessible oils (and fats) such as coconut or sesame oil and lard.

49 Quoted in Cruz Monclova, *Historia de Puerto Rico*, 2:803.

50 Valle Atiles, *Cartilla*, 74.

51 Ibid.

52 Innis, *The Cod Fisheries*, 421–23.

53 Named after its sponsor, Joseph Foraker, a senator from Ohio, the Foraker Act (officially the Organic Act of 1900) established limited popular government on the island, which the United States had annexed following the conclusion of the Spanish-American War.

54 Unlike the United States, Canada exported only salted cod to Puerto Rico, not other salted and pressed fish. In 1895, British territories exported 27,233,987 pounds to Puerto Rico; the figure for the United States—which included salted cod and haddock—was only 1,692,682 pounds. In 1897, these figures were 22,092,936 and 2,149,499 pounds, respectively (this latter total for the United States applied solely to salted cod; it was complemented by 1,988 kilos of preserved shellfish and hake. See CIH, *Balanzas Mercantiles*, 1895, 1897.

55 Consider that the island received supplies totaling 55,319,858 pounds in 1897. The nine countries were: Spain, the United States, Germany, Sweden, Norway, England, France, British overseas possessions, and Italy. See CIH, *Balanzas Mercantiles*, 1897.

56 Ibid.

57 Hill and Noguera, *The Food Supply*, 19.

58 Ibid., 26

59 Díaz Pacheco, *El consumo*, 21.

60 Descartes et al., *Food Consumption*, 55.

61 Ibid., 20.

62 As is commonly known, salted cod is a food that loses considerable volume in the transition from desalting, to cooking, to finally being consumed. Hence the actual amount consumed must have been less than that indicated in the Department of Agriculture's statistics. Furthermore, one should pay particular attention to the data for San Juan as concerns the weekly consumption—0.18 pounds, or an ounce and a half per person—of salted cod. For rural working families, who had many fewer dietary options, the estimated intake of salted cod in 1937 was only fractionally higher—0.20 ounces per person—than the figure for the capital. See Descartes et al., *Food Consumption*, 58; Díaz Pacheco, *El consumo*, 17; and Lang and Morales Otero, "Health and Socio-economic Studies," 123.

63 See Ortíz Cuadra, "1942: El hambre," 122–33.

64 Roberts and Stefani, *Patterns of Living*, 152–53.

65 Morales Otero, "Trastornos de la nutrición," 14.

66 *El cocinero puertorriqueño*, 105–11.

67 Archivo Histórico Diocesano de la Arquidiócesis de San Juan, Fondo Carmelitano, series Cuenta y Datos, January 1862.

68 Ferguson, *Home Making*, 78–79.

69 As examples, see "Reglas generales para la alimentación," 193–99; Torres, "Consideraciones," 252–58; Roberts, "Deficiencias en la dieta," 259–65; Zeijo de Zayas, "El puertorriqueño," 266–81; and "Salud prepara un nuevo plan de nutrición," *El Mundo* (San Juan), 17 January 1952, 12.

70 "Pueblo celebra quinto aniversario el próximo jueves," *El Mundo* (San Juan), 23

April 1960, 30; "En la intersección de la avenida Central y San Francisco inaugurará hoy Supermercado Superama," El Mundo (San Juan), 29 September 1995, 14; "Hoy inaugura nuevo supermercado Pueblo," El Mundo (San Juan), 31 May 1956, 26; "Inauguran Supermercado Todos en Hato Rey," El Mundo (San Juan), 22 March 1957, 3; "Avenida 65 de Infantería: Miles acuden a inaugurar nuevo supermercado Todos," El Mundo (San Juan), 19 November 1958, 5; "Lansing P. Shield: Objetivo de Grand Union es bajar los precios," El Mundo (San Juan), 2 October 1959, 27.

71 Ortíz Cuadra, "La vida buena."

72 Junta de Planificación de Puerto Rico, Consumo de alimentos, 1950/51–1973/74, 3:23.

73 In the 1937–38 study, salted cod, the others in its family, and pressed and smoked fish were subsumed under the general category of salted and smoked fish, for which reason the statistics tend to reflect an overall consumption of salted fish that could well be taken as indicative of the consumption of salted cod proper, although other types of fish clearly figured in the total. Descartes et al., Food Consumption, 59. The total for 1970 is very close to the amount—five pounds—that the wealthiest families in San Juan, those earning more than $3,600 per year, consumed per person in 1937. Families with lower incomes— between 600 and 2,000 dollars—consumed on average ten pounds per family member.

74 The study published by the Planning Commission in 1965 covers the period 1956–57 through 1961–62. The 1978 study covers the period from 1951–52 through 1973–74. See Junta de Planificación, Anuario estadístico, and Junta de Planificación, Consumo de alimentos, 1951–52/1973–74, 3:23.

75 These figures are approximate and derive from the total amount of salted cod imported from abroad without considering any reexportation of the fish. The annual totals have been computed based on the present (2003) overall population (3.8 million) of Puerto Rico.

76 All this history gave rise to the notorious Cod Wars (1958–61, 1971, and 1975– 76), which culminated in the gradual establishment of quotas, set according to time of year, type of fishing boat, and species of cod. Kurlansky, El bacalao, especially the chapter entitled "Tres guerras para cerrar el mar abierto," 149 and passim. The near extinction of the fish resulted from the development of industrial-scale fishing from 1951 on, begun by the British fleets with their enormous "factory-trawlers," equipped with sophisticated technology and machinery developed during the Second World War. Canadian marine scientists have demonstrated that, between 1647 and 1750, 8 million tons of Atlantic cod were fished from the waters. Between twenty-five and forty generations of cod were captured during that period. According to these scientists, since industrialized fishing with trawlers began in 1951, it took only fifteen years to produce these same results, the normal time period for the reproduction of just one generation of cod. See Woodard, "A Run on the Banks," 34 and passim.

77 Some incoming shipments of hake and pollock have had a water content of up to 50 percent, according to documents pertaining to external trade. Beginning in the late 1990s, however, markets have increasingly offered substitutes, coming from the fishing fleets of the Republic of China, including a particular salted fish that is sold in Puerto Rico as cod but is actually something else. In 1999, 187,847 pounds of this substitute fish arrived from China. In 2001, 762,146 pounds of pollock were imported onto the island. Around September 2002, pollock—labeled as salted cod from China—was sold in the Grande supermarkets at $2.89 per pound, a price much lower than that for Atlantic cod from Canada's Gaspé Bay, which at this same time fetched a price of $6.99 per pound. See Grande's sales notice corresponding to the weeks of 18 September to 1 October 2002.

78 Junta de Planificación, Programa de Planificación Económica y Social, Oficina de Análisis Económico, *Shipments of Merchandise from the United States to Puerto Rico by Commodity*, 1996–2010. I am indebted to José Mulero González, of the Department of Agriculture, and to William Galindo, of the Planning Commission, for facilitating my access, electronically, to the data on salted cod, its near relatives, and salted fish from the lengthy chapter on *Fish and Shellfish from External Trade*. The term "gross" is used because these statistics include the total number of imports, from which any portion that is reexported, above all to the Lesser Antilles, is not subtracted.

79 Commonwealth of Puerto Rico, Office of Agricultural Statistics, *Facts and Figures*, 117–21.

80 Junta de Planificación de Puerto Rico, *Imports of Merchandise*.

CHAPTER 5

1 Roberts and Stefani, *Patterns of Living*, 168.

2 For a detailed description of the biochemical properties of Manihot esculenta, see Johns, *With Bitter Herbs*, 52; and McKey and Beckerman, "Chemical Ecology," 83–84.

3 For a description of the process, see Oviedo, *Historia*, book 7, chap. 2, 230.

4 Torres Vargas, "Descripción de la isla y ciudad de Puerto Rico, y de su vecindad y poblaciones, presidio, gobernadores y obispos: Frutos y minerales," 1647, in Fernández Méndez, *Crónicas*, 182. An order of 1515, sent by the monarchy to San Juan's city officials, acknowledged the good that "you did in sending word of the 19,000 bulbs and seedlings of basic foodstuffs that you have ordered be planted, out of the 50,000 that there were." In the same piece, the monarchy issues the following directive: "*Take care that the 30,000 missed by the worm are fertilized.*" Could this be the second plague to which Torres Vargas refers in his letter? See Ballesteros Garbrois, *La idea colonial*, 232. Whatever the case, Torres Vargas copied, almost to the letter, the anecdote about the plague of ants from the *Década segunda* of Antonio de Herrera in the latter's *Crónica General*

de las Indias. See Antonio de Herrera, *Década segunda*, reprinted in Tapia y Rivera, *Biblioteca histórica*, 120.

5 Montanari, *The Culture of Food*, chap. 2, especially the section entitled "Give Us This Day Our Daily Bread," 47 and passim.

6 See Oviedo, *Historia*, 231–32; and López Cantos, *Miguel Henríquez*, 103.

7 *El cocinero puertorriqueño*, 170–71.

8 Johnston, *Staple Food Economies*, 25–26. According to Johnston, Portuguese slavers, during the sixteenth century, took cassava with them with the express purpose of feeding captured slaves who would need to be kept in port prior to being transported across the Atlantic to Brazil. Other scholars note the existence of written sources that record the cultivation of the cassava plant in coastal regions of Angola (Loango, 1608, and Luanda, 1620). See, Von Oppen, "Cassava," 47. More recent studies settle on 1612 as the year when the first written record of cassava was registered in West Africa, in Gabon specifically. Others place the year of the first written record at 1593. See Alpern, "Exotic Plants," 65 and 73; Jones, *Manioc in Africa*, 60; and Karasch, "Manioc," 1:181–86.

9 Von Oppen, "Cassava," 51.

10 De Grosourdy, *El médico*, 472.

11 De Grosourdy, *El médico*, 472 ; and Von Oppen, "Cassava," 43–71. See also O'Hair, "Tropical Roots."

12 "Ordenanzas hechas por el cabildo, justicia y regimiento de esta ciudad de San Juan de Puerto Rico," 11 September 1627, in Real Díaz, *Catálogo de cartas*, 279.

13 It seems somewhat surprising that the same measures of weight that prevailed at the outset of colonization were still being used at the beginning of the seventeenth century. Oviedo had noted, with reference to affairs in Santo Domingo, that during the period of Spanish settlement cassava cakes had sold in loads of "two *arrobas*, which total fifty pounds [consisting] of [fifty cassava cakes, each weighing] sixteen ounces." In 1627, cassava was still sold by the same units in San Juan, in two-arroba loads.

14 "Directorio General que ha mandado formar el Sr. Don Miguel de Muesas," 22 May 1770, in Caro Costa, *Antología de lecturas*, 425.

15 The opinions quoted are from de Acosta, *Historia natural*, 172; "Relación del viaje," 153; "López de Haro," 164; Abad y Lasierra's comments, in his "Viaje a la América," regarding the visit he made to the community of Fajardo beginning on 16 August 1772; and Huerga, *Vida y obras*, 233–34. See also the descriptions of the Italian Antonio de Filangieri, in López Cantos, *Miguel Henríquez*, 117; and "Del Valle Atiles," 73.

16 In 1862, for example, De Grosourdy observed in the islands controlled by France that cassava was planted on plantations "to let the soil rest after the sugarcane was yanked out, and that [this] vianda serves as sustenance for the working class and the poorer elements, and for that reason is little valued by the rich who hardly use it, although it would be most advantageous for those estate owners who have to maintain a large peon workforce." He later advises

that because of its sturdiness in comparison to other food crops it ought to "be effective to have it as a secondary crop, available to supplant other viandas in the event they fail or produce a weak yield." De Grosourdy, El médico, 470–71.

17 El cocinero, 170.

18 Abad, Puerto Rico, 116–18.

19 Wilsey, Tropical Foods, 19–24.

20 According to the 1930 census, the number of square meters planted was: sweet potatoes, 46,061; tannier, 16,683; yams, 8,373; and cassava, 6,072. United States Bureau of the Census, Fifteenth Census, 230.

21 Cook, "History of the First Quarter," 30.

22 As noted earlier, one cuerda equaled 3,929 square meters.

23 Hill and Noguera, The Food Supply, 21.

24 Mauleón Benítez, El español, 85.

25 Rodríguez Juliá, Elogio, 45.

26 I am indebted to the Loiza artist Daniel Lind for organizing my visit with doña Benicia.

27 It is worth noting that cassava was also a source for making a type of honey, vinegar, wine, and dense soups, as well as poison and—using the dry branches of the shrub—fire.

28 Oviedo, Historia, 235.

29 De Grosourdy, El médico, 471.

30 Ferguson, Home Making, 34. Although Ferguson translated the name as "tortillas," these were (and are) commonly known as tortitas.

31 Milán, "Tubérculos," 55.

32 Wilsey and Janer Vilá, Vegetales tropicales.

33 Pérez García, "El cultivo," 779–82; and Cook and Toro, "History of the First Quarter," 3–99.

34 Haddock and Hernández, "Consumer Preferences," 4.

35 Montanari, El hambre, 93–94.

36 Oviedo, Historia, book 7, chap. 4, 234.

37 The fragment in which he refers to tropical fruits reads: "The fruits generally are not good and there are few like those in Spain, but there are some which are incomparably better, the Queen of all and as many as Nature has created is the Pineapple, so called because it is made like no other, the mamón [limoncillo] is excellent, best eaten with a spoon. It is almost like caramel spread, there are sweet potatoes all year round, they are plentiful and better than those in Spain, the plantains, which dot the countryside, are good and excellent when roasted." He later goes on to refer to the imported citruses (bitter and sweet oranges and grapefruit) that had been introduced into the island's agricultural fields. "Carta del señor fray Juan Alonso de Solís Obispo de Puerto Rico a mi señora doña Beatriz Ordóñez de Castro," in Cabanillas, El puertorriqueño, 407–9.

38 "López de Haro," in Fernández Méndez, Crónicas, 165.

39 Oviedo's is the oldest description of techniques for planting and propagating sweet potatoes; see his Historia, book 7, chap. 4, 234–35. For a nineteenth-

century (1863) description, see De Grosourdy, *El médico*, 471–72; and for the twentieth century, see Milán,"Tubérculos," 53–58 and Moscoso, "El cultivo," 126–39.

40 Abad y Lasierra, *Historia geográfica*, 186.
41 Córdoba, *Memorias*, 5:409–11.
42 Vaughn and Geisler, *The New Oxford Book*, 222.
43 Roberts and Stefani, *Patterns of Living*, 55–69, 87–94, 145–66.
44 See two articles by Bascom, "Yoruba Cooking," 124–25; and "Yoruba Food," 41–53.
45 It is not entirely clear just when the yam was introduced into the New World. In book 7 of his *Historia general*, Oviedo mentions that the yam was under cultivation on both the island of Hispaniola and in other parts of the Indies, further noting that the number of plantings had multiplied considerably on the islands on which Spaniards had settled. Although the first nineteen books of the *Historia general* were in Seville, ready to be printed, around 1535, it also happens that between 1535 and 1540 Oviedo revised them, adding a good deal more information. Hence it is not possible to pinpoint just when he made the reference to yams. Oviedo, *Historia general*, 244. For more on the publication dates and Oviedo's revisions, see Pérez de Tudela's critical introduction to the *Historia general*, 122. On the important role played by yams in African cultures prior to the era of European exploration and expansion, see Lewicki, *West African Foods*, 49–52. According to Lewicki, the first Arab reference to yams dates to 1352–53.
46 Lewicki, *West African Foods*, 49–52; Bascom, "Yoruba Food."
47 Bascom, "Yoruba Cooking," 132; Ortíz, "La cocina," 419; *El cocinero de los enfermos, convalecientes y desganados*, 88–89.
48 De Grosourdy, *El médico*, 470; Simons, "El cultivo del ñame," 204.
49 West African cuisine is replete with yam wrapped in banana leaves. An example is *amuyale*, or grated yam that is seasoned and then molded by hand into little balls. These are brushed with water until they are moist and soft, after which they are wrapped in the banana leaves and steam-cooked. Very similar to the amuyale is the *epa*, the difference being that it is made with leftover pieces of boiled yam, which are cut and dried, and later pounded in a mortar so as to obtain a paste that is moistened. The paste is then worked into little balls, which are wrapped in leaves and steamed. Two other versions are the *waiwai* and the *gunni*. These differ in being coarse pieces of leftover grated yam that are then used to make flour. See Bascom, "Yoruba Cooking," 130–31.
50 Oviedo, *Historia*, 248.
51 Braudel, *Civilization and Capitalism*, 177.
52 The most authoritative account, dating to the nineteenth century, is that of the botanist Alphonse de Candolle in his work *Origin of Cultivated Plants* (New York: Appleton, 1885), 306–7. In broad terms, those who have investigated the botanical-geographic origins of the *Musacae* family concur that it developed within the geographic zone that stretches from the northeast of India, through

Burma, Cambodia, parts of southern China, and the islands of Sumatra, Java, Borneo, and the Philippines, to Taiwan. See, among others, George, *The Propagation*; Keep, *The Banana*; and McEwen Dalziel, *Useful Plants*.

53 Indeed, the Arab sources consulted by Lewicki on West Africa during the Middle Ages make no mention of either the plantain or the banana. For the most complete synthesis of hypotheses concerning the movement of the *Musacae* family, and of the oldest references to it in different parts of the world, see Keep, *The Banana*, 19–38.

54 It should be noted, though, that in the culinary terminology of Puerto Rico, unripe ("green," as they are called on the island) bananas that are boiled in salt water are also considered viandas.

55 On the basis of Oviedo's description of how it grew and what it looked like, the first of the *musas* in the Caribbean seems to have been the "paradisiacal, or plantain; though Cabanillas believes it was the banana.

56 On attempts to plant and reproduce nonindigenous fruit trees, see Oviedo, *Historia*, 247.

57 López Tuero, *Plátano*, 23.

58 Ibid., 5.

59 De Acosta, *Historia natural*, 178–80.

60 "Real Cédula a los oficiales reales de la isla de San Juan de Puerto Rico para que lleven cuenta y razón de lo que se hubiere gastado y gastare en una estancia el gobernador Antonio de Mosquera," 1 November 1597, in Cabanillas, *El puertorriqueño*, 400.

61 López Cantos, "La vida cotidiana," 154.

62 Mintz, *Tasting Food*, 36–37. These concerns had been addressed during the seventeenth and eighteenth centuries on French sugar plantations in the Caribbean. French estate owners tried three ways of providing food to their slaves: the distribution of fixed rations, the cultivation of crops by the slaves themselves via their own gardens and plots, and common or communal lands, these consisting of an area on the plantation used expressly for the production of foodstuffs. This last approach came under regulation in the eighteenth century and obligated the estate owner to mark off land for planting in keeping with the number of slaves on his plantation. Although the three approaches were often combined, estate owners in the eighteenth century preferred to let slaves grow their own food. This practice was advantageous to them—since, to the extent that the slaves could maintain their own native gastronomic traditions—the slave owners could avoid having to import food and concern themselves with its storage. Moreover, they could reach mutual agreements on what crops to plant. The record suggests that the three approaches were all used, in combination, in Puerto Rico. It also reveals that as the sugar plantation economy gained ground, a dialogue ensued over the issue of slaves' diets, in which the slave owners made clear that they favored certain foods over others. It likewise reveals the importance of the fixed-rations approach which, as we observed in the complaints raised by the slaves on José Martínez's

hacienda, was a source of many grievances. On the French experience in the Caribbean, see Debien, "La nutrición," 13–16.

63 "Reglamento para la educación, trato y ocupaciones que deben dar a los esclavos sus amos y mayordomos," 1826, 262–73.

64 Ibid.

65 Moreno Fraginals, 3:56–58.

66 López de Haro, in Fernández Méndez, Crónicas, 165.

67 De Grosourdy, El médico, 468.

68 Ibid.

69 Abad y Lasierra, "Diario de viaje," entry for 16 August 1772, describing his visit to Fajardo.

70 "Relación circunstanciada del actual estado de la población frutos y proporciones para el fomento que tiene la isla de San Juan de Puerto Rico, con algunas ocurrencias sobre los medios conducentes a ello," 1765, in Tapia y Rivera, Biblioteca histórica, 526–55.

71 Meléndez Muñoz, "Tirijala," in Cuentos del cedro.

72 I specifically use the expression "again take up" because, as of 1814, the armchair agriculturists who formed part of the editorial board of the Diario Económico de Puerto Rico had advanced the idea of mechanizing the processing of cassava, corn, coconut, and rice. Later apparently, in a development which extended to the end of the century, some of the more prosperous farmers on the island devised ways of speeding up the process, as demonstrated by the example of the Buena Vista hacienda as well as by some of the entries in the Balanzas Mercantiles, which record the importation of equipment for grinding corn. Likewise, the samples of plantain flour, and of starch extracted from different viandas, that were shown at the exposition and trade fair held in Ponce in 1882 hint at attempts to reform agriculture so that domestic foodstuffs could be channeled more effectively toward commercial and industrial ends. See "Máquinas, sus efectos y ventajas," in Diario económico de Puerto Rico, 1814–1815, 1:291–96; Baralt, La buena vista, 64–67; CIHBM; and Abad, Puerto Rico, 112–20.

73 Abad, Puerto Rico, 112–20. In 1882, José Ramón Abad coined the phrase alimentación pública to refer to the diet of the island's overall population, as opposed to the diet of day laborers alone. In Abad's words: "In order of abundance and nutritional value, plantains and bananas are followed by root vegetables, tubers, and rhizomes, which are used as everyday food in the countryside and in hamlets and small settlements. Such plants merit greater consideration than they currently receive from us, because they are a powerful aid to the diet of the general public; the enormous amounts of sweet potatoes, yams, and tannier that are consumed is a matter of record, we are going to have to rely on harvests of these root vegetables to keep our heads above water." It should be stressed that, for Abad, these simple, ordinary plants were front and center among those which deserved "greater attention." Equally important is that, unlike many others who expressed themselves on the matter during the

eighteenth century, he did not set up an opposition, insofar as who consumed these products, between city and countryside. For him, they "are used every day in towns and rural areas." Abad, *Puerto Rico*, 20. A similar concern for the place of crops of basic foodstuffs in the face of an uncertain future of food supplies was voiced by Eugenio Astol: "There is a lot of tobacco, sugar, and coffee, but one doesn't eat these. Of what is consumed—rice, beans, corn, edible tubers, etc., etc [*sic*]—it would be difficult to find even a poorly cultivated *cuerda*. Puerto Rico lacks truck farms like those of Europe, the farmworker does not have granaries, as a result, in cities as well as in rural areas the matter of subsistence is subject to the fluctuations of trade. Stop it completely for two months, and we will die of hunger." Cited in Cruz Monclova, *Historia de Puerto Rico*, 3:283. This concern was reflected in the establishment, in 1880, of the island's first agricultural experiment station, and was addressed as well in the agricultural seminars it sponsored, in the years 1888–1895, under the direction of the agronomist Fernando López Tuero.

74 López Tuero, *Plátano*, 5.

75 López Tuero, *La reforma agrícola*, 201.

76 Asenjo, "Composición química," 281.

77 *Aguinaldo puertorriqueño*, 203.

78 Tapia y Rivera, *La leyenda*, 160.

79 Roqué de Duprey, *Luz y sombra*, 90.

80 Bonafoux Quintero, "El carnaval," 100.

81 Álvarez Nazario, *El elemento*, 266.

82 *El cocinero*, 136.

83 Ibid., 128.

84 Dooley, *Puerto Rican*, 104.

85 Cabanillas, *Cocine a gusto*, 68.

86 For a long time, cookbooks also omitted any recipes for *alcapurria*. This was a dish made with plantains or some other grated vianda—cassava and tannier in particular. These were mashed into a dough that was colored with achiote and filled with spiced meat or land crabs that had been stewed in a strong sofrito sauce. The mixture was then placed on plantain leaves that were folded over into the shape of a pie and fried in hot fat. In the most authentic *freidurías* of Puerto Rico's northeastern coast, the custom is to wrap the filling in the leaves of the seagrape (*cocolobos uvífera*), a shrubby tree that grows along the beach fronts. The first alcapurria recipe in fact appeared in Wilsey and Janer Vilá's 1931 cookbook devoted to the tannier (not the plantain). See their *Vegetales tropicales*, 23.

87 Kennedy, *Las cocinas*, especially the chapter "Tamales y platillos," 73–91; and Mejía Prieto, *Gastronomía*, with special emphasis on the chapter devoted to food and cooking in Chiapas, 97–106. For Colombia, see de Zurek, *Cartagena*, 131. The differences are not great. In Mexico, the tamal, or pastel, is made with a cornmeal dough and is generally steam-cooked. In Cartagena, it is wrapped

in *bijao* leaves (similar to plantain leaves) and boiled, and it is called *hallaca* in Venezuela.

88 The hallacas included by Eliza Dooley were Venezuelan hallacas, made with a base of cornmeal and wrapped in plantain leaves. This last feature, as well as their filling—garbanzos, raisins, pork meat, chili peppers—and their being cooked in boiling water makes them similar to pastel de plátano. Hallacas are not common in Puerto Rico, as they are, during the Christmas season, in Venezuela and the Guyanas. Dooley, *Puerto Rican*, 165.

89 Ibid., 164.

90 Ferguson, *Home Making*, 91, 144–45.

91 Piononos are made by slicing a ripe plantain lengthwise into several strips. These are folded into a circular shape and secured at the edges. The center is stuffed with well-seasoned, chopped, stewed meat. Flour, eggs, and water are blended to make a batter, which is poured over the filling, and the piononos are then deep-fried on both sides. The name of the dish may have been trans-posed to Puerto Rico from Spain, where in the nineteenth century a pastry by the same name, created by the baker Ceferino Ysla in honor of Pope Pius IX (famous for his sweet tooth), became traditional in Santa Fe, a municipality adjacent to the city of Granada. The piononos sold in all of Santa Fe's pastry shops closely resemble the pionono in Puerto Rico—both are rolled into a cylindrical shape.

92 Dooley, *Puerto Rican*, 103–4.

93 Wilsey, *Tropical Foods*.

94 Wilsey and Janer Vilá, *Vegetales tropicales*.

95 Cabanillas, Ginorio, and Quirós, *Cocine a gusto*; and Valldejuli, *Cocina criolla*.

96 In September, the Breadfruit Festival is celebrated in the municipality of Hu-macao. As part of the festivities, there is a cooking contest, one of which fea-tured no less than a version of lasagna made with breadfruit.

97 In this context, Ángel Quintero Rivera has called attention to the proliferation of festivals during the last decade of the twentieth century. He assembled a list, up to 1994, of 179 festivals, 24 of which had as their main purpose the celebra-tion of popular gastronomy. The names of 8 of the festivals, furthermore, were explicitly chosen to commemorate a particular foodstuff. Quintero also noted that the majority of the festivals were associated with food products or dishes that had traditionally been "poor people's fare," or food that was held in low esteem. Of the total number of festivals, 3 were specifically devoted to viandas: the Festival Nacional del Plátano, the Festival de la Pana, and the Festival de La Yuca, held in the municipalities of Dorado, Humacao, and Coamo, respec-tively. See Quintero Rivera, "De la fiesta al festival," 97–107.

98 Bourdieu, *Distinction*, 79.

99 Fischler, *El (h)omnívoro*, 92–93.

100 Ibid., 89.

101 Ibid., 103.

102 Junta de Planificación, External Trade Statistics, *Imports into Puerto Rico . . .* 2000; and Junta de Planificación, External Trade Statistics, *Imports Into Puerto Rico . . . United States.*

103 Estado Libre Asociado de Puerto Rico, Departamento de Agricultura, *Consumo de alimentos farináceos, papas elaboradas,* 1975–2003, Folder 1657b18. The figure for 2003 is preliminary; the count is official up to July.

104 This notion comes from from Pelto and Pelto, "Diet and Delocalization," 507–23. See also Montanari, *The Culture of Food,* 158.

105 Estado Libre Asociado, Departamento de Agricultura, Oficina de Estadísticas Agrícolas, *Consumo de alimentos farináceos, año 2000 y 2001.* Also, Junta de Planificación, *External Trade Statistics . . . 2000 and 2001.*

CHAPTER 6

1 Carroll, *Report,* 98–99.

2 Ibid.

3 "A Rise in the Price of Meat from Europe Is Forecast," *El Nuevo Día,* 15 March 2001, 72.

4 "The Uruguayan Ambassador Arrives to Explain the Situation with Hoof and Mouth Disease," *El Nuevo Día,* 6 July 2001, 63. On the reaction in Europe, see Jesús Contreras Hernández, "The Cultural Aspects of Meat Consumption," 221–46.

5 DRHPR, 142.

6 Ibid., 176.

7 Ibid., 140.

8 Ibid., 142.

9 Ibid., 205–6.

10 Ibid., 172–307.

11 Crosby, *The Columbian Exchange,* 74 and 98.

12 Royal Treasury account books recorded monetary reimbursements for pigs and meat supplied by various Spaniards who had received grants of Indian labor and needed to feed their workers. Although the pigs brought in by private individuals were certainly few in number, they nonetheless may have been critical in helping "sustain" the Indians during their obligatory periods of work in the mining operations. On these payments, see DRHPR, 46–50.

13 Reitz, "Dieta y alimentación," 13–14.

14 Domingo, *La mesa,* 147–48 [part of section entitled "El cerdo, ese viejo cristiano"]. The sheer quantities of salt pork transported from Hispaniola to Puerto Rico, when the search for gold was at its peak, seems to indicate that the salting of meat was not done purely to help meet the food needs of the conquistadores. Between September and December 1512, 2,350 pounds of salt pork were imported onto the island. On 7 February 1513, 1,137 pounds were offloaded from the ship *Espíritu Santo,* and on the following two days, respectively, the island received shipments of 2,387 and 4,424 pounds (the lat-

ter carried by the ship *Gracia de Dios*). This pattern continued unaltered during subsequent years. See DRHPR, 165 and passim. For the reference to salt pork, see ibid., 214.

15 On these and other saline resources, see Sued Badillo, "La valoración de las salinas," 9–26.

16 Badillo, *El Dorado*, 326.

17 Fischler, *El (h)omnívoro*, 110–11.

18 Badillo, *El Dorado*, 325.

19 Crosby, *The Columbian Exchange*, in particular the chapters "New World Foods and Old World Demography," 171; and "Old World Plants and Animals in the New World," 75. In addition, see Oviedo's anecdote about the native islander who went off to hunt wild pigs, in the mountains of Hispaniola, accompanied by domesticated pigs (*de crianza*). Oviedo, Historia, book 6, chap. 51, 221. See also Cadilla de Martínez, "El lechón asado," 399–401.

20 Yáñez's strategy for getting the animals to reproduce seems to have involved releasing "two female pigs and one male pig and a male goat and some female goats" on the island's western coast. See Gil de Bermejo, *Panorama histórico*, 62.

21 Oviedo, *Historia*, book 6, chapter 51, 221.

22 The ordinances are reproduced in Vila Vilar, *Historia de Puerto Rico*, 40–46.

23 Abad y Lasierra, *Historia geográfica*, 213.

24 Lewicki, *West African Food*. On this point Lewicki states: "We can find abundant information in medieval Arabic sources regarding the consumption of meat, fish, etc., by Africans during the Middle Ages. There are also numerous references to the raising of domestic animals for meat, as well as to hunting." Ibid., 79.

25 Martínez, *Pasajeros a Indias*, 58–67.

26 "Memoria sobre la propiedad," 239–310; and Elizaguirre, "Los sistemas," 65.

27 Murga Sanz, *Puerto Rico*, 348. Years later, with the closure of some sugar plantations, working and well-fed cattle were abandoned to their fate, or so an inventory, made around 1570 on behalf of an indebted hacendado and cattle rancher Martín de Aceituno, would seem to suggest. On his property, according to the inventory, there had been "three herds of cows, wild . . . and one that was Pedro Maldonado's and another that was the Church's, and in none of them was even a single cow enclosed." See Caro Costa, *Antología de lecturas*, 162–64.

28 In this idea of Mintz's, which is different from Fischler's concept of a "supplementary food," the new food survives not through the channel of interethnic exchange, but through the force exerted by systems of power. See Mintz, *Tasting Food*, especially the essay entitled "Food and Its Relationship to Concepts of Power," 17–32.

29 Ibid.

30 Montanari, *The Culture of Food*, 74–78.

31 Gonzalez García, "Una comida de gala," 52–55.

32 Consider, for example, the following arguments put forward by San Juan's municipal council: "Owing to the many debts which exist between neighbors

and residents on this island, and the dismal payments made by their creditors, the people who have stores of cassava and meat which they use to feed the slaves and others who extract gold from the mines are loathe to give them out on credit . . . we beseech . . . that all such stores of cassava, meat, and corn to be allotted and sold on credit, be the debts which are paid before any others." See "El cabildo de la ciudad de San Juan a la Emperatriz Doña Isabel: Expone la situación difícil que las tormentas y la compraventa a plazos ha creado en la isla," 18 April 1533, in Murga Sanz, *Historia documental*, 1:22.

33 Ibid.

34 In Europe, between the fourteenth and sixteenth century, the number of days on which the faithful were to abstain from eating meat has been calculated by Montanari as ranging from a low of 40 to a high of 160. Montanari, *The Culture of Food*, 78–81.

35 "El consejo de la Ciudad de San Juan entrega una instrucción de treinta y siete puntos o problemas que Juan de Castellanos, procurador, ha de presenter al Rey," 6 July 1534, in Murga Sanz, *Historia documental*, 1:131. At times [the council] even implies that the Inquisition would use the consumption of meat during Easter as a pretext to accuse someone with whom it is in conflict over some other matter. See the 1536 case involving the excommunication of Dr. Velázquez, who was made the object of an auto-da-fé, because "he had eaten meat during Lent, [despite] being, as he is, a hidalgo." Ibid., 307.

36 "Relación de la jornada de Pedro Menéndez Valdés escrita en forma de diario por el capellán del general Francisco López de Mendoza," in Murga Sanza, *Puerto Rico*, 402.

37 Ibid. Wild cattle used as a source of meat were also found in Hispaniola. It was reported, around 1560, that wild dogs killed 60,000 head of cattle in the mountains. See Hakluyt, *The Principal Navegations*, 7:29–30; and Super, *Food, Conquest*, 26–29.

38 "Relación de viaje a Puerto Rico de la expedición de Sir George Clifford, escrita por el Reverendo John Layfield," 147–48.

39 Some historians have made too much of this letter as providing evidence of the island's material impoverishment, including its lack of supplies of meat, in the mid-seventeenth century. They failed to note that the bishop's observations about food conditions in the colony came in the wake of a hurricane that had battered the island in 1642. In addition, being the dignitary he was, López de Haro was undoubtedly accustomed to having meat on his table regularly; hence his comment that "[finding] meat in the butcher shops every day is not a certainty," but—such uncertainties notwithstanding—he also noted that he had eaten "two or three lamb stews." Reproduced in Fernández Méndez, *Crónicas*, 164. It was common, after a hurricane struck, to hear references to the short supply of meat. López Cantos included some of these in his *Historia de Puerto Rico*, 61–65.

40 "Acusaciones contra," 132.

41 López de Cantos, *Historia de Puerto Rico*, 62. Consider, for example, an order

issued in 1662 by the island's governor, Pérez de Guzmán: "In view of the great need that existed for cattle and pigs, caused by owners of herds disposing of them as barter for clothing and other things, I issued an order that removing them was not to be allowed within this jurisdiction."

42 Ibid., 63.

43 Among other works, see Morales Carrión, *Puerto Rico*, 59 and passim; Brau, *Puerto Rico y su historia*, 117–20; Coll y Toste, "Memoria sobre la propiedad territorial," 239–310; Vila Vilar, *Historia*, 40–46; López Cantos, *Historia de Puerto Rico*, 61–65; Moscoso, *Lucha agraria*, 150–55; Picó, *Historia general*, 58–71 and 92–94; Scarano, *Puerto Rico: Cinco siglos*, 201–5 and 242–66; Quintero Rivera, *Patricios y plebeyos*, above all the chapter entitled "Ponce, la capital alterna."

44 Morales Carrión, *Puerto Rico y la lucha*, 102.

45 In a 1775 report on land ownership, San Juan's municipal council observed: "In the breeding operations there is promotion of the raising of hogs that are fattened in the wild on the fruits of the forest. The hunts are sent out so that those who have a right to them recover this released livestock at not too great a distance, entering these same breeding grounds to move them out with dogs. Since these animals live off the fruits that come down from a great many trees, the land is not considered to be valueless or unused; although they do not put it to agricultural use, those possessing it exploit it for the purposes indicated, and even dedicate it to fund chaplaincies." In the same report, arguing for the value that the herds of cattle have for hauling out wood, the councilors noted that a particular kind of palm tree grew on the land, from which people could make "cuttings of palm, to cover houses in the campo, replacing at no risk and at little cost tile coverings; from these palms they [also] make ropes, containers, and wrappings in which to enclose and carry all the fruit, including such as gets exported; this palm tree also yields fruits in bunches, which is sustenance for the hogs." See "Informe del cabildo de San Juan," 262 and passim.

46 Ibid.

47 López Tuero, *Plátano*.

48 O'Reilly, "Relación circumstanciada, 239–69.

49 Abad y Lasierra, "Diario de viaje," entry for 29 August 1772, corresponding to his stay in Maunabo.

50 Ibid., entry for 17 November 1772, corresponding to Abad y Lasierra's stay in Arecibo.

51 Ibid., entry for 30 September 1772, corresponding to his stay in San Germán.

52 Ibid., from the chapter entitled "Carácter de los habitantes de Puerto Rico." The above-cited passage was rewritten by Abad y Lasierra in his *Historia geográfica, civil y natural*, with the intention of distinguishing between city dwellers, or those who lived on the outskirts of towns and cities, and the rural population, in terms of their respective opportunities for consuming meat. Abad y Lasierra writes in the *Historia*: "Those who live close in to settled communities are accustomed to having fresh beef, from cows killed twice per week. Those

who live far out only get it when they go on hunts; then they eat it gluttonously and they all like the meat not to be well cooked; pig meat especially they like served dripping blood." Abad y Lasierra, it is important to note, makes qualitative distinctions (beef is eaten in the city, pork in the campo), but he does not deny the possibility that meat was available. His assessments about beef typically appearing in the butcher shops only twice a week, and campesinos being able to eat meat only when they went out to hunt pigs, smack more of the disappointment of one accustomed to consuming meat on a daily basis than an outright denial that such food was available to the island's inhabitants. Abad y Lasierra, *Historia*, 186.

53 ACSJBPR, minutes of 16 August 1757, 161–65.

54 Ibid., 163.

55 Ibid., 164.

56 García Colón, "El mercado de tierras," 23–38. See also Moscoso's *Lucha agraria*, which brings out the conflicts between those who owned great herds of cattle and ranchers who operated on a smaller scale concerning areas where cattle could pasture. Also see Scarano, *Puerto Rico*, 242–66.

57 Archivo General de Indias, Audiencia Territorial, Santo Domingo, "Informe del deslindador Julián Díaz de Saravia al gobernador Juan Dabán sobre el desmonte de hatos," 1787, in Centro de Investigaciones Históricas, Universidad de Puerto Rico, microfilm.

58 Caro Costa, *El cabildo*, 2:36–37.

59 Ibid., 38.

60 Ibid., 87.

61 For example, the 1626 ordinances stipulate that "meat from cows and pigs slaughtered in the city be weighed in its butcher shops, it cannot be sold anywhere else and it should be sold by *arreldes* [a unit of measurement for weighing meat] and half-arreldes and each arrelde should be 4 pounds, at 16 ounces [to the pound] . . . with the same requirements in place for cow and pig tripe . . . and salted beef . . . be sold by arrobas and arreldes and that it be dry and lean and well aged." See Real Díaz, *Catálogo de cartas y peticiones*, 280.

62 Ibid., 288–90.

63 Ibid.

64 The opposition of cattle ranchers to the demarcation of boundaries by the state has been interpreted as a class struggle arising from socioeconomic factors, one in which the reorganization of agricultural resources was aimed at dispossessing people of their means of production. This line of interpretation, however, obscures a basic condition of eighteenth-century Puerto Rico: that, more than the means of production, wilderness areas were the means by which the population acquired and consumed food. For more on this phenomenon as class conflict and as a struggle to control the means of production, see Moscoso, *Lucha agraria*, 150–55; and Scarano, *Puerto Rico*, 302–4.

65 In 1767, the cabildo of San Juan had adopted a resolution directed at informing the island's governor of the damage wreaked on cattle by wild dogs. Such was

the cabildo's concern over the situation that it proposed to the *Tenientes a Guerra* (a class of military officers) that they deploy the vecinos in their jurisdiction "to kill the ravaging dogs and to this end each vecino should contribute four heads [dogs' heads, that is] each month that will be delivered to the teniente a guerra of his respective administrative area or [he will have to pay] one silver real for each head he fails to deliver; and, by the same token, the wild dogs on the cattle ranches and in the breeding grounds should be killed, as should any that might be on ranches themselves; furthermore, the owners of said ranches are not allowed more than one dog to guard their houses, the dog is to be tied up by day and released at night." ACSJBPR, 1761–1767, minutes of 31 August 1765, 105–6. Clearly, this resolution—whether it was enforced or not—is evidence of the care that was now to be taken in watching over cattle, pigs, and other domestic animals. San Juan's city fathers were concerned not just with the monteros and runaway slaves but with the packs of wild dogs as well.

66 Torres, *La isla*, 190–94. Torres got this figure from Hostos, and he faults the latter for not citing his source.

67 The figure is obtained via the calculated estimate that each head of cattle yielded 400 pounds of meat. See López Tuero, *Estudios*, 72. It is useful to note that this calculation is in line with the 1764 reparto figure, cited earlier, of 2,400 head of cattle. In addition, it highlights the imbalance in the consumption of meat in San Juan between the civilian population, on the one hand, and the military population, on the other. See Caro Costa, *El cabildo*, 1:87.

68 Cited in Morales Carrión, *Puerto Rico*, 145.

69 López Medrano, "Disertación de la filgtegna gangrenosa de Puerto Rico."

70 Ibid., 44.

71 See Picó, "Deshumanización del trabajo," 187–206; Abad, *Puerto Rico en la Feria*, 102–24 and 288; López Tuero, *La reforma*, 24–25; *Circular sobre que toda cabeza de Ganado*; and Ayuntamiento de San Juan, *Reglamento para la carnicería*. Between 1765 and 1899, the island's population reached the following levels: 1765, 44,883; 1800, 155,426; 1815, 220,892; 1832, 330,051; 1860, 583,308; 1877, 731,648; 1887, 798,565; and 1899, 953,243. See United States Bureau of the Census, *Sixteenth Census*.

72 Cited in Asenjo, *Recuerdos y añoranzas*, 100–101. The moniker *madamas cangrejeras* used by Asenjo refers to women, descended from slaves, who lived in Boca de Cangrejos, an oppressively hot and humid coastal district belonging to the municipality of Carolina, located some six miles from the capital.

73 Méndez Quiñones, "El cuento del matrimonio," 21–37. The poem (whose wit and humor unfortunately get partly lost in translation, because they depend on the rhyming scheme of the original) was published in 1883.

74 Méndez Quiñones, "La triquina," 303–37.

75 AGPR, "Sumaria averiguación . . . Don José Martínez."

76 Harris, *Good to Eat*, especially the chapter entitled "The Abominable Pig," 82–110.

77 The relevant ordinances are cited in Arana Soto, *La sanidad*, 211, 236.

78 Brau, "La campesina," in his Ensayos, 109 and passim. Manuel Zeno takes up the same line of thought in his novel La charca, in the episode in which Juan del Salto, a youthful coffee plantation owner, invites the local curate to lunch with him. "At that moment they let them know that lunch was served. Chatting on, the two friends repaired to the dining room, where, with the meal having been laid out, the steaming dishes had a mouthwatering appeal, and still Father Esteban went on philosophizing . . .—Look here, Father—Juan interrupted, uncovering a dish and spotting a huge piece of meat: here is one of the remedies that this poor sick one needs . . . [the rural peasant]." Zeno Gandía, La charca, 60.

79 Valle Atiles, Cartilla, 64.

80 López Tuero, La reforma, 133.

81 Torres Alba, "Testamentos en Lares," 66–108.

82 Hernández, Adjuntas, 32.

83 López Tuero, La reforma, 133.

84 The pioneering cookbook El cocinero puertorriqueño indicates that, according to how it is treated, meat can remain unspoiled for the following periods: in the summer, beef that is fresh, three days; fried, eight days; and salted, six months. During the same time of year, fresh pork, four days; fried pork, thirty days; and salted pork, six months. See El cocinero, 72.

85 Cabanillas, El puertorriqueño, 433–35.

86 Moreno Fraginals, El ingenio, 3:57–58.

87 Picó, "Deshumanización del trabajo," 188; and his Libertad y servidumbre, 78 and 102.

88 Dávila Cox, Este inmenso comercio, 110. Around 1897, only three countries—Uruguay, Argentina, and the United States—competed in this market. By this time, out of the total of 1,782,861 pounds of dried beef imported into Puerto Rico, Argentina supplied the lion's share, 1,213,753 pounds, or 68 percent. Uruguay, which exported 505,005 pounds, claimed 28 percent of the market, with the United States—at this stage—being no more than a bit player. See CIHBM, 1897.

89 Archivo Histórico Nacional de Madrid, Ultramar, Serie de Fomento, "Impuesto de consumo sobre artículos de comer, beber y arder," legajos 344 and 345, 1893–94, 1894–95; from a microfilm copy in the University of Puerto Rico's Centro de Investigaciones Históricas. A fragmentary part of the record is also reproduced in Cabanillas, El puertorriqueño, 310–11.

90 Reglamento para la carnicería y matadero, 24.

91 "Orden general n° 101, libertad de matanza y venta de carnes," 18 July 1899, in Coll y Toste, Boletín, 6:135.

92 Ferguson, Home Making, 165.

93 In addition to Francisco del Valle Atiles, Fernando López Tuero also sounded this theme, from the ethical point of view, in his essay "La nutrición." For López Tuero, "the nutritive need, or simply nutrition, was one of man's ideals, that is, one of the ends toward which his imagination and the positive satisfac-

tion of this need constantly propel him." He further added that "diet, which, as we see, has so much influence on the physical nature of animals, also has a considerable influence on the moral nature of man; so that every action of human life that springs from our sensibility or reason is a direct function of diet." See López Tuero, El hombre, 28–30.

94 Ashford, Progreso reciente; Del Valle Sarraga, Ideas modernas; and Torres Díaz, "A Preliminary Study."

95 "It was in hotel kitchens, in small pueblos, or in the kitchens of families kind enough to bid me welcome that I learned the art of preparing Puerto Rican dishes." Ferguson, Home Making, 1–2.

96 Ferguson, La organización. Grace Ferguson, who came to Puerto Rico in 1913 with the mission of organizing courses in home economics, remained on the island until 1919, five years after she had edited the manual Home Making and Home Keeping. In 1938, she was invited by the University of Puerto Rico to an event commemorating the founding of its formal program in home economics, recalling, as part of the occasion, that "the home economics students taught women to prepare dishes using substitutes for meat and wheat and to cultivate gardens using the school courtyard." See Archivo Central de la Universidad de Puerto Rico, Fondo de Organizaciones y sus Funciones, Escuela de Economía Doméstica, Recopilación Especial n° 73, caja 25; and Puerto Rico Food Commission, Informe, 3–7; Department of Education, Report of the Commisioner, 518–19.

97 The dishes in which meat was the central ingredient were: (1) stewed liver with potatoes, olives, and capers, white rice, and a banana; (2) beef stew and potatoes, lettuce salad, white rice, and cocoa; (3) meatballs, boiled potatoes, raw cabbage salad, boiled sweet potato, and cocoa; (4) beef hash and baked ground plantain, banana; (5) beef hash with yams, tannier, tender beans, and plantains, and a Valencia orange; (6) stew of pig innards (chopped into little pieces) with chopped potatoes, boiled or baked plantain, fruit salad. See, Department of Education, Manual del comedor, 7–8.

98 See Government of Puerto Rico, Department of Agriculture and Commerce, Annual Book, 14. For example, in 1935, 7,799,462 pounds of canned meats were imported onto the island. See also De Hostos, "The External Trade of Puerto," 22.

99 Descartes et al., Food consumption, 57.

100 U.S. Bureau of the Census, Fifteenth Census, 225.

101 Roberts and Stefani, Patterns of Living, 193.

102 Ibid.

103 Ibid.

104 Ibid.

105 Ibid., 365.

106 Ibid., 196.

107 Indeed, as Jean Jacques Hermandinquer reminds us, in times of scarcity, pigs competed with people for food. Hermandinquer, "The Family Pig," 54.

108 Wolf, "San José: Subcultures," 211.
109 Hitchcock, *Trade*, 45. Government of Puerto Rico, Department of Agriculture and Commerce, Division of Commerce, *Annual Book on Statistics*, Fiscal Year 1934–35, 14.
110 Díaz Pacheco, "La distribución," 3–44.
111 Government of Puerto Rico, Department of Agriculture and Commerce, Division of Commerce, *Annual Book on Statistics*, Fiscal Year 1934–35, 14.
112 Loriana Aponte Rivera, "A Study of the School Lunch," 57. See also Departamento de Instrucción Pública, *Comedores escolares*.
113 Mintz, "Cañamelar," 400.
114 Departamento de Agricultura, Oficina de Estadísticas, *Consumo de carnes en Puerto Rico, 1975–2010*, Folder 1158c9.
115 Ibid., Folder 1159c10.
116 Descartes et al., *Food Consumption*, 54.
117 Fischler, *El (h)omnívoro*, 103.
118 Valle Atiles, *Cartilla*, 63–65.
119 The price of beef and pork continued to go up between the final years of the Great Depression (1937–38) and the mid-1950s. True, the price of inferior cuts (meat used in soup) remained more or less stable, but the cost of better cuts (for example, "round steak," and "stewing meat") increased by nearly forty-eight cents a pound during this period. The same was true for the price of pork, which, by 1953, reached 51 cents a pound. Since 1955, however, the rate of increase in the price of meat has moderated considerably. For example, on 19 September and 2 October 2002, round steak was selling at $1.55 per pound in the supermarket Pitusa, whereas in 1955 it cost 68 cents per pound. The increase is modest in comparison to current price rises. Similarly, the leanest cut of pork sold for 59 cents per pound in 2002, an increase of only 8 cents from its price in 1955. See Descartes et al., *Food Consumption*, 54, and Junta de Planificación, Negociado de Economía y Estadísticas, *Anuario estadístico*, 1955, "Precios al por menor de alimentos seleccionados," 180. See also Pitusa supermarket's sale notice covering the two-week period of 19 September to 2 October 2002.
120 Peggy Ann Bliss, "Eating Animals Kills Warm Fuzzy Feelings," in *Portfolio: The San Juan Star*, 3 September 3001, 35. The radio program *Alternativa natural*, produced by the ideologue of all things natural, Norman González Chacón, and broadcast on Sunday mornings by the station WKAQ to a large audience, is the best example of the diffusion of this new ethic.
121 As exemplified, again, in the thinking of Norman González Chacón, who argues that the excessive intake of meat-based proteins in the current Puerto Rican diet—the *bisté*, as he calls it—is unnecessary, since the common Puerto Rican diet already includes a good many foods, such as beans, which contain them. He also correctly points out that after people reach a certain age, their metabolic system no longer requires such proteins for building and maintaining muscle and body tissue. González Chacón attributes many of the meta-

bolic disorders and diseases that currently afflict people, such as diabetes, cellulitis, and kidney failure, to this excess of meat-based proteins in the body. He makes no attempt, however, to explain the meanings that still attach to the consumption of meat in cultural terms, meanings that—as we have seen—trace back to its virtual disappearance, during a long period of the island's history, from the diet of all but the wealthiest and most advantaged Puerto Ricans. Nor does his argument account for either the organoleptic elements that influence the high consumption of meat or such extra-human factors as the ability of agroindustry to exploit the taste for meat by building in value-added measures that make the product even more attractive (e.g., offering more cuts at modest prices, convenient packaging, and a wide range of canned meats). *Alternativa Natural*, WKAQ, 13 January 2002.

122 The final years of the twentieth century have seen a notable increase in the consumption of turkey: from 0.93 pounds per capita annually in 1975, to 1.85 pounds in 1985, 4.6 pounds in 1995, and 5.31 pounds in 2000. This trend has been aided by several factors, including a greater interest by many people in monitoring, if discreetly, their own nutrition, a huge expansion of the import business, and the price advantage enjoyed by turkey relative to other types of meat. With respect to the latter-most point, an entire turkey, weighing sixteen or more pounds, was selling at seventy-five cents a pound in September 2002. See Departamento de Agricultura, Oficina de Estadísticas Agrícolas, *Consumo de alimentos, consumo de carne de aves, pavo fresco y/o congelado*, 1975–2003, folder 1160c10; and "Hoja de rebajas del hipermercado Pitusa," 19 September to 2 October 2002. On the other hand, the annual per capita consumption of fresh and/or frozen chickens—just chickens, no other poultry—was calculated at 96.8 pounds in 2003, whereas in 1950 the annual per capita consumption of poultry (including turkeys, guinea fowl, chickens, and ducks) was a mere 5.1 pounds. By 1977, total poultry consumption had risen to 53.13 pounds per capita annually. See Departamento de Agricultura, Oficina de Estadísticas Agrícolas, *Consumo de alimentos, carne de aves, pollo fresco y/o congelado*, 1975–2003, folder 1160c9; Miguel Díaz Román, "Favorecida la industria de pollo local," El Nuevo Día, 7 February 2004, and C. M. Ortiz Cuadra, "Pollo picú y quién eres tú," *Diálogo*, September 2002.

CHAPTER 7

1 See Junta de Planificación de Puerto Rico, Negociado de Análisis Económico y Social, *Anuario estadístico*, 1965; and, from the same source, *External Trade, Shipments of Merchandise from the United States Into Puerto Rico*, Fiscal Year 1999 and 2001. To place these figures in historical context, in 1949, out of a sample of 1,044 Puerto Rican families, only 0.9 percent had electric stoves.

2 Although the supermercado and hipermercado are viewed by Puerto Ricans as essentially one and the same, in reality there is a considerable difference between them. Above all, the supermarket is characterized by its sale of food

products at retail cost. Some supermarkets will also have cafeterias, bakeries, and a section of items and meals readymade for heating up and cooking. In contrast, the hipermercado sells food at wholesale in addition to functioning as an ordinary market. It also sells such nonperishable items as clothing, hardware, and home electrical appliances. The tendency to use the two terms interchangeably goes back to the mid-1950s when, financed by U.S. capital and spurred by the island's "modernizing" project, large retail grocery stores began to crop up, with the English-language term "supermarket" mechanically translated into the Spanish supermercado to describe them. See "Más allá de la comida: Los supermercados amplían su variedad de productos y servicios," El Nuevo Día, Suplemento Negocios, 1 November 1998. For the statistics from 1956, see "Auge del supermercado moderno," El Mundo, 27 September 1958, 24. See Ortíz Cuadra, "La 'buena vida,'" 16–30.

3 For the 1960 figures, see Nieves Falcon, Diagnóstico, 256; and for those from 2007, see Colón Reyes, Sobrevivencia, 268–69.

4 "Casi un 40% de la población está bajo el nivel de pobreza en Puerto Rico," Primera Hora, 9 September, 2011, http:www.primerahora.com/casiun40dela poblacionestabajoelniveldepobrezaenpuertorico-550065.html.

5 Ileana Delgado, "Ofensiva contra la obesidad," El Nuevo Día, 8 November 2011.

6 Josean Ramos, "Por el suelo la cultura del agro," Diálogo: Periódico de la Universidad de Puerto Rico, 14, no. 136 (February 2001): 6–7. Looked at from another angle, the agricultural sector in Puerto Rico contributed 24.3 percent of the island's net income in 1950. By the beginning of the 1990s, its share had fallen to less than 1 percent.

7 Departamento de Agricultura de Puerto Rico, Oficina de Estadísticas Agrícolas, Resumen total del consumo de alimentos por grupos alimenticios, 2008.

8 Mennell, All Manners of Food, 317–44.

9 Fischler, El (h)omnívoro, 204 and passim.

10 Montanari, The Culture of Food, 170.

11 Ibid., 171.

12 Ibid., 170.

13 Ibid.

14 Urry, The Tourist Gaze.

15 Ibid., 13–14.

16 Ritzer, La Mcdonalización, 15.

17 Ibid., 129–33.

18 Ibid., 127

19 Ibid., 59–61.

20 Ibid., 111.

21 Ibid., 165.

22 Cook and Crang, "The World," 131–53. It is important to note that Cook and Crang think that "ignorant understandings" (or "ignorances," as they call them)—such as the conditions under which a strange type of food is pro-

duced—are also appropriated. All in all, they believe that in the long run new types of food are turned into fetishes.

23 García Canclini, *Consumidores y ciudadanos*, 16.

24 Pelto and Pelto, "Diet and Delocalization," 507–23.

25 Warde, *Consumption*, 37–38.

26 The geographers David Bell and Gill Valentine develop the idea that the term "community" can be understood today as carrying three meanings: that of locality, with defined lines of social and spatial separation, like those of a neighborhood; that of a network of interrelationships without such spatiality and physical proximity, as in the case of ethnic communities; and that of qualities or particularized kinds of interrelationships, such as exist within a community whose members are bound together by a spirit of reaffirmation (gay, lesbian, vegetarian, and so on). The passage above refers to the first type of community, although the latter two are also observable in the realm of food and culinary practices. Take, for example, the "network" type of community, where Spaniards, Dominicans, Cubans, and Asians—all part of immigrant communities—use their own specialized cuisine as a way of reaffirming their common identity, despite having lost physical proximity to their countries and regions of origin; or vegetarians and vegans, who exemplify the third type of community. Bell and Valentine, *Consuming Geographies*, 94.

27 Appadurai, "How to Make a National Cuisine," 18.

28 Ibid., 5–10.

29 Ibid.

30 The sociologist Ulrich Beck reasons that in contemporary societies, the individualization of human beings leads to their experiencing the sensation of "de-traditionalization." All the same, he contemplates that this experience engenders a countertrend, which he classifies as the "invention of hybrid traditions," for which reason he believes that "it is hardly surprising that various idylls—grandma's apple cake, forget-me-nots, and communitarianism—are experiencing a boom." See Beck, "Living Your Own Life," 165.

31 Hobsbawm, "Introduction: Inventing Traditions," 1–14. Hobsbawm's thesis may be seen to have an element of determinism, in the sense that it possesses an "automatic nature," which for him is part and parcel of the "invention of tradition" with respect to the past. One would have to consider and distinguish the possible differences that the meaning of the past could have in the imagination of those participating in "that" tradition once it is "invented" in the present. Hence at times it is possible to understand these inventions as re-inventions.

32 Bourdieu, *Distinction*, 177. To a critic like Gustavo Tellez Iregui, habitual practice is "the system of dispositions," or—according to the author himself, "attitudes or inclinations for perceiving, feeling, acting, and thinking that are internalized by individuals, beginning with the objective conditions of their existence; acquired, permanent, transferable, allowing [one] to act, perceive,

feel, and think in a particular way. These dispositions are incorporated by social agents as they live their lives, beginning with the prolonged, multi-form business of learning and education . . . the 'habitus' is an 'operator of unconscious calculation' (underscored in the original) that allows us to orient ourselves in a social space with the need for reflection." Iregui, *Pierre Bourdieu*, 205 and 209–10. I am grateful to Carlos Rojas Osorio for bringing this reference to my attention.

33 Bourdieu, *Distinction*, 172.

34 Ibid., 176.

35 Ibid., 185.

36 Levenstein, *Paradox of Plenty*, especially the chapter entitled "The Golden Age of Food Processing," 101–18; and by the same author, "The Perils of Abundance," 518–29. See also Mennell, *The Sociology of Food*, in particular the chapter entitled "Food Technology and Its Impact," 68–74.

37 See Mennell's comments in his *The Sociology of Food*, 11–12.

38 Warde, *Consumption*, 41.

39 The idea of fondas and of restaurancitos criollos is taken from the definitions outlined by Rodríguez Juliá in his *Elogio de la fonda*. For him, the local or native food that is eaten "outside the home" is found in three specific locations: the fonda, which is a modest restaurant characterized by a strong preference for the flavors of home-style cooking, where the food, in both its preparation and presentation, has nothing about it of the impersonal. Above all, the fonda is known for stewing rather than frying its food, although items which are fried can be part of its menu. The second is the *friquitín*, where the opposite is true—all of the dishes are fried. The third location is the "unpretentious small restaurant serving local cuisine." Here the service is personal, but the kitchen and other staff are not necessarily all from the same family or related in some way to each other. This restaurant might be known for a special dish or style of cooking, but in the way it prepares its food and in the character of its meals, there is no sense or feeling that distinctions of social class are being upheld.

40 Warde and Martens, *Eating Out*, 17.

41 Ibid., 14.

42 Warde, *Consumption*, 172.

43 The company most esteemed for its selection of fine foods imported from the United States and Europe was Cerecedo y Cía, which had been founded in San Juan in 1875. As far back as the first years of the twentieth century, it was known and prized among the few "gourmands" in San Juan for its canned foie gras and truffles, along with its exclusive stock of Galician wine from the Avia Valley region. Cerecedo was flanked by the Sobrinos de Luiña company, founded one year later and located on Fortaleza Street in the capital. This company specialized in olives, vinegar, dried sweetmeats, crystallized fruits, and tinned food. See Blanch, *Directorio comercial*. For a reference to the importation of the Galician wine from the Avia Valley, see "The Ladies Aid Society of the First Methodist Church," *The Porto Rican Cook Book*, 1909, in the advertisements

section; and for a reference to the foie gras and truffles purchased in Cerecedo, see Belaval, "Presentación del puertorriqueño," 127.

44 Conditions permitting, the establishment promised "stuffed roast turkeys, and what can truly be called truffles, [or] choose hams served in wine according to your wishes, meat pies of different kinds, especially cold truffle pies, from Príncipe, Bulevar, Persier, filled with French veal." The daily menu offered beefsteak, chateaubriand, and *filet mignon a la rusa*. See *La correspondencia de Puerto Rico*, 8 November 1877; cited by José Luis Díaz de Villegas, who in turn took the information from the "Colección de Teodoro Vidal," in *El Nuevo Día*, Suplemento En Grande, 16 February 1997.

45 Revel, *Un festín*, 207–8.

46 These restaurants, with their respective menus, are listed in Picot, *Gourmet International*.

47 Revel, *Un festín*, 207–8.

48 I use the word "renewal" because the possibility of attaining professional status as a cook or as a worker in some other branch of hostelry also existed in the 1950s with the founding of the Escuela Hotelera. The possibilities that exist today, however, are much greater.

49 Fischler, *El (h)omnívoro*, 219 and 229–30. The large number, frequency, and wide distribution of articles about food and dining that now appear in newspapers, magazines, and other media is a fairly recent phenomemon. This makes perfect sense, since for a long time the average home lacked the resources to lavish attention on dining, and even less could most people afford to cultivate their palate by eating out, although—as we have seen—there were some high-end restaurants, as well as gourmands who could appreciate them. Not surprisingly, columns devoted to matters of food and dining that ran in the periodical press varied in form, content, and the frequency with which they appeared. Although I have only consulted a small number from the early 1900s, it is clear that, as of the mid-1950s, they began to resemble the serialized articles we have today—with their own designated space, fixed schedule of publication, pointed discussion of methods and techniques for cooking, their author's personalized comments on novel ways of preparing dishes, recipes, and food products from around the globe, and—though typically upbeat and uncritical—reviews of local restaurants. Early on in the press, the theme of food and cooking was subsumed under the more general subject of the home, the latter being considered of paramount importance. Furthermore, these columns were generally written by home economists. One of the most long-lasting, launched in the weekly newspaper *Puerto Rico Ilustrado* in January 1939, appeared under the heading "Home Page." The column treated such matters as the rules of common courtesy, how to keep a home clean and tidy, personal hygiene, and home decorating, with a recipe for a meal as a kind of add-on. Beginning in 1946, the column was published under the title "The Cooking Page," so the slant had changed somewhat. See the issues of *Puerto Rico Ilustrado* for January 1939 and December 1946, respectively. The col-

umn "Home Page," which ran in the newspaper El Día and appeared under the byline of Isabel Suárez, was rather different. It is not known exactly when it first appeared or how long it lasted, but on the basis of my reading of four numbers from 1942, it seems that this column—in contrast to that in *Puerto Rico Ilustrado*—focused on cooking rather than on other activities of the home. It included recipes for such gourmet items as avocadoes filled with foie gras, supplemented by menus for meals to serve to close friends. These combined the novel (stuffed beets) with the familiar (rice and chicken); other offerings were eggs in béchamel sauce with roast leg of pork and green plantains and banana fricassee. Súarez, however, simply printed the recipes absent any comments or opinions on her part. See El Día, 11, 18, and 25 April, and 30 May 1942. In this same year, El Día launched a column called "Día del plato criollo," part of a strategy of the administration of Governor Rexford Tugwell to discourage the use of the imported products favored by the well-to-do, in anticipation of the food rationing programs instituted during the Second World War. Direct, simple, and anonymous, the column offered a menu that covered the three meals of the day, each consisting of three servings. Its recipes, calling for the use of products grown on the island, could easily form the heart of a restaurant set up today that aspires to serve authentic local cuisine without the fripperies and showiness of *nouvelle criollo*. See El Día, 16 and 30 April, 1942. A culinary literature that liberated itself from domestic themes began to flourish in the mid-1950s, as restaurants with chefs from abroad, who offered an international cuisine, began to appear under the sponsorship of the Compañía de Fomento de Puerto Rico (the government's development agency). Henceforth, the newspaper El Mundo began to cover the culinary arts in a serious way, with articles that dealt with professional chefs and incorporated the commentary of food critics who visited the island; the bylines belonged to Nory Segarra, Helen Tooker, and Arnaldo Meyners, all three of whom got away from the prescriptive tone of the earlier columns and celebrated the virtues of both foreign cuisines and the positive qualities of local cooking. Segarra, for example, in a column devoted to the then chef of the Caribe Hilton, the Frenchman Henri Souller, featured a recipe for boned chicken stuffed with truffles, accompanied by a desert of local pineapple sprinkled with champagne. See Nory Segarra, "Chef de cocina recomienda preparer mejor comida Boricua," El Mundo, 5 January 1952. Both Meyners and Tooker devoted columns to the visit paid to the island by the food critic for the *New York Herald*, Clementine Paddleford, who stayed in the Caribe Hilton during the spring of 1952. See Arnaldo Meyners, "Clementine Paddleford interesa conocer secretos de la cocina criolla," El Mundo, 7 March 1952; Helen Tooker, "Cocina criolla: La experta del *Herald Tribune* busca recetas en Puerto Rico," El Mundo, 13 March 1952. At present, the four main Puerto Rican newspapers include supplements, every Wednesday, devoted to cooking and dining or related themes. In addition, José Luis Díaz de Villegas (Paco Villón), by far the most widely read food authority in Puerto Rico, contributes to a supplement, *Domingo*, which accompanies the Sunday edition of the paper *El Nuevo Día*. Locally focused weekly newspapers, like *El Oriental* or *La Semana*, published in the municipalities of Humacao and Caguas, respectively, also feature columns on gastronomy.

50 "Los tenedores del milenio," *El Nuevo Día*, Suplemento Domingo, 12 December 1999. "Veinte años del Certamen del Buen Comer," *El Nuevo Día*, Suplemento Domingo, 9 December 2001.

51 "Alrededor del fogón: El 'Gran Cocinamiento' del Bankers Club," *El Nuevo Día*, Suplemento Por Dentro, 2 May 2001.

52 Thus, in an attempt to open up access to the most expensive restaurants, the food critic José Luis Díaz de Villegas (Paco Villón), offered a scheme that would enable one to dine economically in the exclusive San Juan restaurants Compostela and Augusto's, both of which received awards in the 2001 competition. His recommendation was that the diner focus on ordering appetizers or starters, consume only one glass of house wine, and not eat dessert. Even with this strategy, the least expensive meal for one person, in Compostela, would come to $37.30 ($30.00 without a gratuity). The recommended menu included: soup of the day, $6.45; grilled vegetables and goat cheese, $10.95; beans with squid and leeks, $13.95; and a glass of house wine, $5.95. By comparison, $37.50 was the amount that a consumer would pay (at the bottom end) in 1998 to purchase a basket of twenty-five items in a hipermercado. See Paco Villón, "Coma bien y gaste poco," *El Nuevo Día*, Suplemento Domingo, 9 December 2001. On shopping in hipermercados, see "Caro el placer de comer," *El Nuevo Día*, 15 February 1998.

53 See "Chefs de Puerto Rico en Anguila," *El Nuevo Día*, Suplemento Por Dentro, 22 July 2001. This Caribbean island was the site for the creation of the CuisinArt Resort and Spa, a hotel that combines what has come to be called "spa food" with sophisticated gastronomy classes for its guests. Its own grounds include hydroponic greenhouses where the vegetables, fruit, and herbs used in the preparation of its meals are grown. Chefs of international renown are invited to the hotel, to prepare meals and special fare for tasting.

54 Quintero Rivera, "De la fiesta al festival," 97–107.

55 Ibid. *Tablas de contabilización de festivales*, mimeograph, 1988. I am grateful to Quintero Rivera for providing me with a copy of his tabulations.

56 "Loíza en el Hilton," *El Nuevo Día*, Suplemento En Grande, 29 October 1995; and "Competencia de Comida Criolla," *El Nuevo Día*, Suplemento Por Dentro, 18 September 2002.

57 Warde, *Consumption*, 38.

58 For different theories about consumption as it applies specifically to food, see ibid., 7–21.

59 "Cocinan el mofongo más grande del mundo," *El Nuevo Día*, 23 July 2001; "Arropa a Villalba un asopao de gandules," *El Nuevo Día*, 16 December 2001; and "Sabroso superpastel," *Primera Hora*, 7 January 2002.

60 "Cocinan el mofongo más grande del mundo," *El Nuevo Día*, 23 July 2001. Other "invented" elements were also integral to this activity—for example, the *super*

pilón made out of mahogany, which was used for crushing 3,500 plantains. The artisan Neftalí Maldonado was put in charge of this part of the work.

61 Rodríguez Juliá, *Elogio*.

62 Huyke, *La cocina*, 10.

63 Bell and Valentine, *Consuming Geographies*, 19.

64 To feel that one is part of a community is, Alan Warde thinks, a widely held aspiration in modern societies, "in part because modernity is perceived to destroy the natural rootedness and uncomplicated sense of belonging which village life in traditional societies engendered." Warde points out that the concept of community is very difficult to define and has various ramifications. But he thinks that even when certain social groups and institutions lament its disappearance, and believe that community life has led to a better life, the reality is not so obvious. Nor is it so clear "that 'communion,' or the sense of community, necessarily or exclusively derives from dense face to face interaction in limited geographical areas." All the same, he concludes: "The ideal of intense community life continues to inspire individuals, groups, neighbourhoods, and state policy makers. Attempts are constantly being made to restore, re-create, or invent communities." Warde, *Consumption*, 183.

65 Per announcements in 1997 by José Nieves, McDonald's marketing director in Puerto Rico, as appearing in "El reino de las comidas rápidas," *El Nuevo Día*, Suplemento Negocios, 8 June 1997, 5.

66 The campaign was accompanied by the image of a serving of food composed of rice and beans, mofongo, and fried pork, garnished by slices of avocado and fresh coriander leaves. In addition, the plate sits on top of a plantain leaf with a pilón and the ingredients for making sofrito around it—both are emblematic of cookery understood as traditional. See the advertisement, which takes up a full half page, in *El Nuevo Día*, 18 April 2001, 59.

67 Fischler, *El (h)omnívoro*, 189.

68 Consider the following statistics. In 2010, the available supply of meat from poultry, including that produced on the island, was approximately 352 million pounds for a population of 3.9 million; or, in gross terms, 94.6 pounds per person annually. This figure stands in stark contrast to that of 1937, when there were two pounds of poultry meat available per person, for a population on the island of approximately 1.7 million persons. In 2010, the island tallied a supply of pork and beef of approximately 384.7 million pounds, or some 98.6 pounds of the two types of meat, combined, per person annually. In that same year, the amount of beef available actually came to 45.8 pounds per person, and of pork, 53.8 pounds per person whereas in 1937 the corresponding figures were 15 and 6 pounds, respectively. In the case of rice, including short, medium, long, and whole-grain, the available supply around 2010 reached 361.7 million pounds, or, in round terms, 92.7 pounds per person annually. In 1937, the amount of rice available—including both imported and locally produced supplies—was 259.5 million pounds, or the equivalent of 143.1 pounds per person annually. The small increase in the overall amount of rice available in contemporary

Puerto Rico, as compared to the totals in earlier periods, would seem to negate the claim that the island had entered an era of abundance. In fact, however, it corroborates a defining trend among more prosperous countries insofar as food is concerned: namely, that their populations rely much less on food that had been basic to the diet during times of scarcity, as was always the case with rice. Moreover, a statistical comparison between Puerto Rico and some of its Caribbean neighbors confirms the claim of abundance in the former. Around the fiscal year 2009, for example, the supply of poultry per person came to 79.6 pounds in Venezuela, 43.5 pounds in Cuba, and 72.8 pounds in the Dominican Republic, and 107.3 in Jamaica (surpassing Puerto Rico). In that same year, the supply of beef and pork per person in the Dominican Republic was 23.1 and 22.08 pounds, respectively; in Cuba, the comparable figures were 14.5 and 47.9 pounds. Venezuela, on the other hand, recorded a figure similar to that of Puerto Rico for the average amount of beef consumed (53.6 pounds), but not for pork (only 16.7 pounds). In the case of rice, with the notable and understandable exception of Cuba (139.4 pounds), the amount available per person in 2010 in Puerto Rico exceeded that in Venezuela (70.6 pounds) and Jamaica (51.4 pounds), but was surpassed in the Dominican Republic (117.4 pounds). Finally, on an annual basis (as in 1999–2001), the United States supplies 53.8 million pounds of prepared foods (meat, fish, poultry, shellfish, mollusks, etc.), or approximately 14.8 pounds per person, to Puerto Rico, along with 127.4 million pounds of potatoes (33.54 pounds per person) and 20.9 million pounds of "snacks" (5.5 pounds per person). See Departamento de Agricultura, Oficina de Estadísticas Agrícolas, August 2010. See also Junta de Planificación, *External Trade, Shipments of Merchandise from the United States into Puerto Rico*, Fiscal Year 1999 and 2001. For the 1937 figures, see Descartes et al., *Food Consumption*; and Hill and Noguera, *The Food Supply*. Finally, see Food and Agriculture Organization, *Food Balance Sheet*, 2009, at <http://faostat.fao.org/site/368/DesktopDefault.aspx?PageID=368#ancor>.

69 It follows in the train of Fischler's idea of the "dietetic," in the classic sense of "a lifestyle," a "food regimen," a "rational approach toward diet." Fischler himself follows Michel Foucault's idea, emerging from the latter's work on classical medicine, of "diet" as the "practice of health," "an organizing principle of life," "that which governs daily existence,"—part of what permits one to "take control of one's own conduct." In the case of Puerto Rico, this association—at least up to 1948, which saw the publication of the *Puerto Rican Cookbook* by the North American Eliza Dooley—is found in recipes and in peoples' posture and actions vis-à-vis food. An attempt at separating the two took place as early as the mid-nineteenth century, with the publication of the landmark El *cocinero puertorriqueño*, in which a growing gastronomic sensibility can be detected in both the language used in the introduction to the cookbook and in the frequent hedonistic references, made at the end of recipes, to the pleasurable taste they will impart. Similarly, there was a sign, among certain social elements, that greater attention was being paid to the sensory aspects of

food and diet. All the same, *El cocinero puertorriqueño* begins by proffering dishes for people who are ill, and those groups whose position in society allowed them to experience haute cuisine and a food keyed to pleasing the senses did so only occasionally, in circumstances tied, by and large, to private festivities or official public banquets held to honor or commemorate a person or event. The delay in effecting a separation between cooking conceived as an activity designed for pleasure and a narrower outlook on cooking as dietetics was in all likelihood also aided by the limited range of food consumed during the period of the simplification of the diet, combined with the teaching and practice of home economics over the first half of the twentieth century, with its preachy emphasis on balanced nutrition and parallel stress on a form of cooking stripped of the pleasurable and abounding with the morally and nutritionally uplifting. The best examples of this orientation, in the case of nineteenth-century Puerto Rico, are the chapter devoted to food and diet in Francisco del Valle Atiles's *Cartilla de Higiene* and López Tuero's essay, "La nutrición," in his book *El hombre* (San Juan: Imprenta del Boletín Mercantil, 1897). On the use of the term "dietetic" in the sense in which Foucault's employs it, see Fischler, *El (h)omnívoro*, 222. For an interpretation of home economics as the cause of a certain circumspection about food, see Shapiro, *Perfection Salad*, 5–7. The view of the home economist as a woman who developed a "palate without any real life" is shared by the clinical psychologist Catherine Manton, and advanced in her book *Fed Up*, 55–57.

70 Carla Méndez Martí, "Carbohidratos o grasa: Nutrición en la balanza," *El Nuevo Día*, Suplemento Domingo, 22 September 2002, 10–13. See also Sandra Rodríguez Cotto, "Una bomba de tiempo la malnutrición," *El Nuevo Día*, 27 January 2003.

71 The text of the law is found in http://www.lexjuris.com/lexlex/leyes2003/lex12003083.htm.

72 Marian Díaz, "Alza de 8% en el índice de precios al consumidor," *El Nuevo Día*, 2 September 2002. See also Departamento del Trabajo y Recursos Humanos, *Importancia relativa*, 2002.

73 "Más allá de la comida: Los supermercados amplían su variedad de productos y servicios," *El Nuevo Día*, Suplemento Negocios, 1 November 1998.

74 In the previously cited newspaper article, supermarkets are described as having been turned into "minimalls." In Puerto Rico, "BBQ" is the abbreviated form of the American word "barbecue(d)." Cordero Badillo was actually referring to roast chicken.

75 Ibid.

76 "Góndolas vacías: Un gran dolor de cabeza," *El Nuevo Día*, 15 August 2001.

77 As cited by Bell and Valentine, *Consuming Geographies*, 134.

78 Gaither International, in "El reino de las comidas rápidas," *El Nuevo Día*, Suplemento Negocios, 8 June 1997. The data were collected between April 1996 and April 1997.

79 Berríos Figueroa, "McDonald's remozará imagen y atmósfera de restaurantes,"

El *Star*, 17 October 2003. Among Latin American and Caribbean countries of greater physical size, as of July 2002, Mexico was the only one with a roughly equal number of Burger King outlets (164) as Puerto Rico. The Dominican Republic had 28, and McDonald's had only 51 outlets spread over all the islands of the Caribbean as of 2003. See "Burger King Historical Facts Sheet." By 2010, Burger King, McDonald's, and Wendy's had between them 330 Puerto Rican outlets, with Burger King leading (176), followed by McDonald's (112) and Wendy's (40). See Marian Díaz, "Burger King se une a Total," *El Nuevo Día*, 12 August 2010.

80 From the Gaither International study, see note 74.

81 Ibid.

82 Ibid.

83 See in particular Fischler, *El (h)omnívoro*, 213–15; and also his essay "The McDonaldization of Culture," 530–47.

84 See Departamento del Trabajo y Recursos Humanos de Puerto Rico, http://www.net-empleopr.org/almis23sec_empleos.jsp. More recent figures indicate that unemployment has spiked upward, to 16.1 per cent, according to government data and to 20.7 per cent, according to non-government sources. In the first instance, see Departamento del Trabajo y Recursos Humanos de Puerto Rico, "Departamento del Trabajo anuncia estadísticas de empleo y desempleo para el mes de enero 2012," http://www.dtrh.gobierno.pr/det_news.asp?cnt_id=364; and in the second, Ricardo Cortés Chico, "Cifras que no cuadran: Discrepan el gobierno local y el Censo en torno al desempleo," *El Nuevo Día*, 28 September 2012.

85 From the Gaither International study, see note 74.

86 The data are cited by Sandra Rodríguez Cotto in her report, "Acelera el mercado de comidas rápidas," contained in "El reino de las comidas rápidas," *El Nuevo Día*, Suplemento Negocios, 13 January 2002. Rodríguez Cotto notes that the sample group was spread throughout the entire island. In 2000, it was estimated that Puerto Ricans took their meals outside the home thrice per week, or 144 times per year, with a good many of these meals obviously eaten in fast food restaurants or diners. See Martín Díaz Román, "Terror en la industria de alimentos por fast-foods," *El Nuevo Día*, 2 November 2000. Research carried out in 2003 confirmed this pattern, with its estimate that on average Puerto Ricans visited a fast food establishment two or three times per week. See Gaither Marketing and Opinion Research, *Changing Trends in Fast-Food Marketing in Puerto Rico between 1998 and 2003*, 10.

87 Schlosser, *Fast-Food Nation*, 1–28.

88 On the first "Tastee Freeze," see *El Mundo*, 11 February 1959.

89 The Burger King chain was founded in 1954 by the team of James W. McLamore and David Edgerton. In 1957, it introduced its signature hamburger, the "whopper." It is interesting to note, and worthwhile pointing out, that the first two Burger King outlets established outside the United States, in 1963, were located in Puerto Rico. See "Historical Fact Sheet," www.burgerking.com.

90 Héctor Berríos Figueroa, "McDonald's remozará imagen y atmósfera de restaurantes," El Star, 17 October 2003.

91 Schlosser, Fast-Food Nation, 43.

92 In his book Kids as Customers: A Handbook on Marketing to Children (New York: Lexington Books, 1992), James U. McNeal classifies the strategies that children use, when appealing to their parents to buy them something, into seven major categories: "A pleading nag is one accompanied by repetitions of words like 'please,' or 'mom, mom, mom.' A persistent nag involves constant requests for the coveted product and may include the phrase 'I'm gonna ask just one more time.' Forceful nags are extremely pushy and may include subtle threats like 'well, then, I'll go and ask Dad.' Demonstrative nags are the most high risk, often characterized by full-blown tantrums in public places, breath-holding, tears, a refusal to leave the store. Sugar-coated nags promise affection in return for a purchase and may rely on seemingly heartfelt declarations, like 'You're the best dad in the world.' Threatening nags are youthful forms of blackmail, vows of eternal hatred and of running away if something isn't bought. Pity nags claim the child will be heartbroken, teased, or socially stunted if the parent refuses to buy a certain item." Taken from Schlosser, Fast-Food Nation, 42–44.

93 See "TV Strikes Gold as Advertisers Tour Products on P.R. Tube," The San Juan Star, 16 October 1996.

94 Lama Bonilla, "Fast foods invierten millones en publicidad," El Nuevo Día, 5 March 2001. In 2003, their investment in advertising had increased to $30 million. See Gaither Marketing and Opinion Research, Changing Trends in Fast-Food Marketing in Puerto Rico between 1998 and 2003, 14.

95 See "Wendy's invertirá 5 millones en 2002," El Nuevo Día, 30 July 2001. Between 1999 and 2001, the Wendy's chain opened sixteen new outlets in Puerto Rico, giving it a total of forty, spread across the island, by 2002. In terms of annual sales, Burger King topped the market for fast food meals in 2007 ($180 million), followed by McDonald's ($130 million). See Gaither International, Market Barometer, Fast Foods Restaurants, March 2007, 4. In 2010, Burger King expended a combined $6 million on new advertising strategies and opening indoor outlets in gas stations. See Marian Díaz, "Burger King se une a Total," El Nuevo Día, 12 August 2010.

96 Sandra Rodríguez Cotto, "Popular el gusto por comer fuera," in "El reino de las comidas rápidas," El Nuevo Día, Suplemento Negocios, 13 January 2002.

97 Sandra Rodríguez Cotto, "Una bomba de tiempo la malnutrición," El Nuevo Día, 27 January 2003. Medical science considers as obese those individuals whose Body Mass Index (BMI) exceeds thirty. The BMI is a function of weight in relation to height, and—using the metric system—is calculated by dividing weight by height squared (kg/m2). See www.obesity-online.com; Schlosser, Fast-Food Nation, 240.

98 Sandra Rodríguez Cotto, "Una bomba de tiempo la malnutrición," El Nuevo Día, 27 January 2003.

99 According to Schlosser, McDonald's added large French fries to its menu in 1972. Twenty years later, it added the super large French fries, which were three times greater in volume than the original serving. See his *Fast-Food Nation*, 241. Around 2001, the competition among hamburger franchises became so intense that they began to offer hamburgers for only 99 cents. Advertising specialists and the managers of fast food outlets alike stressed that the offers represented an attempt to provide the consumer with a less costly alternative, one that made a real difference to his wallet. As Juan José Jiménez, Burger King's senior vice president for marketing for the Caribbean area, noted in 2001, the special offers "are there to give the consumer an alternative, since various sectors are going through difficult economic times." Jiménez's rationale disguised the real purpose behind these offers—they were meant to serve as "traffic builders," a way of attracting more customers, boosting sales volumes, while maintaining a healthy profit margin. See Lama Bonilla, "Fast foods invierten millones en publicidad," *El Nuevo Día*, 5 March 2001.

100 Sandra Rodríguez Cotto, "Opción real para los Boricuas la educación nutricional," *El Nuevo Día*, 27 January 2003. To give one example, in July 2003, the organization Fast Food Nutrition Explorer estimated that the combination of a regular "Whopper," a small order of French fries, and a small Coke—probably the most popular combination on the Burger King menu—contained 1,100 calories, which represented 55 percent of the recommended daily intake of a diet based on 2,000 calories. In addition, 44 percent of the calories came from fat, almost all of which—80 percent—was saturated fat. The basic McDonald's combination (a regular hamburger, not a "Big Mac," plus a small order of French fries and a small Coke) consumed by a youngster contained 600 calories, 30 percent of which came from fat, a substantial portion of which—28 percent—was saturated fat. One Big Mac (weighing 216 grams) had 590 calories, 53 percent of which were fat calories, with 55 percent of the latter consisting of saturated fat. This total excluded any French fries. A small serving of five pieces of Burger King's "Chicken Tenders" (76 grams) contained 210 calories, 52 percent of which came from fat, and 18 percent from saturated fat. The maximum intake of saturated fat recommended by the American Heart Association and the U.S. Department of Agriculture, which is the standard used in Puerto Rico, puts the upper limit at 30 percent of a person's total caloric intake. For the fat, calorie, and other values of many other fast foods, see http://www.factcalorie.com. On top of the figures already given, the practice followed by hamburger outlets of adding bacon to hamburgers and sandwiches, and by pizzerias of offering extra amounts of cheese and increasing the size of pizzas, also needs to be considered.

101 Sandra Rodríguez Cotto, "Opción real para los boricuas la educación nutricional," *El Nuevo Día*, 27 January 2003.

102 Gaither International, "Perfil del consumidor que come fuera," in Sandra Rodríguez Cotto, "Popular el gusto por comer fuera," *El Nuevo Día*, Suplemento Negocios, 13 January 2002.

103 "Complicaciones de la diabetes," El Nuevo Día, 26 March 2003. See also Schlosser, Fast-Food Nation, 240.

104 Mimi Ortiz, "¿Qué como rápido y saludable?," El Nuevo Día Suplemento Por Dentro, 30 April 2001. See also "Comiendo fuera," Primera Hora, 11 June 2001; and "Fast Foods," El Nuevo Día, Suplemento Domingo, 18 July 1999.

105 See Melba Brugueras, "Como en casa con Giovanna," in the edition of the popular television guide, TV al día, covering the week of 10–16 January 1999. With her characteristic honesty, the corpulent Giovanna Huyke admitted that she had needed to thin down by seventy-five pounds during a nine-month period. Her motivation to do so was a comment by her daughter Valerie, who had stated that she wanted "to eat a lot because she wanted to be really fat like me." She confessed during the interview that her daughter's comment made her frantic.

106 Beck, "Living Your Own Life," 167–68.

107 Christine Ridout, "Ingestión compulsive: El drama diario de la glotonería," El Vocero, 18 February 1998.

108 "Lo que cuesta ser gordo," in Sandra Rodríguez Cotto, "Opción real para los boricuas la educación nutricional," El Nuevo Día, 27 January 2003. Rodríguez Cotto uses the figures compiled by economist Gus Amato, who estimates that in 2002 the outlays related to treatments against obesity (diets, clothing, medication and laboratory tests, payments to physicians, gym memberships, and exercise equipment) came to $312 million, a figure, moreover, that has been growing at an annual rate of 8.8 percent since 1990.

109 Sandra Rodríguez Cotto, "Alto riesgo en el uso de la efedrina," El Nuevo Día, 23 February 2003.

110 But not ignored in Spain, for example. In Barcelona, the Food Studies Group at the University of Barcelona has made solid progress in this regard. See García Arnáiz, "Los trastornos," 350–77.

111 Emily Nelson, "La comida empaquetada avanza más," The Wall Street Journal Americas, reproduced in El Nuevo Día, 21 July 2002.

112 "Ascienden a trescientos mil los diabéticos," El Nuevo Día, 11 October 2002.

113 Carla Méndez Martí, "Carbohidratos o grasa: Nutrición en la balanza," El Nuevo Día, Suplemento Domingo, 22 September 2002, 10–13. For the 2010 data, see Estado Libre Asociado de Puerto Rico, Departamento de Agricultura, Oficina de Estadísticas Agrícolas, Consumo de arroz en Puerto Rico, 1975–2010, Folder 1759b1.

114 See Warde, "Production, Consumption," 185–200.

115 Warde, Consumption, 7.

116 Fernando Zalacaín, "Tendencias en la economía," El Nuevo Día, Suplemento Negocios, 13 January 2002. Zalacaín, an economist, observed that the labor market was very depressed and that total employment had suffered a loss of 20,000 jobs during the preceding twelve months (2001–2002). He estimated that during this same time period 31,000 people had become unemployed. He also noted that in this one year alone the working age population had in-

creased by 30,000 people, without the labor market being able to absorb them. As of July 2003, a total of approximately 173,000 people, or some 13 percent of the active workforce, were unemployed in Puerto Rico. See Junta de Planificación de Puerto Rico, Programa de Planificación Económica y Social, *Informe*, 11 to 15 September 2003.

117 "Guayama rompe record," *El Nuevo Día*, 15 February 1998.

118 See, Departamento del Trabajo y Recursos Humanos, *Índice de precios al consumidor*, August 2002, 2. See also Marian Díaz, "Alza de 8% en el Índice de precios al consumidor," *El Nuevo Día*, 2 September 2002.

119 Marian Díaz Román, "Lo que te cuesta tu compra," *El Nuevo Día*, 18 September 2010.

120 Méndez Martí, "Carbohidratos o grasa: Nutrición en la balanza," *El Nuevo Día*, Suplemento Domingo, 22 September 2002, 10–13. According to the University of Puerto Rico's School of Public Health nutritionist Michael González, "We need to eat less red meat and more fish and white meat, less sugar and more complex carbohydrates like fruit and vegetables."

121 Departamento del Trabajo y Recursos Humanos, *Índice de precios al consumidor*, August 2002, 2.

122 Hipermercado owners tend to play down the importance of data generated from the Consumer Price Index, arguing that the basket of basic food products has changed from what it used to be. While on the face of it this claim is true, it is also true, and quite obvious to anyone paying the slightest attention, that the basket of basic goods is increasingly composed of inexpensive products, above all of food that comes in cans and has a high sugar and flour content, which pumps up a person's energy level and leaves him feeling full. It is via this avenue that the majority of Puerto Ricans appear to have confronted and dealt with prices increases and job insecurity.

123 "Caro el placer de comer," *El Nuevo Día*, 15 February 1998.

124 The demographer Judith Rodríguez estimates that, at present, out of 1,261,325 homes, 589,409 have children under the age of eighteen (46 percent) See "Por las nubes la crianza de un hijo," *El Nuevo Día*, 24 March 2002.

125 "Estiran el dólar en la compra para el mes," *El Nuevo Día*, 3 May 2001.

126 Colón Reyes, *Sobrevivencia*, 109 and 269.

127 "Insisten en que la fórmula 75/25 del PAN perjudica al pequeño comerciante," *El Nuevo Día*, 15 May 2001.

128 Some food critics and writers think that a dissonance is created between the image and the reality of high-end food, as advertised in stories accompanied by glossy photo spreads, versus how the food actually appears when served in these fashionable restaurants themselves. The gap between image and reality causes diners and those cooking at home to experience a continual sense of dissatisfaction and disappointment. The revolution in gastronomic photography is a twentieth-century invention, capable of stirring up fetishistic visions—grounded in falsehood—that go beyond our capacities for smelling, tasting, and feeling, and for reproducing meals in our kitchens. These

observers insist that food, while never before having looked so attractive and appealing, has at the same time never been so inaccessible. See Molly O'Neill, "Delicias para la vista," El Nuevo Día, Suplemento Por Dentro, 3 October 1999.

129 Ángel Ortiz, the chef and owner of La Fonda de Ángelo—an "unpretentious criollo restaurant"—in fact started out as a chef's assistant in the well-known restaurants Swiss Chalet and Top of the First. See Mariel Echegaray, "Una fonda diferente: Placer criollo en cada plato," El Nuevo Día, Suplemento Por Dentro, 28 August 2002.

130 For Gofton and Ness's concrete definition according to Warde's citation of it, see note 80 in chapter 2.

131 Bell and Valentine, Consuming Geographies, 60.

132 Tatiana Pérez Rivera, "Son más las amas de casa," El Nuevo Día, 8 March 2003. Vidal Rodríguez's study, which remains unpublished, is entitled "La mujer en Puerto Rico: Retos, demandas y perspectivas ante un nuevo milenio." Pérez Rivera notes that Vidal Rodríguez uses statistical data from the Departamento del Trabajo, the Procuradía de la Mujer, la Oficina de Planificación y Desarrollo de la Universidad de Puerto Rico, and the portion of the U.S. Census that applies to Puerto Rico.

133 Ibid.

134 That women still carry the burden of fulfilling the traditional core of domestic tasks is something Vidal Rodríguez recognizes in writing that "Although they [women, housewives, or female workers] dedicate themselves to the children, it is good that they pursue other things, stay current in their profession, and share in other ways with their partner." And she concludes: "Change has to start with us and [also has to come] from the [underlying] structures. This is the moment for action."

135 Warde, Consumption, 127. The figure for the number of women in the workforce comes from Zuleika Vidal Rodríguez, as quoted in Tatiana Pérez Rivera, "Son más las amas de casa," El Nuevo Día, 8 March 2003.

136 "Caro el placer de comer," El Nuevo Día, 15 February 1998.

137 "Inundadas de carros las carreteras," El Nuevo Día, Suplemento Negocios, 20 October 2002.

138 "Supermercados vs pantries," El Nuevo Día, 13 September 1999.

139 Ibid.

140 "Se convierten en minimalls los supermercados," El Nuevo Día, 13 September 1999.

141 "Desenfocadas las tiendas con las necesidades de los clientes," El Nuevo Día, 15 August 2001. The respondents considered the variety of products and brands to be most important, followed by the availability of good specials.

142 Warde, Consumption, 129.

143 Francisco Rodríguez Burns, "Comida chatarra fuera de las escuelas," Primera Hora, 29 January 2004; and Camile Roldán Soto, "A mejorar la nutrición en las escuelas," El Nuevo Día, 28 January 2004. It warrants mentioning that there are 1,543 public schools in Puerto Rico with dining halls, where some 300,000

breakfasts and lunches are served daily. There are 649,000 students enrolled in the public school system.

144 In 1999, a commercial with a strong emotional appeal made its appearance on television. The commercial, created to advertise the semi-prepared food products of the company Casera Foods, and playing on the word "casera," had as its central theme, or message "Casera es la unión familiar" (Family togetherness is Casera) The message was delivered around a story in which a middle-class mother had to decide whether to give her children fast food or home-style food after picking them up at school. She opts for the second, and viewers are then treated to a scene that has everyone in the family, at home, happily eating dishes that are typical of the mother's cooking. The commercial also had as a referent the tension which exists in the moment when a decision must be made between the gastronomy and food practices of convenience or those of care.

145 Bell and Valentine, Consuming Geographies, 64.

146 Ibid. In making this point, Bell and Valentine draw on an example from C. Dorfman, "The Garden of Eating: The Carnal Kitchen in Contemporary American Culture," Feminist Issues 12 (1992): 21–38.

147 "Giovanna Huyke, "Cuando vamos a comer en familia," El Nuevo Día, 16 July 1997.

CHAPTER 8

1 Torres Díaz, "A Preliminary Study," 2.

2 Flandrin and Hayman, "Regional Tastes and Cuisines," 221–51.

3 Referenced in González, "La ilusión del paraíso," 281.

4 Fischler, El (h)omnívoro, 197.

5 Díaz de Villegas, Puerto Rico, 40, 96, and 219.

6 The 2000 census puts the estimated number of "legal" Dominicans living in Puerto Rico at 56,146. The number of Cubans was given as 19,793.

7 "Celebrate Christmas All Year with 'Pastelitos del Fogón,'" The San Juan Star, Food and Beverage Supplement, 30 May 1997. Indeed, food industry managers marketed their pastelito by appealing to one of the most traditional culinary operations—and one that enjoyed great favor among those sitting down to eat plantain pasteles—namely, using firewood to soften the leaves in which the pastel was wrapped. See the article "Goya Remains a Fixture of Puerto Rican Homecooking," ibid., 31 July 1997.

8 Eileen Rivera Esquilín, "Redescubre nuestros tesoros: Aprende a confeccionar platos tradicionales de la cocina puertorriqueña," El Nuevo Día, 12 September 2012.

9 Fischler, El (h)omnívoro, 213.

Bibliography

ARCHIVES

Caguas, Puerto Rico
  Archivo Histórico del Municipio de Caguas
San Juan, Puerto Rico
  Archivo Central de la Universidad de Puerto Rico
    Fondo de Organizaciones y sus Funciones, Facultad de Pedagogía,
      Escuela de Economía Doméstica, Recopilación n° 73
    Informales Anuales, Departamento de Economía Doméstica, 1930–1935.
      Archivo General de Puerto Rico
  Archivo Histórico del Arzobispado de San Juan
    Fondo Carmelitano, Serie de Cuenta y Data de las Monjas Carmelitas,
      1861, 1862, 1863
  Universidad de Puerto Rico
    Centro de Investigaciones Históricas de la Universidad de Puerto Rico
  Archivo General de Puerto Rico
    Fondo de Beneficencia, Series del Hospital Municipal, 1864–1930
    Balanzas Mercantiles, 1845–1895
    Fondo de los Gobernadores Españoles de Puerto Rico, Asuntos Políticos o
      Civiles, Libro de Contratos de Libertos, 1873–1874

OFFICIAL DOCUMENTS

Puerto Rico
Ayuntamiento de San Juan. *Reglamento para la carnicería y matadero de esta ciudad.*
  San Juan: Imprenta del Boletín Mercantil, 1894.
Commonwealth of Puerto Rico. Department of Agriculture. Office of Agricultural
  Statistics. *Facts and Figures on Agriculture in Puerto Rico,* 1996. San Juan: Department
  of Agriculture, 1996.
Departamento de Agricultura de Puerto Rico, Oficina de Estadísticas Agrícolas.
  Consumo de alimentos en Puerto Rico, productos pecuarios, 1950/51–1973/74, 1977.
  ———. *Consumo de grasas y aceites, pescado y marisco, sopas y especias,* 1978.
  ———. *Consumo de alimentos en Puerto Rico, Cosechas,* 1979/80–1986/87, 1988.
  ———. *Consumo de alimentos en Puerto Rico, Arroz,* 1975–2003.

———. *Consumo de aves, 1975–2003.*

———. *Consumo de res, 1975–2003.*

———. *Consumo de cerdo, 1975–2003.*

———. *Farináceos, 1975–2003.*

———. *Legumbres, 1975–2003.*

———. *Maíz y sus derivados, 1975–2003.*

Departamento del Interior de Puerto Rico. Oficina de Agricultura y Minas. *Cultivo de arroz en los Estados Unidos.* San Juan: Imprenta del Boletín Mercantil, 1902.

———. Negociado de Agricultura y Minas. *Cultivos de maíz en el sur.* San Juan: Imprenta del Boletín Mercantil, 1903.

Departamento del Trabajo y Recursos Humanos de Puerto Rico. *A Report on Wages and Working Hours in Various Industries and on the Cost of Living in the Island of Puerto Rico.* San Juan: Bureau of Supplies, Printing and Transportation, Bulletin no. 5, 1944.

———. *Índice de Precios al Consumidor.* 1988, 2002.

Estado Libre Asociado de Puerto Rico. Junta de Planificación. Negociado de Economía y Estadísticas. *Anuario Estadístico,* 1955.

Government of Puerto Rico. *Importancia relativa de los artículos y servicios de consumo en el Índice de Precios al Consumidor para todas las familias de Puerto Rico.* June, 2002.

———. Department of Agriculture and Commerce, *Annual Book on Statistics,* 1934–1935.

———. *Annual Book on Statistics,* 1946.

———. Department of Education. *Manual del Comedor Escolar.* San Juan: Negociado de Imprenta, Materiales y Transporte, 1929.

———. *Report of the Comissioner of Education for Porto Rico.* Washington, D.C.: Government Printing Office, San Juan, P.R., 1918. [issued as part of the annual report of the governor of Puerto Rico].

Junta de Planificación, Negociado de Economía y Estadísticas. *Anuario Estadístico, Estadísticas Históricas, Puerto Rico,* 1959.

———. *Anuario Estadístico,* 1955, 1965.

———. *Imports into Puerto Rico from the United States,* Fiscal Year 2000, 2001.

———. *External Trade Statistics. Imports of Merchandise into Puerto Rico from Foreign Countries by Commodity and Country of Origin,* Fiscal Years 1999, 2000, 2001.

———. Oficina de Estadísticas. *External Trade Statistics, Shipments of Merchandise into Puerto Rico from the United States by Commodity,* Fiscal Year 1999, 2001.

———. Programa de Planificación de Puerto Rico, *Programa de Planificación Económica y Social. Informe,* 11–15 September 2003.

Municipio de San Juan. *Actas del Cabildo de San Juan Bautista de Puerto Rico,* 18 vols.

———. *Reglamento para el matadero y carnicería de esta ciudad.* San Juan: Imprenta del Boletín Mercantil, 1894.

Puerto Rico Food Commission. *Informe.* San Juan: Bureau of Supplies, Printing and Transportation, 1918.

United Nations

Food and Agricultural Organization. *Food Balance Sheet*, 1999, at http://faostat.fao
   .org.
———. *Rice and Rice Diets: A Nutritional Survey*. Rev. ed. Rome: Stabilimento
   Tipográfico Fausto Failli, 1954.

United States

U.S. Bureau of the Census. *Census of Agriculture, Puerto Rico, 1998*. Washington,
   D.C.: Government Printing Office, 1999.
———. *Fifteenth Census, Outlying Territories and Possessions*. Washington, D.C.:
   Government Printing Office, 1930.
———. *Sixteenth Census of the United States*. San Juan, 1943.
U.S. Department of Agriculture. *Sixteenth Annual Report of the Bureau of Animal
   Industry for the Year 1900*. Washington, D.C.: Government Printing Office, 1900.
United States Government. *Annual Report of the Governor of Puerto Rico*. Washington,
   D.C.: Government Printing Office, 1930.
War Food Administration. *Report of Operations of the Caribbean Emergency Program,
   July 1942–December 1943*. Washington, D.C.: War Food Administration, Office
   of Distribution, 1944.

NEWSPAPERS, NEWS WEEKLIES, AND MAGAZINES

Diario Económico de Puerto Rico
E: The Environmental Magazine
El Día
El Mundo (San Juan)
El Nuevo Día
El Star

El Vocero
Puerto Rico Ilustrado
Primera Hora (San Juan)
Noticiero Teleonce
The San Juan Star

COOKING MANUALS AND COOKBOOKS

Busó de Casas, Carmen. *777 aventuras de cocina*. Río Piedras: Editorial Cultural,
   1978.
Cabanillas de Rodríguez, Berta, Carmen Ginorio, and Carmen Quirós de
   Mercado. *Cocine a gusto*. Barcelona: Ediciones Rumbos, 1950.
de la Mata, Juan. *Arte de repostería*. Facsimile ed. Burgos: Editorial La Olmeda, 1992.
Cocina desde mi pueblo: Tres años de cocina puertorriqueña. [San Juan: Concepto
   Creativo], 1998.
Dooley, Eliza Bellows King. *Puerto Rican Cookbook*. Richmond, Va.: Dietz Press,
   1948.
El cocinero de los enfermos, convalecientes y desganados. Havana: Imprenta y Librería
   La Cubana, 1862.

El cocinero puertorriqueño o formulario para preparar toda clase de alimentos, dulces y pasteles conforme a los preceptos de la química y la higiene y las circunstancias especiales del clima y de las costumbres puertorriqueñas. 3rd ed. San Juan: Imprenta de Acosta.

Ferguson, Grace J. *Home Making and Home Keeping: A Textbook for the First Two Years' Work on Home Economics in the Public Schools of Porto Rico.* San Juan: Department of Education, 1915.

Hernández, Zenny. *Sabores de ayer en la cocina de hoy.* n.p.: n.p., 1999.

Huyke, Giovanna. *La cocina puertorriqueña de hoy.* Río Piedras: Esmaco Printers, 1993.

Kennedy, Diana. *Las cocinas de México.* New York: Harper and Row, 1982.

Lugo Lugo, Herminio. *Las recetas de ayer de Puerto Rico son el gourmet de hoy: Cuentos y recetas.* San Juan: Agencia de Publicaciones de Puerto Rico, 2001.

Mejía Prieto, Jorge. *Gastronomía de las fronteras.* Mexico City: Consejo Nacional para la Cultura y las Artes, 1990.

Nola, Ruperto de. *Libro de cocina.* Facsimile of 1525 ed. Madrid: Taurus, 1982.

Ortiz, Yvonne. *A Taste of Puerto Rico: Traditional and New Dishes from the Puerto Rican Community.* New York: Penguin Books, 1994.

Porter, Virginia E. *The Canned Food Cookbook.* New York: Doubleday, 1939.

Quintero, Elizabeth N., and Marie L. Tolosa. *Recuerdos y recetas de Borinquen.* San Juan: E.N. Quintero and M.L. Tolosa, 1996.

Román de Zurek, Teresita, Amparo Román de Vélez, and Olga Román Vélez. *Cartagena de Indias en la olla.* Bogotá: Ediciones Gamma, 1988.

Romano, Dora R. *Cocine conmigo.* San Juan: Editorial Edil, 1981.

Sororidad Mu Jota Alpha. *Delicias del paladar mayauezano.* 3rd ed. n.p.: Mornes Press, 1996.

The Ladies of the First Methodist Church of Puerto Rico. *Porto Rican Cook Book.* San Juan: Imprenta de M. Burillo, n.d.

Valldejuli, Carmen Aboy. *Cocina criolla.* Santurce: Valldejulí, 1977.

Vergés, Virginia, and Iván Soto, eds. *Cocina desde mi pueblo: Compilación de recetas de cocina del programa Desde mi pueblo.* San Juan: Editorial Concepto Creativo, 1998.

Willsey, Elsie Mae. *Tropical Foods: Arracacha, Bread Fruit, Cassava, Lerén, Malanga.* Río Piedras: Department of Home Economics, University of Puerto Rico, 1929.

Willsey, Elsie Mae, and Carmen Janer Vilá. *Vegetales tropicales: Yautía.* Publication/ University of Puerto Rico, College of Education, no. 11. Río Piedras: Department of Home Economics, University of Puerto Rico.

OTHER WORKS

Abad, José Ramón. *Puerto Rico en la Feria Exposición de Ponce en 1882.* Facsimile ed. San Juan: Editorial Coquí, 1967.

Abad y Lasierra, Iñigo. "Diario del viaje a la América." *Boletín de la Academia Puertorriqueña de la Historia* 5, no. 18 (1 July 1977): n.p.

———. *Historia geográfica, civil y natural de la isla de San Juan Bautista de Puerto Rico.* Río Piedras: Ediciones de la Universidad de Puerto Rico, 1956.

"Acusaciones contra el Gobernador Capitán General Don Gerónimo de Velasco durante su juicio de residencia [1670]." *Revista del Centro de Estudios Avanzados de Puerto Rico y el Caribe* 5 (July-December 1987): 129–39.

Aguinaldo puertorriqueño de 1843: Colección de producciones originales en prosa y verso. Puerto Rico: Imprenta Gimbernat y Dalmau, 1843.

Alegría, Ricardo. "Notas sobre la procedencia cultural de los esclavos negros de Puerto Rico durante la segunda mitad del siglo XVI." *Revista del Centro de Estudios Avanzados de Puerto Rico y el Caribe* (July-December 1985): 58–79.

Alfaro Santiago, Pablo. *De Barcelona a Coamo; Carta privada a los señores Don Ernesto Brusi, Don Venancio Abella, Don Domingo Santos y Don José Clotilde Aponte.* Puerto Rico: Tipografía de González, 1890.

"Alimentación adecuada para el Pueblo de Puerto Rico." *Noticias del Departamento del Trabajo* 3 (15 July 1943): 6–8.

Allston Pringle, Elizabeth. *A Woman Rice Planter.* 6th ed. New York: Macmillan, 1922.

Alonso, Manuel. *El jíbaro.* Facsimile ed. San Juan: Editorial Cultural, 1974.

Alpern, Stanley P. "Exotic Plants of Western Africa: Where They Came From and When." *History in Africa* 35 (2008): 63–102.

Álvarez Curbelo, Silvia, and Mary Frances Gallarty. *Los arcos de la memoria: El 98 y los pueblos puertorriqueños.* San Juan: Editorial Postdata; Mayagüez: Asociación Puertorriqueña de historiadores, 1998.

Álvarez Nazario, Manuel. *El elemento afronegroide en el español de Puerto Rico: Una contribución al estudio del negro en América.* San Juan: Instituto de Cultura Puertorriqueña, 1961.

———. "El vocabulario canario y sus resonancias en Puerto Rico; Vida material: Léxico de comidas, dulcería y bebidas." *Revista del Instituto de Cultura Puertorriqueña* 8, no. 27 (April-June 1965): 26–29.

Aponte Rivera, Luz Loriana. "A Study of the School Lunch and Nutrition Educational Program in the Schools of Puerto Rico." M.A. thesis, University of Texas at Austin, 1947.

Appadurai, Arjun. "How to Make a National Cuisine: Cookbooks in Contemporary India." *Comparative Studies in Society and History* 30 (1988): 3–24.

Arana Soto, Salvador. *La sanidad en Puerto Rico hasta 1898.* San Juan: Academia Puertorriqueña de Historia, 1978.

Ariès, Philippe, and Georges Duby, eds. *Historia de la vida privada.* 5 vols. Madrid: Editorial Taurus, 1988.

"Arropa a Villalba un asopao de gandules." *Primera Hora,* 7 January 2002.

Asenjo, Conrado F. "Composición química de los principales frutos de las antillas." *Revista de Agricultura de Puerto Rico* 43 (January-June 1952): 279–88.

———. *Recuerdos y añoranzas de mi viejo San Juan.* San Juan: Imprenta Venezuela, 1961.

———. "Tabla de composición de alimentos." *Revista de Agricultura de Puerto Rico* 43 (January-July 1952): 279–81.

Ashford, Bailey K. "Anemia in Puerto Rico." *Porto Rico Journal of Public Health and Tropical Medicine* 7 (1931–32).

———. "El tratamiento dietética del esprú." *Porto Rico Journal of Public Health and Tropical Medicine* 7 (1931–32).

———. *Progreso reciente en los problemas de la nutrición.* San Juan: Tipografía La Correspondencia, n.d.

Atkins, Peter, and Ian B. Bowler. *Food in Society: Economy, Culture, Geography.* London: Arnold Publishers, 2001.

"Auge del supermercado modern." *El Mundo*, 27 September 1958.

Ayala Rivera, Vladimir. "Elasticidad—precio de la demanda de arroz en Puerto Rico, 1980–1988." M.A. thesis, University of Puerto Rico, 1989.

Aymard, Maurice. "The History of Nutrition and Economic History." *The Journal of European Economic History* 2 (1973).

———. "Towards the History of Nutrition: Some Methodological Remarks." In *Food and Drink in History: Selections from the Annales*, edited by Robert Foster and Orest Ranum, 1–16. Baltimore: Johns Hopkins University Press, 1979.

Badillo, Jalil Sued. *El Dorado borincano: La economía de la conquista, 1510–1550.* San Juan: Ediciones Puerto, 2001.

Ballesteros Garbrois, Manuel. *La idea colonial de Juan Ponce de León.* San Juan: Instituto de Cultura Puertorriqueña, 1960.

Barthes, Roland. "Pour une psyco-sociologie de l'alimentation contemporaine." *Annales E.S.C.* 16 (1961).

Baralt, Guillermo. *La buena vista: Estancia de frutos menores, fábrica de harinas y hacienda cafetalera, 1833–1904.* San Juan: Fideicomiso de Conservación de Puerto Rico, 1988.

Barrios Román, Ángel de. *Antropología socio-económica en el Caribe: Puerto Rico-Mayagüez, 1840–1875.* [Santo Domingo]: Editorial Cultural, 1974.

Bascom, William. "Yoruba Cooking." *Africa* 21, no. 2 (April 1951): 124–25.

———. "Yoruba Food." *Africa* 21, no. 1 (January 1951): 41–53.

Beardsworth, Alan, and Teresa Keil. *Sociology on the Menu: An Invitation to the Study of Food and Society.* London: Routledge, 1997.

Beck, Ulrich. "Living Your Own Life in a Runaway World: Individualisation, Globalisation, and Politics." In *Global Capitalism*, edited by Will Hutton and Anthony Giddens, 164–74. New York: The New Press, 2000.

Belasco, Warren. "Food Matters: Perspectives on an Emerging Field." In *Food Nations: Selling Taste in Consumer Societies*, edited by Warren Belasco and Philippe Scranton, 2–23. New York: Routledge, 1974.

Belasco, Warren, and Philippe Scranton, eds. *Food Nations: Selling Taste in Consumer Societies.* New York: Routledge, 1974.

Beleval, Emilio. "Presentación del puertorriqueño José S. Alegría." *La Revista del Centro de Estudios Avanzados de Puerto Rico y el Caribe* (July-December 1986): 123–32.

Bell, David, and Gill Valentine. *Consuming Geographies: We Are Where We Eat.* London: Routledge, 1997.

Benevides Barajas, L. *Al-Andalus: La cocina y su historia.* Motril: Ediciones Dulcinea, 1992.

Biasin, Gian-Paolo, ed. *Flavors of Modernity: Food and the Novel*. Princeton: Princeton University Press, 1993.

Blanch, José. *Directorio Comercial e Industrial de la Isla de Puerto Rico para 1894.* Mayagüez: Tipografía El Vapor de la Correspondencia, 1894.

Blanco, Ana Teresa. *Nutrition Studies in Puerto Rico.* Río Piedras: Social Sciences Research Center, University of Puerto Rico, 1946.

Blanco y Fernández de Caleya, Paloma, et al. *Exploración botánica de las islas de Barlovento: Cuba y Puerto Rico, siglo XVIII; La obra de Martín de Sessé y José Estévez.* Theatrum naturae. Serie Textos clásicos. Aranjuez: Ediciones Doce Calles; Madrid: Consejo Superior de Investigaciones Científicas, 1998.

Bonafoux Quintero, Luis. "El carnaval de las Antillas." In *La sátira en la obra de Luis Bonafoux Quintero*, edited by Eduardo Cautiño Jordán, 97–112. San Juan: Instituto de Cultura Puertorriqueño, 1985.

Bourdieu, Pierrre. *Distinction: A Social Critique of the Judgment of Taste.* Cambridge: Harvard University Press, 1984.

Bourne, Dorothy, et al. *Rural Life in Puerto Rico.* [San Juan]: Government of Puerto Rico, Department of Education, 1933.

Brau, Salvador. *Las clases jornaleras de Puerto Rico.* Facsimile ed. Río Piedras: Editorial Edil, 1972.

———. *La colonización de Puerto Rico desde el descubrimiento de la isla hasta la reversión a la corona española de los privilegios de Colón.* 4th ed. Annotated by Isabel Gutiérrez de Arroyo. San Juan: Instituto de Cultura Puertorriqueña, 1969.

———. *Ensayos: Disquisiciones sociológicas.* Colección Poética EDIL. San Juan: Editorial Edil, 1972.

———. *Puerto Rico y su historia.* San Juan: Editorial Coquí, 1974.

Braudel, Fernand. *Civilization and Capitalism, 15th–18th Centuries: The Structures of Everyday Life; the Limits of the Possible.* New York: Harper and Row, 1981.

Brown, Lester P. *Cómo aumentar la producción mundial de alimentos.* Manuales UTEHA. Agricultura y Ganadería, no. 344/344a. Mexico City: Unión Tipografía Hispanoamericana, 1966.

Bryson, Norman. *Looking at the Overlooked: Four Essays on Still Life Painting.* London: Reaktion Books, 2001.

"Burger King Historical Facts Sheet." In Burger King Online Press Room, http://www.burgerking.com.

Caballero Balseiro, Josefina. *Bajo el vuelo de los alcatraces.* Madrid: Ediciones Ensayos, 1956.

Cabanillas de Rodríguez, Berta. *El folklore en la alimentación puertorriqueña.* Río Piedras: Editorial de la Universidad de Puerto Rico, 1983.

———. *El puertorriqueño y su alimentación a través de su historia (siglos XVI al XIX).* Colección Documental. San Juan: Instituto de Cultura Puertorriqueña, 1973.

Ca da Mosto. *Relation des voyages à la Cote d'Afrique de Álvise de Ca'da Mosto, 1455–1457.* Paris: E. Leroux, 1895.

Cadilla de Martínez, María. "Breves apuntes sobre el cultivo y consumo de arroz en Puerto Rico." *Revista de Agricultura de Puerto Rico* 31 (January-March 1939).

————. "Del maíz y el gofio." *Revista de Agricultura de Puerto Rico* 30 (April-June 1938): 291–95.

————. El lechón asado." *Revista de Agricultura de Puerto Rico* 32 (1940): 399–401.

Camporesi, Piero. *The Anatomy of the Senses: Natural Symbols in Medieval and Early Modern Italy.* Cambridge: Polity Press, 1994.

————. *Bread of Dreams: Food and Fantasy in Early Modern Europe.* Chicago: University of Chicago Press, 1989.

————. *The Magic Harvest: Food, Folklore, and Society.* London: Polity Press, 1993.

Candolle, Alphonse de. *Origins of Cultivated Plants.* New York: Appleton, 1885.

Capó, Claudio, comp. *Guía general de Puerto Rico, 1931–1932.* [San Juan: Imprenta Venezuela], 1931.

Carney, Judith. "The Role of African Rice and Slaves in the History of Rice Cultivation in the Americas." *Human Ecology* 26, no. 4 (1998): 525–45.

Caro Costa, Aida. *Antología de lecturas de historia de Puerto Rico.* San Juan: Instituto de Cultura Puertorriqueña, 1980.

————. *El cabildo o régimen municipal puertorriqueño en el siglo XVIII.* 2 vols. San Juan: Instituto de Cultura Puertorriqueña, 1980.

Carreño, Manuel Antonio. *Compendio del Manual de urbanidad y buenas maneras para el uso de las escuelas públicas de Puerto Rico.* San Juan: Imprenta del Boletín Mercantil, 1894.

Carroll, Henry King. *Report on the Island of Porto Rico.* Washington, D.C.: Government Printing Office, 1899.

Cautiño, Jordán, Eduardo. *La sátira en la obra de Luis Bonafoux Quintero.* San Juan: Instituto de Cultura Puertorriqueña, 1985.

"Celebrate Christmas All Year with 'Pastelitos del Fogón.'" *The San Juan Star,* Food and Beverage Supplement, 30 May 1997.

Certeau, Michel de. *The Practice of Everyday Life.* Berkeley: University of California Press, 1984.

Cervantes Saavedra, Miguel de. *Don Quijote de la Mancha.* Edición Conmemorativa. n.p.: Afrodisio Aguado Editores, 1958.

Chandler, José Vicente, et al. *Cultivo intensivo y perspectivas del arroz en Puerto Rico.* Río Piedras: Universidad de Puerto Rico, Colegio de Ciencias Agrícolas, 1977.

Cifre de Loubriel, Estela. *La formación del pueblo puertorriqueño: La contribución de los isleño-canarios.* San Juan: Centro de Estudios Avanzados de Puerto Rico y el Caribe, 1995.

Circular sobre que toda cabeza de Ganado que exista en esta Provincia, deberá encontrarse empadronada y provistos sus dueños de las respectivas matrículas con las formalidades prescritas. San Juan: n.p., 1888.

Clark, Victor S., et al. *Porto Rico and Its Problems.* Washington, D.C.: Brookings Institution, 1930.

"Cocinan el mofongo más grande del mundo." *El Nuevo Día,* 23 July 2001.

Cofradía Extremeña de Gastronomía. *Recetario de cocina extremeña y estudio de sus orígenes.* Biblioteca Básica Extremeña. Badajoz: Universitas Editorial, 1985.

Coll y Toste, Cayetano, ed. *Boletín histórico de Puerto Rico*. 14 vols. San Juan: Tipografía Cantero Fernández, 1914–27.

Collins, James. H. *The Story of Canned Foods*. New York: E. P. Dutton, 1924.

Colombán Rosario, José. "The Porto Rican Peasant and His Historical Antecedents." In *Porto Rico and Its Problems*, written and edited by Victor S. Clark et al., 537–75. Washington, D.C.: Brookings Institution, 1930.

Colón, Emilio M., ed. *El cocinero puertorriqueño*. San Juan: Editorial Coquí, 1971.

Colón Reyes, Linda. *Sobrevivencia, pobreza, y "mantengo": La política asistencialista estadounidense en Puerto Rico; el PAN y el TANF*. San Juan: Ediciones Callejón, 2011.

Comité de Nutrición de Puerto Rico. *Historia y reglamentación*. San Juan: Departamento de Instrucción Pública.

Conde Millet, Mario L. "El cultivo de maíz en Puerto Rico." *Revista de Agricultura de Puerto Rico* 37 (1946): 145.

Contreras Hernández, José. "Los aspectos culturales en el consumo de carne." In *Somos lo que comemos: Estudios de alimentación y cultura en España*, edited by Mabel García Arnáiz, 221–46. Barcelona: Ariel, 2002.

Cook, Donald H., et al. "Nutritional Studies of the Foodstuffs Used in Puerto Rican Dietary." *Puerto Rico Journal of Public Health and Tropical Medicine* 16 (1940–41).

———. "Preliminary Studies of a Common Puerto Rican Diet." *Porto Rico Journal of Public Health and Tropical Medicine* 4 (1928).

———. "A Study of the Diets in Three Insular Institutions: Tuberculosis Sanatorium, Leprosarium, and Insane Hospital." *Porto Rico Review of Public Health and Tropical Medicine* 3 (1927).

Cook, Donald H., and T. Rivera. "Rice and Beans as an Adequate Diet." *Porto Rico Journal of Public Health and Tropical Medicine* 5 (1929).

Cook, Ian, and Philip Crang. "The World on a Plate: Culinary Culture, Displacement, and Geographical Knowledges." *Journal of Material Culture* 1, no. 2 (1996): 131–53.

Cook, Melville Thurston, José Idilio Otero, and Francisco Antonio López Domínguez. *History of the First Quarter of a Century of the Agricultural Experiment Station at Río Piedras, Puerto Rico*. University of Puerto Rico Agricultural Experiment Station, Bulletin no. 44. Río Piedras: University of Puerto Rico, 1937.

Cook, Oratio Fuller. *The Economic Plants of Puerto Rico*. Washington, D.C.: Government Printing Office, 1903.

Cooper, Eugene. "Chinese Table Manners: You Are How You Eat." *Human Organization* 45, no. 2 (Summer 1996): 179–84.

Córdoba, Pedro Tomás de, comp. and ed. *Memorias geográficas, históricas, económicas y estadísticas de la isla de Puerto Rico*. 6 vols. Facsimile ed. San Juan: Editorial Coquí/Instituto de Cultura Puertorriqueña, 1968.

Correa, Alberto. "El cultivo de arroz en Puerto Rico." *Revista de Agricultura de Puerto Rico* 34 (March 1942): 28–36.

Counihan, Carole, and Penny Van Esterik, eds. *Food and Culture: A Reader.*
London: Routledge, 1997.

Cowan Schwartz, Ruth. *More Work for Mother: The Ironies of Household Technology
from the Open Hearth to the Microwave.* New York: Basic Books, 1983.

Crosby, Alfred W. *The Columbian Exchange: Biological and Cultural Consequences of 1492.*
Contributions in American Studies no. 2. Westport, Conn.: Greenwood Press,
1972.

Cruz Monclova, Lidio. *Historia de Puerto Rico en el siglo XIX.* 5 vols. Río Piedras:
Editorial de La Universidad de Puerto Rico, 1957.

Cubero, J. I. "Traditional Varieties of Grain Legumes for Human Consumption."
In *Neglected Crops: 1492 from a Different Perspective,* edited by J. E. Hernando
Bermejo and J. León, 289–301. Plant Production and Protection Series no. 26.
Rome: Food and Agriculture Organization of the United Nations, 1994.

Dalziel, John McEwen. *Useful Plants of West Tropical Africa.* 4 vols. London: Royal
Botanical Gardens, 1985.

Dávila Cox, Emma. *Este inmenso comercio: Las relaciones mercantiles entre Puerto Rico y
Gran Bretaña, 1844–1898.* Río Piedras: Editorial de la Universidad de Puerto Rico/
Instituto de Cultura Puertorriqueña, 1996.

Dawdy, Shannon Lee. "La Comida Mambisa: Food, Farming, and Cuban
Identity." *New West Indian Guide* 76, nos. 1–2 (2002): 45–80.

De Acosta, Joseph. *Historia natural y moral de las Indias: En que se tratan de las cosas
notables del cielo, elementos, metales, plantas y animales dellas, y los ritos, y ceremonias,
leyes y gobierno de los indios.* Edited by Edmundo O'Gorman. Biblioteca
Americana. Serie de Cronistas de Indias no. 38. 2nd rev. ed. Mexico City:
Fondo de Cultura Económica, 1962.

Debouck, D. G. "Early Beans (phaseolus vulgaris L. and P. lunnatus)
Domesticated for Their Aesthetic Value?" In *Annual Report,* vol. 38, of the
International Board for Plant Genetic Resources. Rome: IBPGR, 1989.

Debien, Gabriel. "La nutrición de los esclavos en las plantaciones de las Antillas
francesas en Los siglos XVII y XVIII." *Caribbean Studies* 4, no. 2 (1964): 13–16.

De Grosourdy, René. *El médico botánico criollo: Parte primera, Flora médica y útil a
las Antillas y de la parte correspondiente al Continente Americano.* Paris: Librería de
Francisco Brachet, 1864.

De la Mata, Juan. *Arte de Repostería.* Facsimile ed. Burgos: La Olmeda, 1992.

"Del Valle Atiles." In *Crónicas de Puerto Rico: Desde el siglo XVI hasta nuestros días,*
edited by Eugenio Fernández Méndez, 73. San Juan: Universidad de Puerto
Rico, 1968.

Del Valle Sárraga, Rafael. *Ideas modernas acerca de nuestra ración alimentaria.* San Juan:
Tipografía el Compás, 1921.

Departamento de Instrucción Pública. *Comedores escolares: Diez años de servicio para
el bienestar de nuestros niños.* San Juan: División de Comedores Escolares, 1956.

Descartes Sol, Luis, Santiago Díaz Pacheco, and José R. Noguera. *Food
Consumption Studies in Puerto Rico.* University of Puerto Rico Agricultural

Experiment Station, Bulletin no. 59. Río Piedras: Agricultural Experiment Station, 1941.

"Desenfocadas las tiendas con las necesidades de los clientes." *El Nuevo Día*, 15 August 2001.

Diario Económico de Puerto Rico, 1814–1815. 2 vols. San Juan: Instituto de Cultura Puertorriqueña, 1972.

Díaz, Marian. "Pelea 'grande' en la red." *El Nuevo Día*, 20 August 1999.

Díaz de Villegas, José. L. *Puerto Rico: La gran cocina del Caribe*. Río Piedras: Editorial de la Universidad de Puerto Rico, 2004.

Díaz Pacheco, Santiago. *Consumo de alimentos en la zona urbana de Puerto Rico*. Universidad de Puerto Rico. Estación Experimental Agrícola, Bulletin no. 52. Río Piedras: Estación Experimental Agrícola, 1940.

———. *La distribución de carnes en Puerto Rico*. San Juan: Negociado de Materiales, Imprenta y Transportes, 1942.

Díaz Soler, Luis M. *Historia de la esclavitud negra en Puerto Rico*. Río Piedras: Editorial de la Universidad de Puerto Rico, 1953.

Documentos de la Real Hacienda de Puerto Rico, 1510–1519. Vol. 1 of *Documentos de la Real Hacienda de Puerto Rico, 1510–1545*. Translated and compiled by Aurelio Tanodi et al. Río Piedras: Centro de Investigaciones Históricas, Universidad de Puerto Rico, 1971–2009.

Domingo, Xavier. *La mesa del buscón: En homenaje a Don Francisco de Quevedo y Villegas con ocasión de su centenario*. Los 5 Sentidos no. 10. Barcelona: Tusquets, 1981.

Duby, Georges, and Michelle Perrot, eds. *Historia de las mujeres*. 5 vols. Madrid: Editorial Taurus, 1992.

Du Vall, Nell. *Domestic Technology: A Chronology of Developments*. Boston: G.K. Hall, 1988.

Eizaguirre, José M. "Los sistemas en el régimen de abasto de carnes a San Juan en la primera parte del siglo XIX." M.A. thesis, Universidad de Puerto Rico, 1974.

"El cultivo de legumbres en Puerto Rico." *Boletín [de la] Estación Experimental Agrícola de Puerto Rico*, no. 1 (1903): 7–64.

"El Panapén y sus frutos." *Revista de Agricultura de Puerto Rico* 28 (1937).

"El reino de las comidas rápidas." *El Nuevo Día*, Suplemento Negocios, 8 June 1997.

Elías, Norbert. *The History of Manners*. Vol. 1 of *The Civilizing Process*. New York: Pantheon Books, 1982.

Fage, J. D., and Roland Oliver, comps. *Papers in African Prehistory*. Cambridge: Cambridge University Press, 1970.

Ferguson, Grace J. *La organización de los cursos de economía doméstica*. [San Juan]: n.p., 1938.

Ferguson, Leland. *Uncommon Ground: Archaeology and Early African America, 1650–1800*. Washington, D.C.: Smithsonian Institution Press, 1992.

Fernández de Oviedo, Gonzalo. *Historia general y natural de las Indias*. Edición y estudio preliminar de Juan Pérez de Tudela Bueso. Madrid: Editorial Atlas, 1959.

Fernández Méndez, Eugenio, ed. *Crónicas de Puerto Rico: Desde el siglo XVI hasta nuestros días*. San Juan: Universidad de Puerto Rico, 1968.

Figueroa, C. A. "Los gandules en Puerto Rico." *Revista de Agricultura de Puerto Rico* 11 (1923).

Fischler, Claude. *El (h)omnívoro: El gusto, la cocina y el cuerpo*. Barcelona: Editorial Anagrama, 1995.

———. "The McDonaldization of Culture." In *Food: A Culinary History from Antiquity to the Present*, edited by Jean-Louis Flandrin, Massimo Montanari, and Albert Sonnenfeld, 530–47. New York: Columbia University Press, 1999.

Flandrin, Jean-Louis. "Le gout et la necessité: Sur l'usage des graisses dans les cuisines d'Europe occidentale (XIV–XVII siècle)." *Annales E.S.C.* 38 (1983).

Flandrin, Jean-Louis, and Philip Hayman. "Regional Tastes and Cuisines: Problems, Documents, and Discourses on Food in Southern France in the Sixteenth and Seventeenth Centuries." *Food and Foodways* 1, no. 1 (1986): 221–51.

Flandrin, Jean-Louis, Massimo Montanari, and Albert Sonnenfeld, eds. *Food: A Culinary History from Antiquity to the Present*. New York: Columbia University Press, 1999.

Fleagle, Fred K. *Social Problems in Puerto Rico*. New York: D.C. Heath, 1917.

Forster, Elborg, and Robert Forster, eds. *European Diet from Preindustrial Times to Modern Times*. Basic Conditions of Life. New York: Harper and Row, 1975.

Forster, Robert, and Orest Ranum, eds. *Food and Drink in History: Selections from the Annales, Economies, Societies, Civilizations*. Baltimore: Johns Hopkins University Press, 1979.

Freyre, Gilberto. *Azúcar: Uma sociologia do doce, con recetas do bolos e doces do Nordeste do Brasil*. São Paulo: Companhia das Letras, 1997.

Gaither International. *Changing Trends in Fast-Food Marketing [in] Puerto Rico between 1998 and 2003*. [San Juan]: Gaither International Marketing and Opinion Research, [2003].

García Arnaíz, Mabel. "La alimentación en el umbral del siglo 21: Una agenda para la investigación sociocultural en España." In *Somos lo que comemos: Estudios de alimentación y cultura en España*, edited by Mabel García Arnaíz, 15–38. Barcelona: Ariel, 2002.

———. "Los trastornos alimentarios como trastornos culturales: La construcción social de la Anorexia nerviosa." In *Somos lo que comemos: Estudios de alimentación y cultura en España*, edited by Mabel García Arnaíz, 350–77. Barcelona: Ariel, 2002.

García Canclini, Néstor. *Consumidores y ciudadanos: Conflictos multiculturales de la globalización*. Barcelona: Grijalbo, 1998.

García Colon, Pablo. "El mercado de tierras en la jurisdicción administrativa de San Juan durante las décadas centrales del setecientos." *Revista Exégesis* 8, no. 2 (1995): 23–38.

García Fuentes, Lutgardo. *El comercio español con América*. Seville: Diputación Provincial y Escuela de Estudios Hispanoamericanos, 1980.

García Leduc, José Manuel. *Apuntes para una historia breve de Puerto Rico*. Río Piedras: Isla Negra, 2002.

García Pomales, Cándido. "Política pública del gobierno de Puerto Rico respecto al control de precios del arroz." M.A. thesis, University of Puerto Rico, 1970.

Garrida Arranda, Antonio, comp. *Cultura alimentaria de España y América*. Córdoba: Editorial La Val de Onsera, 1995.

Gelder, G. J. H. van. *Of Dishes and Discourse: Classical Arabic Literary Representations of Food*. Curzon Studies in Arabic and Middle Eastern Literatures no. 3. Richmond, Surrey: Curzon, 2000.

Gil de Bermejo, Juana. *Panorama histórico de la agricultura en Puerto Rico*. Publicaciones de la Escuela de Estudios Hispano-Americanos no. 189. Seville: Consejo Superior de Investigaciones Superiores, 1970.

Girón, Socorro. *Vida y obra de Ramón Méndez Quiñones*. San Juan: Instituto de Cultura Puertorriqueña, 1991.

Gispert Cruels, Montserrat. "Las plantas americanas que revolucionaron los guisos, aderezos y repostería de la comida occidental." In *Los sabores de España y América*, edited by Antonio Garrido Aranda, 213–30. Huesca: Editorial la Val de Onsera, 1999.

"Góndolas vacías: Un gran dolor de cabeza." *El Nuevo Día*, 15 August 2001.

González, Libia M. "La ilusión del paraíso: Fotografías y relatos de viajeros sobre Puerto Rico, 1898–1900." In *Los arcos de la memoria: El 98 y los pueblos puertorriqueños*, edited by Silvia Álvarez Curbelo, Mary Frances Gallart, and Carmen Raffucci de García, 281. San Juan: Universidad de Puerto Rico, 1998.

———. "Pintueles y Compañía: Una casa asturiana en el comercio de café." *Revista del Centro de Estudios Avanzados de Puerto Rico y el Caribe* 12 (January-June 1991): 96–107.

González García, Sebastián. "Una comida de gala en la Fortaleza hace 200 años." *Revista del Instituto de Cultura Puertorriqueña* 9 (January–March 1966): 52–55.

González Ríos, Pedro. "El mejoramiento de la habichuelas en Puerto Rico." *Revista de Agricultura de Puerto Rico* 43 (1952): 140–42.

González Turmo, Isabel. *Comida de rico, comida de pobre: Evolución de los hábitos alimentarios en el Occidente andaluz*. Seville: Universidad de Sevilla, 1995.

Goody, Jack. *Cooking, Cuisine, and Class: A Study in Comparative Sociology*. 4th ed. Cambridge: Cambridge University Press, 1991.

Granja Santamaría, Fernando de la. *La cocina arábigoandaluza según un manuscrito inédito*. Madrid: Universidad de Madrid, 1960. [extract of author's doctoral dissertation of the same title.]

Haddock, Daniel, and Leslie Hernández. *Consumer Preferences for Tanniers (Xanthosoma ssp.) in Puerto Rico, 1949–1950*. Agricultural Experiment Station, Bulletin no. 103. Río Piedras: Agricultural Experiment Station, 1952.

Hakluyt, Richard. *The Principal Navigations, Voyages, Traffiques, and Discoveries of the English Nation*. 8 vols. London: J. M. Dent, 1927–28.

Hamm, Margherita. *Porto Rico and the West Indies.* London: F.T. Neeley, 1899.

Hardyment, Cristina. *From Mangle to Microwave: The Mechanization of Household Work.* Cambridge: Polity Press, 1988.

Harris, Marvin. *Good to Eat: Riddles of Food and Culture.* New York: Simon and Schuster, 1985.

Hayman, Philip, and Mary Hayman. "Printing the Kitchen: French Cookbooks, 1480–1800." In *Food: A Culinary History from Antiquity to the Present,* edited by Jean-Louis Flandrin, Massimo Montanari, and Albert Sonnenfeld, 394. New York: Columbia University Press, 1999.

Henricksen, Henry C. *El cultivo de legumbres en Puerto Rico.* Agricultural Experiment Station, Bulletin no. 7. Mayagüez: Agricultural Experiment Station, 1903.

Hérmandinquer, Jean-Jacques. "The Family Pig of the Ancient Regime: Myth or Fact." In *Food and Drink in History: Selections from the Annales,* edited by Robert Forster and Orest Ranum, 50–72. Baltimore: Johns Hopkins University Press, 1979.

Hernández, Elías. "El cultivo de arroz en Puerto Rico." *Revista de Agricultura de Puerto Rico* 30 (1938): 282–85.

Hernández, Wilhem. *Adjuntas: Notas para su historia.* San Juan: Comité de Historia de los Pueblos, 1985.

Hernández Bernejo, Esteban. "El papel de los jardines botánicos en la introducción e intercambio de especies alimentarias." In *Cultura alimentaria de España y América,* edited by Antonio Garrida Aranda, 225–78. Huesca: Editorial la Val de Onsera, 1995.

Herrera, Antonio de. "Década segunda." In *Biblioteca Histórica de Puerto Rico que contiene varios documentos de los siglos XV, XVI, XVII y XVIII,* coordinated and annotated by Alejandro Tapia y Rivera, 120. 2nd ed. San Juan: Publicaciones del Instituto de Literatura Puertorriqueña, 1945.

Higman, Barry. "Cookbooks and Caribbean Cultural Identity: An English Language Hors d'Oeuvre." *New West Indian Guide* 72, nos. 1–2 (1998): 77–95.

Hill, Elton B., and José R. Noguera. *The Food Supply of Puerto Rico.* University of Puerto Rico Agricultural Experiment Station, Bulletin no. 55. Río Piedras: Agricultural Experiment Station, 1940.

Hitchcock, Frank H. *Trade of Puerto Rico.* United States Department of Agriculture, Section of Foreign Markets, Bulletin no. 13. Washington, D.C.: Government Printing Office, 1898.

Hobsbawm, Eric. "Introduction: Inventing Traditions." In *The Invention of Tradition,* edited by Eric Hobsbawm and Terence Ranger, 1–14. Cambridge: Cambridge University Press, 1992.

Hopkins, Anthony G. *An Economic History of West Africa.* The Columbia Economic History of the Modern World. New York: Columbia University Press, 1973.

Hostos, Felipe de. "The External Trade of Puerto Rico." *Boletín Oficial de la Cámara de Comercio de Puerto Rico* 10, no. 6 (September 1934): 22.

Hudders, Sidney M. "Consideraciones sobre la utilización de tierras en Puerto Rico." *Revista de Agricultura de Puerto Rico* 37 (1946).

Huerga, A. *Vida y obras de Fray Bartolomé de las Casas.* Madrid: Alianza, 1999.

Hui, Y. H., ed. *Encyclopedia of Food Science and Technology.* 4 vols. Singapore: John Wiley, 1992.

Huici, Ambrosio. "La cocina hispanomagrebí durante la época almohade." *Revista del Instituto de Estudios Islámicos de Madrid* 5 (1957): 137–55.

Hurd Green, Carol, and Barbara Sicherman. *Notable American Women: The Modern Period; A Biographical Dictionary.* Cambridge: Belknap Press of Harvard University Press, 1980.

Huyke, Giovanna. "Cuando vamos a comer en familia." *El Nuevo Día,* 16 July 1997.

Iggers, Jeremy. *The Garden of Eating: Food, Sex, and the Hunger for Meaning.* New York: Basic Books, 1996.

Iglesias, César Andreu. *El Derrumbe.* [San Juan?]: Editorial El Club del Libro, 1960.

"Informe del Cabildo de San Juan al Rey, dándole noticia de la situación de la propiedad en la Isla [1775]." In *Boletín histórico de Puerto Rico,* edited by Cayetano Coll y Toste, 262. San Juan: Tipografía Cantero Fernández, 1914–27.

Innis, Harold A. *The Cod Fisheries: The History of an International Economy. The Relations of Canada and the United States.* New Haven: Yale University Press; Toronto: Ryerson Press, for the Carnegie Endowment for International Peace, 1940.

Iranzo, Carmen, ed. *Libro de cocina de Ruperto de Nola.* Facsimile ed. Madrid: Taurus, 1982.

Jacob, François. *La lógica de lo viviente: Una historia de la herencia.* Barcelona: Editorial Laia, 1973.

Jaret, Peter. "Things Go Better with Beans." *Health* 7, no. 6 (October 1993): 32–35.

Johns, Timothy. *With Bitter Herbs They Shall Eat It: Chemistry Ecology and the Origins of Human Diet and Medicine.* Tucson: University of Arizona Press, 1990.

Johnston, Bruce F. *The Staple Food Economies of Western Tropical Africa.* Studies in Tropical Development. Stanford: Stanford University Press, 1958.

Jones, William O. *Manioc in Africa.* Palo Alto: Stanford University Press, 1959.

Kaplan, L., and L. N. Kaplan. "Phaseolus in Archaeology." In *Genetic Resources of Phaseolus Beans,* edited by P. Gepts, 124–42. Dordrecht, the Netherlands: Kluwer Academic Press, 1988.

Karasch, Mary. "Manioc." In *The Cambridge World History of Food,* edited by Kenneth F. Kipple and Kriemhild C. Ornelas, 1:181–86. Cambridge: Cambridge University Press, 2000.

Kirkland, Edward. *Historia económica de Estados Unidos.* Mexico City: Fondo de Cultura Económica, 1941.

Khoo, Tony, et al. *El gran libro del arroz: Historia, cultivo, variedades, práctica culinaria y recetas.* n.p.: Everest, 1999.

Korsmeyer, Carolyn. *El sentido del gusto: Comida, estética y filosofía.* Barcelona: Paidós, 2002.

Kurlansky, Mark. *El bacalao: Biografía del pez que cambió el mundo*. Barcelona: Península, 1999.

Kutzinski, Vera M. *Sugar's Secrets: Race and the Erotics of Cuban Nationalism*. New World Studies. Charlottesville: University of Virginia Press, 1993.

Lang, Rita, and Pablo Morales Otero. "Health and Socio-economic Studies in Puerto Rico III: Nutritional Studies in the Rural Regions of Puerto Rico." *Porto Rico Journal of Public Health and Tropical Medicine* 31 (April 1939): 113–33.

"La valoración de las salinas en la colonización de Puerto Rico." *Revista de Historia* 1, no. 1 (January–June 1985): 9–26.

Legrand, Julio. "El maíz." *Revista de Agricultura de Puerto Rico* 11 (July 1923): 25–30.

Lentz, Carola, ed. *Changing Food Habits: Case Studies from Africa, South America, and Europe*. Vol. 2 of *Food in History and Culture*. Amsterdam: Harwood Academic Publishers, 1999.

Levenstein, Harvey A. *Paradox of Plenty: A Social History of Eating in Modern America*. New York: Oxford University Press, 1993.

―――. *Revolution at the Table: The Transformation of the American Diet*. New York: Oxford University Press, 1988.

Lévi-Strauss, Claude. *Mitológicas I: Lo crudo y lo cocido*. Mexico City: Fondo de Cultura Económica, 1968.

Lewicki, Tadeusz. *West African Food in the Middle Ages According to Arabic Sources*. Cambridge: Cambridge University Press, 1974.

Linares, Olga F. "African Rice (Oryza glaberrima): History and Future Potential." *Proceedings of the National Academy of Sciences* 99, no. 25 (10 December 2002): 16360–365.

Lizardi Pollock, Jorge L. "Mercados, mercaderes y sociedad: Puerto Rico, 1508–1535." M.A. thesis, Universidad de Puerto Rico, 1997.

"Loíza en el Hilton." *El Nuevo Día*, Suplemento En Grande, 29 October 1995.

Long Solís, Janet. "El tomate: De hierba silvestre de las Américas a denominador común de las cocinas mediterráneas." In *Cultura alimentaria de España y América*, edited by Antonio Garrida Aranda, 215–37. Huesca: Editorial la Val de Onsera, 1995.

López Cantos, Ángel. *Historia de Puerto Rico (1650–1700)*. Publicaciones de la Escuela de Estudios Hispano-Americanos no. 231. Seville: Escuela de Estudios Hispano-Americanos, Consejo Superior de Investigaciones Científicas, 1975.

―――. *Miguel Enríquez: Corsario boricua del siglo XVIII*. San Juan: Ediciones Puerto, 1994.

―――. "La vida cotidiana del negro en Puerto Rico en el siglo XVIII: Alimentación." *Revista del Centro de Estudios Avanzados de Puerto Rico y el Caribe* 4 (January-June 1987): 147–55.

"López de Haro." In *Crónicas de Puerto Rico: Desde el siglo XVI hasta nuestros días*, edited by Eugenio Fernández Méndez, 164. San Juan: Universidad de Puerto Rico, 1968.

López Medrano, Andrés. "Disertación de la Filgtegna gangrenosa de Puerto Rico, o historia de todo lo que sin ser ella, llamaron la Llaguita, a consecuencia

de la mortandad del ganado vacuno en el barrio del Algarrobo, partido
de Mayagüez, con la exposición de lo que aclara la materia." In *Memorias
geográficas, históricas, económicas y estadísticas de la isla de Puerto Rico*, compiled and
edited by Pedro Tomás de Córdoba, 5:38–39. Facsimile ed. San Juan: Editorial
Coquí/Instituto Puertorriqueño de Cultura, 1968.

López Tuero, Fernando. *Café y piña de América*. San Juan: Imprenta del Boletín
Mercantil, 1891.

———. *Cultivos perfeccionados: Arroz y cacao*. [San Juan]: Imprenta de Acosta,
1889.

———. *Cultivos perfeccionados: Maíz y tabaco*. [San Juan]: Imprenta y Librería de
Acosta, 1890.

———. *Estado moral de los factores de la producción en Cuba y Puerto Rico*. Madrid:
Librería De F. Fe, 1896.

———. *Estudios de economía rural*. San Juan: Imprenta del Boletín Mercantil,
1893.

———. *El hombre*. San Juan: Imprenta del Boletín Mercantil, 1897.

———. *La mujer*. San Juan: Tipografía del Boletín Mercantil, 1893.

———. *Plátano y palma de coco*. [San Juan]: Imprenta del Boletín Mercantil, 1892.

———. *La reforma agrícola*. [San Juan]: Imprenta del Boletín Mercantil, 1891.

"Los tenedores del milenio." *El Nuevo Día*, Suplemento Domingo, 12 December
1999.

Lovera, José Rafael. *Historia de la alimentación en Venezuela*. Caracas: Monte Avila
Editores, 1988.

Mahbir, Noor Kumar. *Medicinal and Edible Plants Used by East Indians of Trinidad and
Tobago*. Trinidad: Chackra Publishing House, 1991.

Malaret, Augusto. *Diccionario de americanismos, con un índice científico de fauna y flora*.
Mayagüez: Editorial R. Carrero, 1925.

———. *Lexicón de fauna y flora*. San Juan: Comisión Permanente de la Asociación
de Académicos de la Lengua Española, 1970.

Mangelsdorf, Christoph. *Corn: Its Origin, Evolution and Improvement*. Cambridge:
Belknap Press of Harvard University Press, 1974.

Manton, Catherine. *Fed Up: Women and Food in America*. Westport, Conn.: Bergin
and Garvey, 1999.

Martin, Ethel Austin. "The Life Work of Lydia Jane Roberts." *Journal of the American
Dietetic Association* (October 1966): 299–302.

Martínez, José Luis. *Pasajeros a Indias: Viajes transatlánticos en el siglo XVI*. Madrid:
Alianza Editorial, 1983.

"Más allá de la comida: Los supermercados amplían la variedad de productos y
servicios." *El Nuevo Día*, Suplemento Negocios, 1 November 1998.

Mauleón Benítez, Carmen. *El español de Loíza Aldea*. Madrid: Ediciones Partenón,
1974.

Mayo Santana, Raúl, Mariano Negrón Portillo, and Manuel Mayo López. *Cadenas
de esclavitud . . . y de solidaridad: Esclavos y libertos en San Juan, siglo XIX*. Río Piedras:
Centro de Investigaciones Sociales, Universidad de Puerto Rico, 1997.

McKey, Doyle, and Stephen Beckerman. "Chemical Ecology, Plant Evolution, and Traditional Manioc Cultivation." In *Tropical Forests, People and Food: Biocultural Interactions and Applications to Development*. Paris: UNESCO, 1983.

Medina Molera, Antonio. *Diccionario andaluz: Biográfico y terminológico*. Seville: Biblioteca de Ediciones Andaluzas, 1980.

Mejías, Félix. *Condiciones de vida de las clases jornaleras de Puerto Rico*. Río Piedras: Junta Editora de la Universidad de Puerto Rico, 1946.

"Memoria de la primera Feria Exposición de Puerto Rico [1854]." In *Boletín histórico de Puerto Rico*, edited by Cayetano Coll y Toste, 3:178. San Juan: Tipografía Cantero Fernández, 1914–27.

"Memoria sobre la propiedad territorial en la isla de Puerto Rico." In *Boletín histórico de Puerto Rico*, edited by Cayetano Coll y Toste, 1:239–310. San Juan: Tipografía Cantero Fernández, 1914–27.

Méndez Quiñones, Ramón. "El cuento del matrimonio." In *La actualidad del jíbaro*, edited by Antonio S. Pedreira, 21–37. Río Piedras: Universidad de Puerto Rico, 1935.

———. "La Triquina." In *Vida y obra de Ramón Méndez Quiñones*, edited by Socorro Girón, 303–37. 3rd ed. San Juan: Instituto de Cultura Puertorriqueña, 1991.

Mennell, Stephen. *All Manners of Food: Eating and Taste in England and France from the Middle Ages to the Present*. Oxford: Basil Blackwell, 1985.

———. "Divergences and Convergences in the Development of Culinary Cultures." In *European Food History: A Research Review*, edited by Hans J. Teuteberg, 278–86. Leicester: Leicester University Press, 1992.

Mennell, Stephen, Murcott, Ann, and Anneka H. van Otterloo. *The Sociology of Food: Eating, Diet, and Culture*. [Originally published in *Current Sociology* 40, no. 2.] Newbury Park, Calif.: Sage Publications, 1992.

Messer, E. "Maize." In *The Cambridge World History of Food*, edited by K. Kiple and K. Conèe Ornelas, 97–112. Cambridge: Cambridge University Press, 2001.

Milán, Fernando. "Tubérculos." *Revista de Agricultura de Puerto Rico* 1 (August–May1918): 53–58.

Mintz, Sidney. "Cañamelar: The Subculture of a Rural Sugar Plantation Proletariat." In *The People of Puerto Rico: A Study of Social Anthropology*, edited by Julian Steward, 315–417. San Juan: University of Puerto Rico; Urbana-Champaign: University of Illinois Press, 1969.

———. "Eating Communities: The Mixed Appeal of Sodality." In *Eating Culture: The Poetics and Politics of Food*, edited by Tobias Doring, Markus Heide, and Sussanne Muhleisen, 1934. Heidelberg: Winter, 2003.

———. *Sweetness and Power: The Place of Sugar in Modern History*. New York: Viking, 1985.

———. *Tasting Food, Tasting Freedom: Excursions into Eating, Culture, and the Past*. Boston: Beacon Press, 1996.

Molins, José Elías de. *Las admisiones temporales de arroces de la India y Filipinas*. Barcelona: Editorial Barcelonesa, 1883.

Montanari, Massimo. "La cocina, lugar de la identidad y del intercambio."
In *El mundo en la cocina: Historia, identidad, intercambios*, compiled by Massimo
Montanari, 11–15. Barcelona: Paidós, 2003.

———. *The Culture of Food. The Making of Europe*. Oxford: Blackwell, 1994.

———. *El hambre y la abundancia: Historia y cultura de la alimentación en Europa*.
Barcelona: Editorial Crítica, 1993.

———. "Historia, alimentación, historia de la alimentación." In *Problemas
actuales de la historia*, edited by José María Sánchez et al., 24–25. Salamanca:
Universidad de Salamanca, 1994.

———, comp. *El mundo en la cocina: Historia, identidad, intercambio*. Barcelona:
Paidós, 2003.

Montanari, Massimo, Jean-Louis Flandrin, and Albert Sonnenfeld, eds. *Food:
A Culinary History: From Antiquity to the Present*. New York: Columbia University
Press, 1999.

Morales Carrión, Arturo. *Puerto Rico y la lucha por la hegemonía en el Caribe:
Colonialismo y contrabando, siglos XVI-XVIII*. Río Piedras: Centro de
Investigaciones, Universidad de Puerto Rico, 1995.

Morales Otero, Pablo, et al. "La anemia del jíbaro." *Boletín de la Asociación Médica
de Puerto Rico* 24 (1932).

———. "Health and Socio-economic Conditions in Puerto Rico: I, Health and
Socio-economic Conditions in the Tobacco, Coffee, and Fruit Regions." *Porto
Rico Journal of Public Health and Tropical Medicine* 14 (1939).

———. *Health and Socio-economic Studies in Puerto Rico, 1937–1940*. San Juan:
[Puerto Rico Reconstruction Administration], 1940.

———. "Health and Socio-economic Studies in Puerto Rico: I, Health and
Socio-economic Conditions on a Sugar Cane Plantation." *Porto Rico Journal of
Public Health and Tropical Medicine* 12 (1937).

———. "Trastornos de la nutrición." In *Enfermedades de la nutrición, la digestión y
el metabolismo*, 14. San Juan: Departamento de Instrucción Pública, 1954.

Moreno Fraginals, Manuel. *El ingenio: El complejo económico social cubano del azúcar*.
3 vols. Havana: Editorial de las Ciencias Sociales. 1978.

Moreno Fraginals, Manuel, and Manuel A. Pérez. "Health and Socio-economic
Conditions in Puerto Rico: IV, Physical Measurements of Agricultural
Workers." *Porto Rico Journal of Public Health and Tropical Medicine* 14 (1939).

———. "Health and Socio-economic Studies in Puerto Rico: IV, Physical
Impairments of Adult Life among Agricultural Workers." *Porto Rico Journal of
Public Health and Tropical Medicine* 15 (1940).

Moscoso, Carlos G. "El cultivo de la batata mameya." *Revista de Agricultura de
Puerto Rico* 43 (January–June 1952): 126–39.

Moscoso, Francisco. *Lucha agraria en Puerto Rico, 1541–1545: Un ensayo de historia*.
San Juan: Instituto de Cultura Puertorriqueña/Ediciones Puerto, 1997.

———. *Sociedad y economía de los taínos*. San Juan: Editorial Edil, 1999.

Municipio de San Juan. *Actas del Cabildo de San Juan Bautista de Puerto Rico*. 18 vols.
San Juan: Publicación Oficial del Municipio de San Juan, 1968.

Murga Sanz, Vicente. *Historia documental de Puerto Rico*. 3 vols. Río Piedras: Plus Ultra; Santander: Aldus; Río Piedras: Editorial de la Universidad de Puerto Rico, 1956–61.

———. *Puerto Rico en los manuscritos de Juan Bautista Muñoz*. Río Piedras: Editorial de la Universidad de Puerto Rico, 1960.

Muro Carratalá, Ángel. *Diccionario general de cocina*. 2 vols. Madrid: Editorial José María Faquineto, 1892.

———. *El practicón*. 2nd facsimile ed. Barcelona: Editorial Tusquets, 1997.

Newman, Lucile F., et al. *Hunger in History: Food Shortage, Poverty, and Deprivation*. Oxford: Basil Blackwell, 1995.

Nieves Falcón, Luis. *Diagnóstico de Puerto Rico*. San Juan: Editorial Edil, 1972.

Oddy, Derek J., and Catherine Giesler, eds. *Food, Diet, and Economic Change: Past and Present*. Leicester: Leicester University Press, 1993.

O'Hair, Stephen K. "Tropical Roots and Tubers Crops." http://newcrop.hort.purdue.edu/newcrop/default.html.

Oliver, Ángel. "El árbol de pan en Puerto Rico." *Revista de Agricultura de Puerto Rico* 26 (1931).

Oppenheimer, Santiago. *Impresiones de un viaje a Hawaii*. Havana: Imprenta Pérez Sierra y Compañía, 1931.

O'Reilly, Alejandro. "Relación circunstanciada del actual estado de la población, frutos y proporciones para fomento que tiene la Isla de San Juan de Puerto Rico, con algunas ocurrencias sobre los medios conducentes a ello." In *Crónicas de Puerto Rico: Desde el siglo XVI hasta nuestros días*, edited by Eugenio Fernández Méndez, 239–69. San Juan: Universidad de Puerto Rico, 1968.

Ormaechea, Darío. "Memoria acerca de la agricultura, el comercio y las rentas internas de la isla de Puerto Rico." In *Boletín histórico de Puerto Rico*, edited by Cayetano Coll y Toste, 2:226. San Juan: Tipografía Cantero Fernández, 1914–27.

Ortiz Cuadra, Cruz Miguel. "La 'buena vida' no es 'vida buena': Disquisiciones muñocistas sobre nutrición y consumo, 1948–1964." *Exégesis* 18, no. 52 (2005): 16–30.

———. "1942: El hambre que engordó la guerra." In *Historias vivas, historiografía puertorriqueña contemporánea*, 123–33. [San Juan?]: Editorial Posdata, 1996.

———. "Somos lo que comimos: Incursión a la historia sociocultural de los alimentos, la cocina and la alimentación en Puerto Rico; desde el siglo XVI a las primeras décadas del siglo XX." Ph.D. diss., University of Puerto Rico, 1999.

———. "La vida buena: Adecuada nutrición y nuevos consumos en los discursos de Luis Muñoz Marín, 1948–1960." Paper delivered at the Segundo Foro sobre los Discursos de Luis Muñoz Marín, Fundación Luis Muñoz Marín, [San Juan], 23–24 February 2001.

Ortiz, Fernando. "La cocina afrocubana." *Revista Bimestre Cubana* 18, no. 6 (November–December 1923): 84–94.

Oviedo, Gonzalo Fernández. *Historia general y natural de las Indias*. Edited by Juan Pérez de Tudela Buesa. Madrid: Editorial Atlas, 1959.

Payne, G. C., et al. "Heights and Weights of Children in Three Communities of Puerto Rico." *Porto Rico Journal of Public Health and Tropical Medicine* 5 (1930).

Pedreira, Antonio S, ed. *La actualidad del jíbaro.* Río Piedras: Universidad de Puerto Rico, 1935.

Pelto, Gretel, and Pertti Pelto. "Diet and Delocalization: Dietary Changes since 1750." *Journal of Interdisciplinary History* 14, no. 2 (1983): 507–23.

Pérez García, Antonio. "El cultivo de la yautía." *Revista de Agricultura de Puerto Rico* 28 (1932): 779–82.

Picó, Fernando. "Deshumanización del trabajo, cosificación de la naturaleza: Los comienzos del auge del café en Utuado." In *Inmigración y clases sociales en el Puerto Rico del siglo XIX*, edited by Francisco Scarano, 187–206. Río Piedras: Editorial Huracán, 1981.

———. *El día menos pensado: Historia de los presidiaros en Puerto Rico.* Río Piedras: Editorial Huracán, 1994.

———. *La guerra después de la guerra.* Río Piedras: Editorial Huracán, 1987.

———. *Historia general de Puerto Rico.* Río Piedras: Editorial Huracán, 1986.

———. *Libertad y servidumbre en el Puerto Rico del siglo XIX: Los jornaleros utuadeños en vísperas del auge del café.* Río Piedras: Editorial Huracán, 1979.

Picot, Leonce, and Al Kocab. *Gourmet International's Recommended Restaurants of Puerto Rico.* Fort Lauderdale, Fla.: Research Unlimited, 1961.

Pilcher, Jeffrey M. "Tamales or Timbales: Cuisine and the Formation of Mexican National Identity, 1821–1911." *Americas* 53, no. 2 (October 1996): 193–216.

"Preveen alza en precios de carnes de Europa." *El Nuevo Día*, 15 March 2001.

Quintero Rivera, Ángel. "De la fiesta al festival: Los movimientos sociales para el disfrute de la vida en Puerto Rico." *Diálogos de la Comunicación: Revista Teórica de la Federación de Facultades de Comunicación Social*, no. 38 (January 1994): 97–107.

———. *Patricios y plebeyos: Burgueses, artesanos, hacendados y obreros; Las relaciones de clase en el Puerto Rico de cambio de siglo.* Río Piedras: Ediciones Huracán, 1988.

———. "Tablas de contabilización de festivales." Mimeograph. 1988.

Ramcharan, Christopher. "Culantro: A Much Utilized, Little Understood Herb." In *Perspectives on New Crops and New Uses*, edited by Jules Janick, 506–09. Alexandria, Va.: ASHS Press, 1999.

Ramos, Josean. "Por el suelo la cultura del agro." *Diálogo*, February 2001.

Ramos, Luz M., and Dorothy Bourne. *Rural Life in Puerto Rico.* San Juan: Department of Education, 1933.

Real Academia Española. *Diccionario de autoridades.* Facsimile ed. of 1726. 3 vols. Madrid: Editorial Gredos, 1963.

Real Díaz, José J., comp. *Catálogo de cartas y peticiones del cabildo de San Juan Bautista de Puerto Rico en el Archivo General de Indias, siglos XVI al XVIII.* San Juan: Municipio de San Juan/Instituto de Cultura Puertorriqueña, 1968.

Redon, Odile, et al. *Delicias de la gastronomía medieval.* Madrid: Anaya and Mario Muchnick, 1996.

"Reglamento sobre la educación, trato y ocupación que deben dar a los esclavos sus amos o mayordomos." 1825, 1826. In *Boletín histórico de Puerto Rico*, edited by Cayetano Coll y Toste, 10:262–73. San Juan: Tipografía Cantero Fernández, 1914–27.

"Reglas generales para la alimentación." *Revista de Agricultura de Puerto Rico* 41 (1950): 193–99.

Reitz, Elizabeth J. "Dieta y alimentación hispanoamericana en el Caribe y Florida." *Revista de Indias* 51, no. 191 (1991): 13–14.

"Relación del viaje a Puerto Rico de la expedición de Sir George Clifford." In *Crónicas de Puerto Rico: Desde el siglo XVI hasta nuestros días*, edited by Eugenio Fernández Méndez, 153. San Juan: Universidad de Puerto Rico, 1968.

"Relación del viaje a Puerto Rico de la expedición de Sir George Clifford, Tercer Conde de Cumberland, escrita por el Reverendo Doctor John Layfield, capellán de la expedición." In *Boletín histórico de Puerto Rico*, edited by Cayetano Coll y Toste, 5:49–70. San Juan: Tipografía Cantero Fernández, 1914–27.

Revel, Jean-François. *Un festín en palabras: Historia literaria de la sensibilidad gastronómica desde la antigüedad hasta nuestro días*. 3rd ed. [Madrid]: Editorial Tusquets, 1996.

Reynolds, Philip Keep. *The Banana: Its History, Cultivation, and Place among Staple Foods*. Boston: Houghton Mifflin, 1927.

Riollano, Arturo. "El cultivo de maíz dulce en Puerto Rico." *Revista de Agricultura de Puerto Rico* 37 (1946): 78.

———. "Maíz y arroz." *Revista de Agricultura de Puerto Rico* 30 (1938): 382.

Ritzer, George. *La McDonalización de la sociedad: Un análisis de la racionalización en la vida cotidiana*. Barcelona: Ariel, 2002.

Rivera Rivera, Antonia. *El Estado español y la beneficencia en el Puerto Rico del siglo XIX*. [Santo Domingo]: Editorial El Cuervo Dorado, 1995.

Roberts, Lydia Jane. "Deficiencias en la dieta típica y cómo corregirlas." *Revista de Agricultura de Puerto Rico* 43 (1952): 259–65.

———. *Mejor arroz, mejor salud*. San Juan: Departamento de Instrucción Pública, 1951.

———. "Nutrition in Puerto Rico." *Journal of the American Dietetics Association* 29 (1944): 298–304.

Roberts, Lydia Jane, and Rosa Luisa Stefani. *Patterns of Living in Puerto Rican Families*. The Puerto Rican Experience. New York: Arnos Press, 1975. [reprint of the 1949 ed. published by the University of Puerto Rico]

Robinson, Albert Gardner. *The Porto Rico of Today: Pen Pictures of the People and the Country*. New York: Charles Scribners and Sons, 1899.

Rodríguez de Zapata, Lillian. *Aceptación por el consumidor del arroz de grano largo producido localmente*. Río Piedras: Estación Experimental Agrícola de la Universidad de Puerto Rico, 1976.

———. *¿Qué patrones caracterizan a la familia puertorriqueña al comprar alimentos?* Río Piedras: Estación Experimental Agrícola, Recinto de Mayagüez, 1968.

Rodríguez Juliá, Edgardo. *Elogio de la fonda*. San Juan: Plaza Mayor, 2001.

Rodríguez Pacheco, Everlidys. "La siembra comercial de arroz en Puerto Rico." M.A. thesis, University of Puerto Rico, 1976.

Rodríguez Pastor, Julio. *Enfermedades de la nutrición, la digestión y el metabolismo.* San Juan: Departamento de Instrucción Pública, 1954.

Roqué de Duprey, Ana. *Luz y sombra.* Edited by Lizbeth Paravisin-Gebert. San Juan: Instituto de Cultura Puertorriqueña/Universidad de Puerto Rico, 1994.

Rosario Natal, Carmelo. *Los pobres y el 98 puertorriqueño: Lo que le pasó a la gente.* San Juan: Ediciones Históricas, 1998.

Russell Perkins, Janet. *The Leguminosae of Porto Rico.* Contributions from the United States National Herbarium, v. 10, pt. 4. Washington, D.C.: Government Printing Office, 1907.

Sama, Manuel María. *Bibliografía puertorriqueña.* Mayagüez: Tipografía Comercial, 1887.

Sanjur, Diva. *Social and Cultural Perspectives in Nutrition.* Englewood Cliffs, N.J.: Prentice-Hall, 1982.

Santana Rabel, Leonardo. *Historia de Vega Alta de Espinosa.* Santurce: Editorial La Torre del Viejo, 1988.

Scarano, Francisco. *Puerto Rico: Cinco siglos de historia.* San Juan: McGraw-Hill, 1993.

———. *Sugar and Slavery in Puerto Rico: The Plantation Economy of Ponce, 1800–1850.* Madison: University of Wisconsin Press, 1984.

Schlosser, Eric. *Fast-Food Nation: The Dark Side of the All-American Meal.* Boston: Houghton Mifflin, 2001.

Shapiro, Laura. *Perfection Salad: Women and Cooking at the Turn of the Century.* New York: Farrar, Straus and Giroux, 1995.

Sherman, Paul W., and Jennifer Billing. "Darwinian Gastronomy: Why We Use Spices." *Bio-Science* 40, no. 6 (June 1999): 453–63.

Simons, Julio S. "El cultivo del ñame en Puerto Rico." *Revista de Agricultura de Puerto Rico* 26 (1931): 204.

———. "Yautías y malangas: Su cultivo y producción para el mercado." *Revista de Agricultura de Puerto Rico* 25 (1930).

Stahl, Agustín. *Estudios sobre la flora de Puerto Rico.* 2nd ed. 3 vols. San Juan: Imprenta Venezuela, 1937.

Suárez, Ramón M. *Palabras e ideas: Artículos, ensayos, discursos y conferencias médico sociales, 1929–1965.* n.p.: n.p., n.d.

———. "Studies of the Nutritional Problem of Puerto Rico." *Porto Rico Journal of Public Health and Tropical Medicine* 19 (1943).

Sued Badillo, Jalil. "La valoración de las Salinas en la colonización de Puerto Rico." *Revista de Historia* 1, no. 1 (January-June 1985): 9–26.

"Sumaria averiguación instruida por orden de Su Excelencia por queja producida por cuatro siervos propiedad de Don José Martínez Díaz, hacendado de Guaynabo." *Anales de Investigación Histórica* 3, no. 1 (January-June 1976): 80–83.

Super, John C. *Food, Conquest, and Colonization in Sixteenth-Century Spanish America.* Albuquerque: University of New Mexico Press, 1988.

"Supermercados vs 'pantries.'" *El Nuevo Día,* 13 September, 1999.

Tannahill, Reay. *Food in History.* 4th ed. New York: Stein and Day, 1984.

Tapia y Rivera, Alejandro. *La leyenda de los veinte años: A orillas de rhin*. 6th ed. Colección Literaria Cervantes. Mexico City: Editorial Orión, 1967.

———, ed. *Biblioteca histórica de Puerto Rico, que contiene varios documentos de los siglos XV, XVI, XVII, XVIII*. San Juan: Imprenta de Márquez, 1854.

———, ed. *Mis memorias, o, San Juan como lo encontré y como lo dejo*. New York: DeLaisne and Rossboro, 1928.

Taylor, Clara Mae. *Foundations of Nutrition*. 6th ed. New York: Macmillan, 1966.

Téllez Iregui, Gustavo. *Pierre Bourdieu: Conceptos básicos y construccion socioeducativa, claves para su lectura*. Bogotá: Universidad Pedagógica Nacional, 2002.

Teuteberg, Hans, ed. *European Food History: A Research Review*. Leicester: Leicester University Press, 1992.

Tibbles, William. *Foods: Their Origin, Composition, and Manufacture*. London: Ballière, Tindall, and Cox, 1912.

Torres, Bibiano. *La isla de Puerto Rico, 1765–1800*. San Juan: Instituto de Cultura Puertorriqueña, 1969.

Torres, Rosa Marina. "Consideraciones acerca de los problemas de nutrición en un programa de producción de alimentos." *Revista de Agricultura de Puerto Rico* 43 (1952): 253–65.

———. *Tablas de dietética de un libro en preparación*. Río Piedras: Universidad de Puerto Rico, 1937.

Torres de Alba, María Luisa. "Testamentos en Lares, 1849–1899." *Anales de Investigación Histórica* 3, no. 1 (January-June 1976): 64–108.

Torres Díaz, Luis. "A Preliminary Study of Common Puerto Rican Diet." M.A. thesis, University of Puerto Rico, 1930.

Torres Vargas, Diego de. "Descripción de la isla y ciudad de Puerto Rico, y de su vecindad y poblaciones, presidio, gobernadores y obispos: Frutos y minerales." In *Crónicas de Puerto Rico: Desde el siglo XVI hasta nuestros días*, edited by Eugenio Fernández Méndez, 182. San Juan: Universidad de Puerto Rico, 1968.

Toussaint-Samat, Maguelonne. *A History of Food*. Oxford: Blackwell, 1992.

Trinidad, Pablo J. "Persiste el alza del costo de vida en la isla." *El Nuevo Día*, 27 April 1999.

Urry, John. *The Tourist Gaze: Leisure and Travel in Contemporary Societies*. 8th ed. London: Sage Publications, 1998.

Valldejuli, Carmen Aboy. *Cocina criolla*. [Boston?]: Alpine Press, 1954.

Valle Atiles, Francisco del. *Cartilla de Higiene*. [San Juan?]: Imprenta de José González Font, 1886.

Vaughan, J. G., and Catherine A. Geissler. *The New Oxford Book of Food Plants: A Guide to the Fruit, Vegetables, Herbs, and Spices of the World*. Oxford: Oxford University Press, 1997.

"Veinte años del Certamen del Buen Comer." *El Nuevo Día*, Suplemento Domingo, 9 December 2001.

Vila Vilar, Enriqueta. *Historia de Puerto Rico, 1600–1650*. Publicaciones de la Escuela de Estudios Hispano-Americanos no. 223. Seville: Escuela de Estudios Hispano-Americanos, 1974.

Villapol, Nitza. "Hábitos alimentarios africanos en América Latina." In África en América Latina, edited by Manuel Moreno Fraginals, 325–36. Mexico City: Siglo XXI, 1977.

Von Oppen, Achim. "Cassava: The 'Lazy Man's' Food? Indigenous Agricultural Innovation and Dietary Change in Northwestern Zambia, ca. 1650–1970." In Changing Food Habits: Case Studies from Africa, South America, and Europe, edited by Carola Lentz, 43–71. Amsterdam: Harwood Academic Publishers, 1999.

Walsh, Rob. "Untropical Fish: How the Coldwater Cod Became a Caribbean Staple." Natural History 105, no. 5 (May 1996).

Ward, Artemas. Encyclopedia of Food: The Stories of Foods by Which We Live, How and Where They Grow and Are Marketed, Their Comparative Values, and How Best to Use and Enjoy Them. New York: Baker and Taylor, 1923.

Warde, Alan. Consumption, Food, and Taste: Culinary Antinomies and Commodity Culture. London: Sage Publications, 1997.

———. "Production, Consumption, and Cultural 'Economy.'" In Cultural Economy: Cultural Analysis and Commercial Life, edited by Paul Du Gay and Michale Pryke, 185–200. Thousand Oaks, Calif.: Sage Publications, 2002.

———, and Lydia Martens. Eating Out: Social Differentiation, Consumption, and Pleasure. Cambridge: Cambridge University Press, 2000.

Watson Oliver, George. The Propagation of Tropical Food Trees and Other Plants. Washington, D.C.: Government Printing Office, 1903.

Wilk, Richard R. "Food and Nationalism: The Origins of 'Belizean' Food." In Food Nations: Selling Taste in Consumer Societies, edited by Warren Belasco and Philip Scranton, 67–87. New York: Routledge: 2002.

Willsey, Elsie Mae. Tropical Foods. University of Puerto Rico, Department of Home Economics, Bulletin no. 1. San Juan: Bureau of Supplies, Printing, and Transportation, 1925.

Wolf, Eric. "San José: Subcultures of a Traditional Coffee Municipality." In The People of Puerto Rico: A Study of Social Anthropology, edited by Julian Steward, 171–264. San Juan: University of Puerto Rico; Urbana-Champaign: University of Illinois Press, 1969.

Zeijo de Zayas, Esther. "El puertorriqueño puede alimentarse mejor." Revista de Agricultura de Puerto Rico 43 (1952): 256–79.

Zeno, Francisco Manuel. Historia de la capital de Puerto Rico, San Juan. Vol. 1. [San Juan]: Publicación Oficial del Gobierno de la Capital, 1951.

Zeno Gandía, Manuel. La charca. Biblioteca Popular. San Juan: Instituto de Cultura Puertorriqueña, 1968.

Index

Alegría, Ricardo, 288 (n. 13)
Alegrías de maíz, 84
Alfajor, 130, 262
Alfeñiques, 136, 262–63
Almojábanas, 16, 36, 263
Almuerzo, 263–64
Alonso, Manuel, 30
Álvarez Nazario, Manuel, 79, 88, 149, 270, 299 (n. 45)
Amarillos fritos, 157
Amato, Gus, 338 (n. 108)
American Heart Association, 337 (n. 100)
American South, 22
Amogolla'o (gummy), 27, 264
Amuyale, 311 (n. 49)
Anchovies, 107
Andalusian traditions: and almojábanas, 16, 36, 263; and rice pudding, 33; and sofrito, 62; and sweets, 83; and cornmeal cooking methods, 83–84; and fish, 101; and alboronía, 261; and alcapurrias, 262
Anexionismo jíbaro, 1
Annatto seeds: and rice casseroles, 28, 29; and sofrito, 61; and traditional foods, 245; and alcapurria, 262
Apastela'o, 218, 264–65
Apio (arracacha), 154
Aplatanarse, 145
Aponte, Luz Loriana, 194–95
Appadurai, Arjun, 208, 211, 279 (n. 21)
Arañitas, 147, 153, 157
Arawak population, 17, 126, 136, 261, 265, 269, 270
Archuri, Ortuño de, 163
Arepas, 95
Arepitas, 153
Argentina, 49, 189, 268, 322 (n. 88)
Arrieta, Raymond, 1
Arroces compuestos (rice casseroles), 28–31, 49, 218
Arroces húmedos dulces, 32–36, 44
Arroz apastela'o, 28–29
Arroz blanco criollo, 27, 247
Arroz con bacalao, 96
Arroz con coco (coconut rice), 34–35, 36
Arroz con dulce, 35, 84, 152, 257
Arroz con jueyes, 271
Arroz con leche (rice milk), 36

Arroz con perico, 35
Arroz con salchichas, 275
Arvejas (snap peas), 65
Asenjo, Conrado F., 293 (n. 66)
Asian colonies, rice cultivation in, 39, 284 (n. 59)
Asopao, 31, 32, 44, 49, 219, 265, 275
Astol, Eugenio, 314 (n. 73)
Ata, 62
Atlantic cod (Gadus morhua), 98–99, 101, 106, 118, 247, 307 (n. 76), 308 (n. 77)
Ayala, Alfredo, 236
Aymard, Maurice, 299–300 (n. 51)

Bacalaítos, 96, 254, 269
Bacalao guisado (codfish stew), 107
Badillo, Jalil Sued, 165–66
Balanzas Mercantiles, 107, 250, 313 (n. 72)
Banana leaves: and tamales, 78; and yams, 138, 311 (n. 49); and pastel, 150–51
Bananas. See Plantains and bananas
Bankers Club, 215
Baralt, Guillermo, 304 (n. 33)
Bash, Edward J., 41–42
Basque people, 96, 98, 101
Batata política, 137
Battuta, al-Qazwini e Ibn, 55
Bean and legume cooking methods: seasoning of, 51; and sofrito, 51, 59–65, 75–76, 291 (nn. 50, 52); stewing, 60, 289 (n. 31); and red beans, 65–71, 248; soaking, 69–70, 76, 248, 257; and cooking time, 73, 74
Bean and legume cultivation: and Taíno people, 51, 52–54, 55; and African-origin communities, 51, 54–56, 57, 59, 75; and soil enrichment, 54, 57; in South America, 56–57; and tobacco cultivation, 57, 289 (n. 24); and domestic use, 58–59; local production, 66, 67–68, 71, 73, 75, 147, 248, 292 (n. 58); red beans, 66, 67–68, 248
Beans and legumes: red or kidney beans, 4, 51, 65–75, 76, 248, 272, 273, 294–95 (n. 84); as standard food item, 5, 39, 40, 50, 51, 65, 75, 245, 332 (n. 66); and rice casseroles, 30; and dietary habits, 51, 52–53, 56–57, 58, 59; importing of, 52–53,

66, 67, 68, 71, 73, 75, 76; and food insecurity, 53; storage and distribution of,
53; consumption of, 55, 66–67, 69, 71–75,
252, 253, 292 (n. 62), 292–93 (n. 65); and
dietary simplification, 66; nutritional
content of, 67, 69, 70–71, 74, 112, 231, 293
(n. 66); and flatulence, 69, 293 (n. 69).
See also Rice and beans
Beck, Ulrich, 229–30, 327 (n. 30)
Beef: as standard food item, 5, 39; jerked,
81, 88, 108, 268; nutritional value of,
112; salted, 164, 322 (n. 84); cured, 168,
189–90, 268; and contraband market,
173, 319 (n. 41); availability of, 184, 185,
186–87, 332 (n. 68); superiority of, 187;
imports of, 189, 190, 322 (n. 88); price of,
191, 324 (n. 119); consumption of, 192,
195, 196, 246, 333 (n. 68); corned, 255,
260, 267–68
Beer, consumption of, 50–51
Belasco, Warren, 11, 279 (n. 23)
Bell, David, 242, 260, 327 (n. 26)
Bergara, Diego de, 163
Berrios, Rubén, 1
Biasin, Gian-Paolo, 281–82 (n. 32)
Billing, Jennifer, 289–90 (n. 33)
Bizcos (cross-eyed), 55
Black beans, 76, 294–95 (n. 84)
Bocadito de batata, 156
Bocado de batata, 136, 266
Body Mass Index (BMI), 336 (n. 97)
Bolitas, 36, 156
Bonafoux Quintero, Luis, 87–88, 149, 298
(n. 30), 298–99 (n. 40)
Bonanza restaurant chain, 221, 332 (n. 66)
Borínquen (red bean), 71, 293 (n. 72)
Boronía, 261
Bourdieu, Pierre, 155, 157, 209–10, 213
Brau, Salvador, 109
Braudel, Ferdinand, 138
Brazil, 127, 189, 268, 309 (n. 8)
Bread: from corn, 80, 81, 246, 295 (n. 13);
from cassava, 124–25, 126, 127, 128–29,
130, 132, 246, 309 (n. 13); fufu resem-
bling, 137; price of, 161; food products
producing, 295 (n. 13)
Breadfruit (*Artocarpus altilis*), 99, 116, 122,
124, 154, 269

Breadfruit Festival, 219, 315 (n. 96)
Bricolage-cuisine, 9, 61
British Antilles, 103, 106, 107
Brookings Institution, 289 (n. 24)
Budín de arroz, 33
Budín de yuca, 130
Buñeulitos, 156
Buñuelo de maíz veracruzano, 84
Buñuelos, 84, 136
Buñuelos de arroz (rice fritters), 36
Burén, 126, 127, 131, 265
Burger King, 221, 225, 226, 227, 335 (nn. 79,
89), 336 (n. 95), 337 (nn. 99, 100)
Burgos, Norma, 1

Caballero, Pepita, 85
Cabanillas, Berta, 12, 46, 65, 150, 154,
281 (n. 25), 282 (n. 45), 291 (n. 52), 297
(n. 28), 312 (n. 55)
Ca da Mosto, Luis, 55
Cajeta de piña cubana, 136
Campeche, José, 101
Campesinos: and bean and legume cultivation, 58, 59, 68; and cornmeal cooking
methods, 85, 88, 109; and codfish, 107,
108–9, 115; sweet potato cultivation,
134–35; and plantains, 143–44, 145,
146–47; and viandas, 160; and open
lands, 180; and pigs as livestock, 185–86;
and pork, 185–86, 188–89; and beef, 187;
and meat consumption, 194, 320 (n. 52);
corn cultivation, 296 (n. 19)
Canada, 110, 111, 306 (n. 54), 307 (n. 76),
308 (n. 77)
Canary Islands, 83, 138, 164, 173, 270, 297
(n. 24)
Candelario, Blas, 187
Candolle, Alphonse de, 311 (n. 52)
Cannecatim, Bernarde María de, 299 (n. 45)
Capers, 61, 62
Capitalism: consumer capitalism, 199;
disorganized form of, 203–4; and hybrid
cultural practices, 207
Capsicum annum (green pepper), 61
Capsicum chinense (sweet pepper), 61
Caribbean: and identity, 76; trade in,
102–3, 104, 106–7; tourism of, 213–14;
traditional foodstuffs of, 245; ships

Coconut oil: cornmeal combined with, 81, 82; and codfish, 305 (n. 48)

Coconuts: cultivation of, 146, 147; mechanizing processing of, 313 (n. 72)

Codfish, salted: introduction of, 3–4, 254; as standard food item, 5, 39, 96, 99–103, 110, 114, 120, 246–47; as supplementary food, 5, 100, 101, 103, 113, 115, 278 (n. 11); and brothy rice dishes, 32; and guanimes, 78, 270; and funche, 81, 87–88, 116, 296 (n. 17); cornmeal combined with, 81–82; consumption of, 96–97, 103, 111–15, 116, 117–20, 245, 246–47, 267, 306 (n. 62), 307 (n. 73); nutritional value of, 97, 99, 103–4, 109, 112; imports of, 97, 104–5, 108, 110–11, 112, 113, 117, 118–19, 120, 306 (nn. 54, 55); colloquial expressions related to, 97, 105, 162, 304–5 (n. 37); commercial cod trade, 98, 102–3, 104, 105–7, 110–11; species of, 98–99, 105–7, 118–19, 305 (n. 41); drying, 99, 105, 106; convenience of use factor, 100–101; as peripheral food, 108–10, 112, 113, 115, 247; and dietary simplification, 110; as condiment, 113–14; and social differences, 215–16

Codfish cooking methods: and alboronía, 96; codfish stew, 96, 107, 119; serenata, 96, 107, 119, 120; salted cod a la vizcaína, 96, 115, 119; desalting, 96, 305 (n. 48), 306 (n. 62); seasoning, 107–8, 115; marinating in oil, 115; salted cod in cream sauce, 115

Cod Wars, 307 (n. 76)

Coffee cultivation: effect on rice cultivation, 39; and large-scale agriculture, 104, 146; effect on wild pigs, 184

Colmados (grocery stores), 267, 292–93 (n. 65)

Colombia, 152, 159, 263, 273, 314–15 (n. 87)

Colón, Bartolomé, 163

Colón, Diego, 165

Colón, Emilio M., 281 (n. 25)

Colonial model: and exportation of food products, 5; food and cooking in relation to, 9; and gold mining, 18, 19, 52, 287 (n. 5)

Colorá (red or kidney beans), 4, 51, 65–75, 76, 248, 294–95 (n. 84)

Columbus, Christopher, 137, 163

Comidas Puertorriqueñas (festival), 219

Committee on Nutrition, 44, 46

Community: national community, 208; meaning of, 327 (n. 26)

Compañía de Fomento de Puerto Rico, 330 (n. 49)

Competencia de Comida Criolla, 219

Complementary foods: definition of, 5, 99–100, 278 (n. 10); cassava adopted in Africa, 19, 280 (n. 8); and rice, 48, 100, 142, 286 (n. 90); and codfish, 121; and cornmeal, 142

ConAgra, 231

Conchillos, Lope, 166

Congrí, 257

Consumer capitalism, 199

Consumer price index, 233, 339 (n. 122)

Consumption: and individualization, 203, 204, 205, 210, 212; and market segments, 203–4. See also Food consumption patterns; and specific types of foods

Convenience foods, 73, 294 (n. 80)

Cook, Ian, 206, 326–27 (n. 22)

Cook, Oratio Fuller, 144

Cooking: and definition of cuisine, 7–8; women as distinguished cooks, 32–33, 35–36, 85–86, 88, 189, 219; specialization of, 200; professionalization of, 211, 214, 219, 329 (n. 48); loss of basic ideas and principles of, 221; and dietetics, 222–23, 333–34 (n. 69); elements of, 242, 249. See also Bean and legume cooking methods; Codfish cooking methods; Cornmeal cooking methods; Rice cooking methods; Traditional home cooking

Coquí (tree frog), 47

Cordero Badillo, Atilano, 224, 239

Córdoba, Pedro Tomás de, 132, 299 (n. 48)

Core-fringe-legume matrix, 5, 108, 278–79 (n. 12)

Corn: as standard food item, 5, 79, 80–81, 93, 100, 109, 140, 245; as rations in African slave trade, 19; storage and distribution of, 53; representations of, 77–78; types of, 79; bread from, 80, 81, 246, 295 (n. 13); and dietary simplification, 81; for feeding domestic fowl and animals, 82; mechanizing processing of, 313 (n. 72)

Dogs, wild cattle killed by, 318 (n. 37), 320–21 (n. 65)

Dolores, José, 31

Dominican Republic, 159, 160, 256–57, 333 (n. 68), 335 (n. 79), 341 (n. 6)

Domino's Pizza, 225

Dooley, Eliza, 34, 85–86, 150, 152, 154, 282 (nn. 38, 45), 290 (n. 35), 297 (n. 28), 298 (n. 33), 315 (n. 88), 333 (n. 69)

Double commodity fetishism, 206

Dulce de coco, 84, 297 (n. 30)

Dulce de jícama, 136

Easter Holy Week, 120

Economic differences: food and cooking in relation to, 6, 12, 209, 245; and rice cooking methods, 26, 27, 29, 30, 33, 34–35, 37; and sofrito, 61, 76; and cornmeal, 78, 81–82; and cornmeal cooking methods, 87–92, 93, 301 (n. 61); and codfish, 104, 105–6, 107, 109, 111, 114–16, 119–20, 247; and plantains, 140; and meat consumption, 183, 186, 191, 197, 246; and food distribution, 201; and food consumption patterns, 232–36

Economic Society of Friends of the Country, 146

Ecuador, 159

Edgerton, David, 335 (n. 89)

Egypt, 49

El Certamen del Buen Comer (Fine Dining Contest), 215

El cocinero puertorriqueño: on rice preparation, 25, 38; manjar blanco criollo, 33, 34, 282 (n. 42); on bean and legume cooking methods, 65; and majarete, 86–87, 282 (n. 45), 297 (n. 28), 298 (n. 37); and codfish cooking methods, 115; and cassava, 129; and tannier, 133; and sweet potatoes, 136; and plantains, 148, 149–50; and mofongo, 149–50; editions of, 250–51; and cazuela, 266; dating of first edition, 281 (n. 25); and sofrito, 290 (n. 35); and preservation of meat, 322 (n. 84); and dietetics, 333–34 (n. 69)

El Día, 330 (n. 49)

Electric stoves, 199

Elite: and rice casseroles, 29, 247; and codfish, 107, 115–16, 307 (n. 73); and viandas, 123; and cassava, 129; and plantains, 140, 145–46, 147, 148; and meat consumption, 191; and novelty in food consumption, 213; and haute cuisine, 215–16; and food consumption patterns, 235–36, 250; and beans and legumes, 293 (n. 69)

El Jibarito, San Juan, 254

El Mundo, 330 (n. 49)

El Nuevo Día, 1, 2, 330–31 (n. 49)

El Universal (restaurant), 213, 329 (n. 44)

Encomienda, 163–64, 165, 287 (nn. 5, 6)

England, 102–3, 104, 106, 107, 216, 247

Enlightenment, 101, 141

Enslaved African labor: role in food production, 9, 18, 19, 20, 63; rice as basic food for, 17, 19–20, 37, 90, 141, 142, 283 (n. 52); and rice cultivation, 18, 19, 20, 21, 54, 247; food rations of, 19, 88, 90, 137, 141–42, 168, 170, 177, 186–87, 245, 246, 249, 269, 274, 312–13 (n. 62), 318 (n. 32); work ethic of, 21; plots and gardens of, 22, 55, 90, 141, 312 (n. 62); and indigenous population, 54, 55–56, 75; and sugar cultivation, 54, 81, 89, 103, 168, 186–87, 312–13 (n. 62); population of, 54, 141, 297 (n. 24), 299 (n. 46); and bean and legume cultivation, 54–56; and sofrito, 63; corn as basic food for, 81, 318 (n. 32); and cornmeal, 88, 89–90, 93, 142; codfish in diet of, 100, 103–4, 108, 141, 142, 247, 304 (n. 33); cassava as basic food for, 127, 318 (n. 32); plantains as basic food for, 140, 141, 142, 143, 149; meat as basic food for, 141, 142, 170, 186–87, 318 (n. 32); productivity of, 141–42; and cattle, 168; and gold mining labor, 170, 318 (n. 32). See also Runaway slaves

Epa, 311 (n. 49)

Ephedrine, 230

Escuela Hotelera, 214, 329 (n. 48)

Estenós, Felipe Ramírez de, 177

Estévez, Domingo, 21

Estrada, Epifania, 91, 300 (n. 57)

Exercise, 230, 338 (n. 108)

Fabes (fava beans), 52

Fano, Vicente A., 146

Fast Food Nutrition Explorer, 337 (n. 100)
Fast food restaurant culture: emergence of, 200, 204–5; Mcdonalización, 204–6, 218, 221, 243, 272; and efficiency, 205; self-service offered by, 205, 226; and public school dining halls, 220; and indulgence, 224–25; proliferation of, 225, 227, 335 (n. 79); meals taken in, 226, 335 (n. 86); marketing strategy, 226–27, 228, 229, 336 (n. 94), 337 (n. 99); and social identity, 228; and supersizing portions, 228, 337 (n. 99); nutritional shortcomings of, 228–29; prices of, 234

Favichiela, 52

Federal Emergency Relief Act, 300 (n. 58)

Ferguson, Grace J., 31, 129, 133, 150, 153, 191, 266, 323 (n. 96)

Fésoles, 52, 59

Festival de Comida Típica de Loíza, 219

Festival de la Pana, 315 (n. 97)

Festival de La Yuca, 315 (n. 97)

Festival Nacional del Plátano, 315 (n. 97)

Festivals: and rice casseroles, 30–32; and meat consumption, 186, 193–94; and traditional foods, 218–19; and pork, 219, 246; and apastela'o, 265; and viandas, 315 (nn. 96, 97)

Festive gatherings: rice cooking methods, 29–32; and cornmeal cooking methods, 84–85, 87; and pork, 183, 185, 188–89, 193–94, 246

Fischler, Claude: definition of cuisine, 7–8; on mothers' cuisine, 37, 156–57; on complementary foods, 99–100, 278 (n. 10); on meat consumption, 197; on food autonomy, 202; and homogeneity, 207; on culinary terminology, 215; on food critics, 215; on high-end effect, 215, 216, 257; on dietetics, 222, 333–34 (n. 69); on time spent eating, 225–26; on home dining table, 242; on culinary influences, 255–56, 258; on supplementary foods, 278 (n. 11), 317 (n. 28); on decline of characteristic foods, 286 (n. 89)

Fish: and ciguatera, 92, 266–67; fresh, 100, 102, 104, 111, 112; availability of, 171, 173; price of, 234. *See also specific types of fish*

Flan de coco (caramelized coconut custard), 50

Flandrin, Jean-Louis, 251, 279 (n. 23)

Fondas, 268, 275, 328 (n. 39)

Fondo de cocina (seasoning base), 60, 63

Food: and representation of social reality, 1–2, 209; as representation of history, 2, 3, 208; definition of, 4, 241; historiography of, 10–14, 279 (n. 23); prices of, 161, 191, 193, 233–35, 324 (n. 119), 324 (n. 122); distribution of, 201–2; social and spatial contexts of, 206, 209–10, 219

Food and Foodways, 10

Food consumption patterns: historiography of, 10–14; indicators of, 11; studies of, 12; theories of, 56–57, 108, 200, 201–12; and social and material progress, 191–92, 322–23 (n. 93); democratization of, 196–97, 198; cultural influence on, 197–98; and traditional foodstuff, 200, 208, 216–21, 231–32, 233, 236, 241, 243, 252, 253, 327 (nn. 30, 31); continuity in, 201, 257; cultural and material differences in, 209; and novelty, 213–21, 329–31 (n. 49); imagined culinary pasts, 217, 219; and health and indulgence, 220, 221–32, 234, 235, 240, 333–34 (n. 69); and economy and ostentation, 232–36, 240, 339 (n. 122), 339–40 (n. 128); and convenience and care, 236–44, 341 (n. 144)

Food critics, 215, 329–31 (n. 49), 331 (n. 52), 339–40 (n. 128)

Foodies, 216

Food-importation market: food and cooking in relation to, 6; and rice, 17–18, 38, 39, 43, 45, 46, 47–48, 49, 111, 247–48, 280 (n. 3), 284 (n. 59); and rice cooking methods, 35, 37, 38; and beans and legumes, 52–53, 66, 67, 68, 71, 73, 75, 76; and snack foods, 94, 333 (n. 68); and codfish, 97, 104–5, 108, 110–11, 112, 113, 117, 118–19, 120, 306 (nn. 54, 55); and mackerel, 101, 106, 107, 171; and shrimp, 120; and viandas, 123, 159, 160; and potatoes, 157; and beef, 189, 190, 322 (n. 88); dependence on, 200, 213; and tradition in food consumption, 220; and novelty in food

165, 287 (n. 5), 288 (nn. 7, 10); indigenous peoples as laborers in, 164, 165–66, 316 (n. 12); and food insecurity, 165, 166; role in New World, 168, 303 (n. 27); and enslaved African labor, 170, 318 (n. 32)

González, Gaspar, 183

González, Michael, 339 (n. 120)

González, Velda, 1

González Chacón, Norman, 324 (n. 120), 324–25 (n. 121)

González Dávila, Gil, 125

Goody, Jack, 279 (n. 21)

Goya Foods, 94–95

Gran Cocinamiento (Great Cookoff), 215

Granitos, 16, 36

Great Depression, 41, 68, 324 (n. 119)

Greater Antilles, 138

Guanimes, 78, 91, 95, 130, 246, 257, 270

Guariquitén, 126, 269

Guía de política pública para la vente de alimentos en las escuelas (Public Policy Guide for the Sale of Food in the Schools), 241

Gunni, 311 (n. 49)

Gutiérrez, Elías, 16

Habichuela blanca, 60

Habichuelas, 51, 52, 68, 287 (n. 1)

Habichuelas guisadas ablandadas (soaked stewed beans), 257

Haddock (Melanogrammus aeglefinus), 98, 99, 117, 118–19

Hake (Urophicis chuss), 98, 106, 107, 117, 118, 308 (n. 77)

Hallacas, 152, 315 (nn. 87, 88)

Hamm, Margherita, 63, 64

Hanseatic League, 303 (n. 14)

Harris, Marvin, 5, 56

Haute cuisine, 213–16, 221–22, 236, 250–51, 329–31 (n. 49), 331 (n. 52), 334 (n. 69), 339–40 (n. 128)

Health consequences of food choices: guidelines for, 16, 71, 207, 231, 234, 245; and obesity, 200, 203, 222, 228, 229–31, 232, 336 (n. 97), 338 (n. 108); and food consumption patterns, 220, 221–32, 234, 235, 240, 333–34 (n. 69)

Henríquez, Miguel, 126, 250

Henry, Guy V., 161

Hermandinquer, Jean Jacques, 323 (n. 107)

Herrera, Antonio de, 308–9 (n. 4)

Herring: and funche, 81; and cornmeal, 82; as supplementary food, 100; market for, 106, 107, 303 (n. 14); as cured fish, 109; as import, 171

Hervor de sonrisa (gentle boil), 60

Higman, Barry, 10, 279 (n. 21)

Hipermarcados, 5, 92, 93, 199, 216, 224–25, 239, 267, 325–26 (n. 2), 339 (n. 122)

Hispaniola, 52, 53, 164, 311 (n. 45), 318 (n. 37)

History: food as representation of, 2, 3, 208; and historiography of food, 10–14, 279 (n. 23)

Hobsbawm, Eric, 208–9, 217–18, 327 (n. 31)

Home Making (Ferguson): and cassava, 129; and tannier, 133; and mofongo, 150; and plantains, 153; and meat consumption, 191; and cazuela, 266

Horses, and Spanish colonists, 164, 171

Hospital patients, rice in diet of, 37, 283 (n. 52)

Human body, aesthetic of, 229–30, 259

Hurricanes, 41, 139, 174–75, 266, 318 (n. 39)

Huyke, Giovanna, 220, 229, 243–44, 338 (n. 105)

Identity: food and cooking as vehicle for self-representation of, 2, 3, 9; and abstention from meat, 100; social, 228. See also National identity

Income levels, 200, 223

India, 208

Indigenous peoples: agriculture of, 17, 18, 52–54, 288 (n. 7); and corn cultivation, 18, 52, 75, 79, 288 (n. 7); and cassava cultivation, 18, 52, 124–25, 130, 288 (n. 7); women of, 53, 288 (nn. 7, 10); and enslaved African labor, 54, 55–56, 75; and bean and legume cultivation, 54, 56–57, 75; and bean and legume cooking methods, 61–62; and sweet potatoes, 132; and tannier, 132; as laborers in gold mining, 164, 165–66, 316 (n. 12); culinary knowledge of, 249

Infants. See Children

Infiernillo, 87, 298 (n. 37)

Manso, Alonso, 18, 125, 250, 280 (n. 4)

Mantengo (maintenance), 91

Manton, Catherine, 334 (n. 69)

Manual del comedor escolar, 192, 284 (n. 53), 323 (n. 97)

Manzanillo, 29

Marifinga, 92, 252, 271, 301 (n. 64)

Maroon communities, 20. *See also* Runaway slaves

Marota, 92, 252, 271–72, 301 (n. 64)

Marriage customs, 30

Martens, Lydia, 211–12

Martin, Ricky, 1

Martínez, José, 187, 283 (n. 52), 312–13 (n. 62)

Mata, Juan de la, *Arte de repostería*, 282 (n. 42)

Matahambre, 144

Mata puercos, 194

Matos, Alejo, 184

Matrimonio, 72, 272

Mazamorra, 92, 272, 297 (n. 28), 301 (n. 64)

McDonald's, 221, 225, 226, 227, 272, 332 (n. 65), 335 (n. 79), 336 (n. 95), 337 (nn. 99, 100)

Mcdonalización, 204–6, 218, 221, 243, 272

McLamore, James W., 335 (n. 89)

McNeal, James U., 336 (n. 92)

Meat: and changes in rural environment, 4, 161–62; as standard food item, 10; beliefs toward consumption of, 13; and brothy rice dishes, 32; abstention from, 33, 35, 97, 100, 101–2, 103, 104, 120, 171, 173, 275, 303 (n. 22), 318 (n. 34); canned, 46, 116, 163, 192, 194, 195, 255, 275, 323 (n. 98); and food preferences, 56; preservation of, 61, 117, 164–65, 171, 172, 192, 289–90 (n. 33), 322 (n. 84); cornmeal combined with, 81; and funche, 90; in core-fringe-legume matrix, 108, 279 (n. 12); food ordinances on, 128, 296 (n. 13); in food rations for enslaved African labor, 141, 142, 170, 186–87, 318 (n. 32); and plantains, 153; and viandas, 155; price of, 161, 191, 193, 234, 324 (n. 119); and popular sayings, 162; consumption of, 162–63, 167, 169–73, 176–77, 183–92, 193, 194–98, 216, 246, 318 (nn. 35, 39), 323 (n. 97); as supplementary food, 169; availability of, 176–77, 184, 187, 188–89, 193, 197, 198, 246; contamination of, 183–84, 186, 187–88; as desired food, 183–89, 196, 197, 198; imports of, 189, 190, 194, 332 (n. 88); progress associated with, 191–92, 196–97, 198; substitutes for, 192, 323 (n. 96); and mixta, 273. *See also* Beef; Pork; Poultry

Medalla brewery commercial, 50–51

Medicinal use of plants, 61

Medina Molera, Antonio, 262

Melao (sugarcane syrup), 82, 272–73

Meléndez Muñoz, Miguel, 146

Memory. *See* Palate's memories

Men: and women as distinguished cooks, 36; beer consumption of, 50; and women's use of sofrito, 60–61; and women associated with meat, 162; as professional chefs, 214

Méndez, Sarah, 297 (n. 28)

Méndez Quiñones, Ramón, 30, 297–98 (n. 30), 321 (n. 73)

Menéndez Valdés, Pedro, 171

Mennell, Stephen, 6–7, 8, 201–2, 205, 209, 210

Menudencias, 128, 296 (n. 13)

Mestizos: and rice cooking methods, 25; and arroces húmedos dulces, 35; and bean and legume cultivation, 55, 57, 58, 59; and cassava bread, 125; and cassava cultivation, 127; seasonings in cooking, 136; and plantains, 148, 153; and corn-meal cooking methods, 246, 298 (n. 40)

Mexico, 152, 262, 314–15 (n. 87), 335 (n. 79)

Meyners, Arnaldo, 330 (n. 49)

Milk, consumption of, 193

Millstones, 82

Mintz, Sidney: definition of cuisine, 7, 8–10; on regional cooking, 9, 256; on rice, 19–20; on inventiveness, 63, 169, 317 (n. 28); on matrix of food consumption, 108, 112; on public school dining halls, 195

Mixta, 273

Mofongo, 137, 149–50, 155, 157, 219, 266, 273–74, 332 (n. 66)

Molinos de Puerto Rico, 94–95

Mona, 52

Monoculture, and exportation of food products, 5, 184, 249

Montanari, Massimo: on inventions and influences, 2; on archival material, 11; on historiography of food, 12, 279 (n. 23); on culture of fear of famine, 13–14, 223; on food security/insecurity, 202; on nutritional excess, 202–3; on diet, 203, 222; on symbolic role of food, 295 (n. 13); on codfish, 303 (n. 14); on abstention from meat, 318 (n. 34)

Morales Otero, Pablo, 292 (n. 62), 296 (n. 17)

Moscoso, Francisco, 320 (n. 56)

Mosquera, Antonio de, 80, 140

Mothers' cuisine, 37, 46, 155–57, 211, 220

Mountains: unbranded hogs in, 167–68, 174, 184, 245; and wild cattle, 168–69, 171, 174, 245, 318 (n. 37); and outlaw population, 174; hunting in, 175, 178, 180, 320 (n. 64); as source of foodstuffs for urban areas, 177

Moya Pons, Frank, 304 (n. 27)

Mozárabes, 52

Muesas, Miguel de, 128, 182

Mulatto descendants: of aboriginal population, 25; of slaves, 90

al-Mullabi, 55

Mundo nuevo, 84–86, 94, 297 (nn. 28, 30), 301 (n. 64)

Muñoz, Vicente, 161, 162

Musacae family, 138, 311–12 (n. 52), 312 (nn. 53, 55). See also Plantains and bananas

Music, "Arroz con leche" song, 36

Ñame, 124

National identity: food associated with, 1, 2, 231, 252, 258, 260; and rice, 47; and puertorriqueñidad, 64, 152; and beans and rice, 74–75; and codfish, 121; and plantains, 148–50; and viandas, 160

Newfoundland, 101, 102, 106, 110, 303 (n. 14)

Ngfungi, 89–90

Nicaragua, 273

Nieves, José, 332 (n. 65)

Nísperos de batata, 136

Nola, Ruperto de, Libro de cocina, 34, 282 (n. 42)

Norway, 107

Nouvelle criollo, 222, 330 (n. 49)

Nouvelle cuisine, 236

Nuevo caribe, 158

Nuevo criollo cooking, 92, 222

Nuevo latino, 158

Nutritional assistance programs, 91, 199, 212, 258, 268, 275

Nutritional disorders, 230, 231

Nutrition Assistance Program (PAN), 16, 235, 241

Obesity, 200, 203, 222, 228, 229–31, 232, 336 (n. 97), 338 (n. 108)

Olive oil, 305 (n. 48)

Oller, Francisco, El velorio (The Wake), 77–78

Oranges, 147

O'Reilly, Alejandro, 145, 175–76

Organoleptic factors: and rice casseroles, 28; and codfish, 113; and meat consumption, 325 (n. 121)

Ortiz, Ángel, 340 (n. 129)

Ortíz, Fernando, 92

Ortiz, Secundina, 92, 301 (n. 61)

Oryza glaberrima, cultivation of, 18, 19, 20, 54

Oryza sativa, 17, 19, 20–21

Outlaw population, 174

Oviedo, Fernández de: on beans, 52, 59; on corn, 80; on cassava, 126, 309 (n. 13); on tannier, 132; on sweet potatoes, 134, 310 (n. 39); on yams, 137, 311 (n. 45); on pigs, 166, 167, 317 (n. 19); on gold mining, 287 (n. 5), 288 (n. 7); on plantains, 312 (n. 55)

Pacheco, Xavier, 257

Paddleford, Clementine, 330 (n. 49)

Palate's memories: and bond with food and diet, 2–3, 51; and sofrito, 61; and immigration, 65, 75; and cornmeal cooking methods, 85; and sweets, 85; and World War II food rationing, 90–91; and funche, 91, 92, 117; and codfish, 117, 120; and serenata, 121; and cassava, 131; and viandas, 156; influences on, 220, 253, 255–58

Palm oil (Elaeis guineensis), 62, 261

Palm trees, 319 (n. 45)

160; salted, 164–65, 189–90, 194, 316–17 (n. 14), 322 (n. 84); consumption of, 166, 184, 185, 186, 192–93, 195, 196, 246, 333 (n. 68); cured, 168; and contraband market, 173, 319 (n. 41); and festive gatherings, 183, 185, 188–89, 193–94, 246; imports of, 190; and festivals, 219, 246; price of, 324 (n. 119); availability of, 332 (n. 68)

The Porto Rican Cookbook: and cassava, 129; and tannier, 133; and plantains, 153

Portugal, 102, 106, 127, 309 (n. 8)

Potatoes: viandas compared to, 157, 216; and plantains, 158; as complement food, 286 (n. 90). See also Sweet potatoes

Poultry: consumption of, 155, 198, 325 (n. 122); raising of, 193; price of, 234; availability of, 332 (n. 68). See also Chicken; Turkey, consumption of

Power relations: and meat consumption, 170, 186, 194; and new foods, 317 (n. 28)

Power y Giralt, Ramón, 101

Prisoners: rice in diet of, 37, 283 (n. 52), 284 (n. 53); cassava in diet of, 140; plantains in diet of, 140

Professional Market Research, 226, 239

Public schools: cooking classes, 30–31, 115, 129, 133, 154, 191, 323 (n. 95); dining halls, 46, 75, 90, 115–16, 192, 194–95, 212, 220, 241, 268, 275, 283 (n. 52), 294 (n. 82), 340–41 (n. 143); social etiquette, 88; home economics curriculum, 191–92, 323 (n. 96)

Publish Records Inc., 227

Pudín de maíz seco, 84

Pueblo International, 224

Puerto Rican Cookbook (Dooley): and majarete, 86, 152, 297 (n. 28); and cassava, 130; and mofongo, 150; and pastel, 152; and viandas, 154; and sofrito, 290 (n. 35); and dietetics, 333 (n. 69)

Puerto Rican cookery: development of, 9; changes and continuities in, 13, 250, 251–58, 260; sofrito's role in, 28, 64, 65. See also Bean and legume cooking methods; Codfish cooking methods; Cornmeal cooking methods; Rice cooking methods; Traditional home cooking

Puerto Rican culinary culture: formation of, 6, 8; and rice cooking methods, 25–26; nutritional value of, 231, 249; preferences for, 232, 252–53; factors shaping, 249–53, 258–60; introduction of non-Caribbean dishes, 254; traditional foodstuffs in, 255–58, 260; suspension effect, 256, 257, 258; immigrants' contributions to, 256–57; and generational differences, 258; and eating outside the home, 259

Puerto Rico: population of, 39, 104, 170, 177, 184, 256, 284 (n. 60), 297 (n. 24), 341 (n. 6); shipping routes, 102, 103, 124, 168, 173, 303–4 (n. 27); as colony of United States, 110, 191, 306 (n. 53); as military post, 168, 249; modernizing project, 326 (n. 2)

Puerto Rico Emergency Relief Administration (PRERA), 91, 300 (n. 58)

Puerto Rico Food Commission, 285 (n. 68)

Puerto Rico Ilustrado, 329–30 (n. 49)

Puerto Rico: La grand cocina del Caribe, 256

Puertorriqueña de navidades, 16

Puertorriqueñidad, 64, 152

Pumpkin (Cucúrbitae pepo), 265–66

Quebec, 110

Quintero Rivera, Ángel, 217, 218–19, 299 (n. 40), 315 (n. 97)

Race and race relations: and funche, 90, 298–99 (n. 40); and cassava, 126; and yams, 137

Ramcharan, Christopher, 290 (n. 37)

Recao, 61, 62, 63, 261, 274–75, 290 (nn. 35, 37)

Refrigerators and refrigeration, 97, 111, 116, 191, 192, 197, 199, 290 (n. 33)

Republic of China, 49, 308 (n. 77)

Restaurancitos criollos, 211–12, 328 (n. 39)

Revel, Jean-François, 214

Rey, César, 294 (n. 82)

Rhizobium genus, 57

Rice: as standard food item, 5, 10, 15–17, 23, 25, 32, 37, 39, 40, 41–42, 43, 46, 47–49, 50, 51, 99, 100, 120, 245, 284 (n. 59), 332 (n. 66); and food insecurity, 17, 37–38, 40, 41, 42, 247; imports of, 17–18, 38, 39, 43,

meat consumption, 169–73; food culture of, 250; and almuerzo, 263–64

Squash, as standard food item, 25, 135

Standard of living, 197, 223

Suárez, Isabel, 330 (n. 49)

Sugar: moscabada, 7, 33, 86; and moist sweetmeats, 32, 33, 34–35; brown sugar, 34–35; and cornmeal, 82

Sugar cultivation: first era of in Puerto Rico, 19, 20; in wetlands and marshy areas, 20; and large-scale agriculture, 38–39, 104, 146, 147, 247; and enslaved African labor, 54, 81, 89, 103, 168, 186–87, 312–13 (n. 62); and cattle, 168; reductions in, 173, 317 (n. 27); and tiempo muerto, 276

Super asopao de gandules, 219

Supermarkets, 117, 197, 199, 210, 236, 239, 268, 325–26 (n. 2), 334 (n. 74)

Supermofongo, 219

Superpastel, 219

Supplementary foods: codfish as, 5, 100, 101, 103, 113, 115, 278 (n. 11); definition of, 5, 100, 278 (n. 11); meat as, 169

Sweet potatoes (Ipomeas batatas): as standard food item, 5, 25, 100, 109, 130, 135, 245; storage and distribution of, 53; as vianda, 122, 135; consumption of, 130, 131, 155; cultivation of, 130, 134, 135, 159, 310 (nn. 20, 39); preserves, 134, 310 (n. 37); cooking methods, 135–37, 158; and cazuela, 265–66

Sweets: arroces húmedos dulces, 32–36, 44; majarete, 34, 84–87, 94, 271, 282 (n. 45), 297 (n. 28), 297–98 (n. 30); and cornmeal, 83–84; mazamorra, 92, 272, 297 (n. 28), 301 (n. 64); gofio, 94, 270; cazuela, 136, 152, 265–66; alfeñiques, 136, 262–63; and nutritional guidelines, 231; traditional, 253; alfajor, 262; frangollo, 269, 301 (n. 64)

Taíno people: and bean cultivation, 51, 52–54, 55; and gold mining, 52, 53, 165, 287 (n. 5), 288 (nn. 7, 10); and encomienda, 53, 287 (nn. 5, 6); women, 53–54, 288 (nn. 7, 10); and cassava flour, 124; and pigs, 165–66; population of, 287 (n. 5)

Tamal de maíz, 152, 314–15 (n. 87)

Tamales, and guanimes, 78

Tannier (Xanthosoma sagitifolium): as standard food item, 5, 100, 130, 133, 245; preparation of, 64, 132–33, 154; as vianda, 122, 123; consumption of, 130, 131, 134; cultivation of, 130, 132, 134, 159, 310 (n. 20); and pastel, 151, 152; alcapurrias, 262; and cazuela, 265

Tañón, Olga, 75, 294 (n. 83)

Tapia y Rivera, Alejandro, 149

Tapioca, 130

Tastee Freeze Carrol's, 226

A Taste of Puerto Rico, and funche, 92–93

Three Kings Day, 31, 85, 149, 152

Tiempo muerto, 276

Tobacco cultivation, and bean and legume cultivation, 57, 289 (n. 24)

Tocinero, 164–65

Tomatoes (Lycopersicum esculentum), 61, 62

Tooker, Helen, 330 (n. 49)

Torres, Bibiano, 181

Torres Díaz, Luis, 249, 291 (n. 50)

Torres Vargas, Diego de, 125–26, 308–9 (n. 4)

Tortilla (sweet confection), 131

Tortillitas, 156

Tortillitas de camarones (crisp shrimp fritters), 96

Tortitas (small cakes), 36, 133, 137, 156

Tortitas de maíz, 84

Tostones, 147, 153, 157, 254

Tourist industry: as object of consumption, 203; and novelty in food consumption, 213–14; gastro-therapeutic tourism, 216, 331 (n. 53); and traditional foods, 219

Traditional home cooking: representations of, 3, 208, 222, 256, 257–58, 327 (n. 30); and mothers' cuisine, 37, 46, 155–57, 211, 220; invention of traditions, 208–9, 217–19, 220, 331–32 (n. 60); familiarity of, 217; and imagined authenticity, 220–21; and sense of community, 221, 332 (n. 64); manual skills grounded in, 253; and nutritional assistance programs, 258

Traffic density, 238–39

Treaty of Utrecht (1713), 103

Trichinosis, 187, 188

Tripleta (baguette sandwich), 260

Tropical Foods (Wilsey): and cassava, 130, 154; and tannier, 154; and viandas, 154; and alcapurria, 314 (n. 86)

Tubers: as standard food item, 23, 90, 111, 124; cultivation of, 54, 135, 147; cooking methods, 135–36, 152; consumption of, 157, 158. *See also* Cassava; Sweet potatoes; Tannier

Tugwell, Rexford, 330 (n. 49)

Turkey, consumption of, 155, 254, 325 (n. 122)

Type II diabetes, 222

Underclass, and rice casseroles, 29

Unemployment rate, 226, 233, 335 (n. 84), 338–39 (n. 116)

United States: South, 22; rice cultivation in, 39, 46, 49, 247; and nuyoricans, 65; beans imported from, 66, 67, 68, 71, 76; and codfish, 107, 110, 111, 306 (n. 54); Puerto Rico as colony of, 110, 191, 306 (n. 53); beef imported from, 190, 322 (n. 88); meat imported from, 194; kitchen appliances imported from, 199; fast food restaurants in, 226; prepared foods imported from, 333 (n. 68); Department of Agriculture, 337 (n. 100)

University of Puerto Rico, 42–45, 64, 70, 133, 153–54, 221, 323 (n. 96); School of Tropical Medicine, 44–45; School of Home Economics, 64, 70, 133, 153–54, 323 (n. 96)

Urban areas: and beans and legumes, 55; and cornmeal, 93; and codfish, 100, 107, 111, 114; and viandas, 153; and meat, 161–62, 167, 176–83, 185, 187, 193, 198; and livestock, 193; food culture of, 200; cosmopolitanism of, 251

Urry, John, 203–4, 205

Uruguay, 189, 268, 322 (n. 88)

Valentine, Gil, 242, 260, 327 (n. 26)

Valldejuli, Carmen Aboy, 154, 282 (nn. 45, 46), 291–92 (n. 52), 297 (n. 28)

Valle Atiles, Francisco del, 109, 187, 322 (n. 93), 334 (n. 69)

Vegetarianism, 198, 221–22, 231, 324 (n. 120), 324–25 (n. 121)

Venezuela, 152, 315 (n. 87), 333 (n. 68)

Vergara de Lupo, Marcos, 170

Viandas: role in diet, 4, 122–23, 153–56, 158, 192, 216, 246, 252; tubers as, 23, 90, 111, 124; and funche, 88, 296 (n. 17); and codfish, 96; consumption of, 112, 155, 158–59, 160, 252, 259; cultivation of, 123, 159–60; as comforting mothers' cuisine, 155–57; and globalization of food, 157–60; nutritional value of, 231; and alcapurrias, 262; and sweets, 265–66; and serenata, 275; in core-fringe-legume matrix, 279 (n. 12). *See also* Cassava; Plantains and bananas; Sweet potatoes; Tannier; Yams

Viandas sancochás (parboiled viandas), 122

Vidal Rodríguez, Zuleika, 237, 340 (nn. 132, 134, 135)

Vignas, 55–56

Vigna unguiculata, 55–56, 59, 60, 75

Vigo, José, 184

Violence, and food insecurity, 41, 285 (n. 68)

Waiwai, 311 (n. 49)

Warde, Alan: culinary antinomies model, 200, 212–13; and homogeneity, 207–8, 211, 221; and food consumption tendencies, 210–11, 232, 233; contemporary food provision, 211–12, 238; and tourism, 219; on community, 332 (n. 64)

War Food Administration, 41–42

Wendy's, 227, 335 (n. 79), 336 (n. 95)

West Africa: rice cultivation in, 18–19, 20; bean and legume cultivation in, 54–55; and seasoning, 62; and corn, 83, 89; and cassava, 127; and fufu, 137; yams in, 137–38, 311 (n. 49)

Wetlands, rice cultivated in, 17, 20–23, 247

Wheat and wheat flour, 79–81, 83, 124, 126, 128, 129, 216, 246, 263, 295 (n. 13)

White beans, 60, 65, 67, 68, 69, 72, 248

Whiting, 106

Wild coriander (*Eryngium foetidum*), 61, 62, 245, 257, 274–75, 290 (nn. 35, 37)

Wilsey, Elsie Mae, 64, 130, 154, 314 (n. 86)

Wolf, Eric, 194

www.ingramcontent.com/pod-product-compliance
Lightning Source LLC
Chambersburg PA
CBHW022346280326
41935CB00007B/90